Core Curriculum for
FORENSIC
NURSING

Core Curriculum for

FORENSIC
NURSING

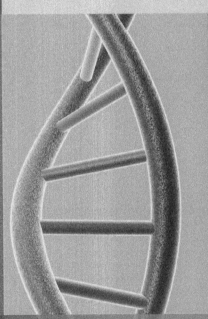

Bonnie Price, DNP, RN, SANE-A, SANE-P, AFN-BC
Director
Bon Secours Richmond Health System
Forensic Nurse Program
Richmond, Virginia

Kathleen Maguire, JD, BSN, BS, RN
Director of Certification
Managing Editor, *Journal of Forensic Nursing*
International Association of Forensic Nurses
Elkridge, Maryland

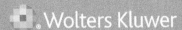. Wolters Kluwer

Philadelphia • Baltimore • New York • London
Buenos Aires • Hong Kong • Sydney • Tokyo

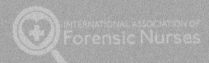
INTERNATIONAL ASSOCIATION OF
Forensic Nurses

Executive Editor: Shannon W. Magee
Product Development Editor: Maria M. McAvey
Senior Marketing Manager: Mark Wiragh
Senior Production Project Manager: Cynthia Rudy
Design Coordinators: Doug Smock and Elaine Kasmer
Manufacturing Coordinator: Kathleen Brown
Prepress Vendor: Aptara, Inc.

9 8 7 6 5 4 3

Printed in the United States of America

Library of Congress Cataloging-in-Publication Data

Core curriculum for forensic nursing / [edited by] Bonnie Price, Kathleen Maguire. – 1e.
　　p. ; cm.
Includes bibliographical references and index.
ISBN 978-1-4511-9323-7 (alk. paper)
I. Price, Bonnie, editor. II. Maguire, Kathleen (Forensic nurse), editor.
[DNLM: 1. Outlines. 2. Forensic Nursing. WY 18.2]
RA1151
614'.1–dc23

2015024156

LWW.com

Contributors

Catherine J. Carter-Snell, PhD, RN, ENC-C, SANE-A
Nurse Education Scholar/Associate Professor
School of Nursing and Midwifery
Mount Royal University
Calgary, Alberta, Canada

Cyndi Leahy, MSN, RN, SANE-A, SANE-P
Forensic Nurse Examiner Program
    Coordinator, Clinical Manager
Winchester Medical Center
Winchester, Virginia

Annie Lewis-O'Connor, PhD, MPH, NP, FAAN
Senior Nurse Scientist; Director, C.A.R.E. Clinic
Brigham and Women's Hospital
Boston, Massachusetts

Judy Malmgren, BSN, RN, PHN, SANE-A, CFN
Forensic Nurse Examiner, Consultant, and
    Expert Witness
Public Health Department, SART Program
Santa Barbara, California

MaryAnne C. Murray, EdD, DNP, FNP-BC, PMHNP-BC, SANE-A
Medical Provider
Willapa Behavioral Health
Long Beach, Washington

Karen S. Neill, PhD, RN, SANE-A
Professor, Associate Director for Graduate Studies
School of Nursing, Idaho State University
Pocatello, Idaho

Bobbi Jo O'Neal, RN, BSN, F-ABMDI
Chief Deputy Coroner
Charleston County Coroner's Office
North Charleston, South Carolina

Michelle Ortiz, RN, MSN, SANE-A, AFN-BC
Forensic Healthcare Coordinator and SAFE
    Program Manager
Emergency Medicine Department
Naval Medical Center Portsmouth
Portsmouth, Virginia

Georgia L. Perdue, DNP, FNP-BC, AFN-BC, CCHP
Nurse Practitioner
Post-Acute Physician Partners
Institutions
Maryland and Delaware

Wesley A. Rivera, RN, MSN, FN
Medical Administrator
La Plata County Jail
Durango, Colorado

Donna Sabella, M.Ed, MSN, PhD, PMHNP-BC
Director of Global Studies and Director of the
    Office of Human Trafficking
College of Nursing and Health Professions
Drexel University
Philadelphia, Pennsylvania

Ashley N. Smith, BScPN, RPN, SANE-A, SANE-P
Sexual Assault Nurse Examiner
Coordinator of the Sexual Assault Nurse
    Examiner Program
Winnipeg Health Sciences Centre
Winnipeg, Manitoba, Canada

Norah (Nodie) Sullivan, MSN, ARNP, ANP-BC, CNS–BC, AFN-BC
Nurse Practitioner, Addictions
Addictions Treatment Center
Puget Sound VA Healthcare System
Seattle, Washington

Pamela D. Tabor, DNP-Forensics, AFN-BC
Director of Arkansas Infant and Child Death
    Review Program
Injury Prevention Center
Arkansas Children's Hospital and University
    of Arkansas for Medical Sciences
Little Rock, Arkansas

Judy Waldman, MN, RN, SANE-A, SANE-P
Judy Waldman Counselling
Toronto, Ontario, Canada

Reviewers

Evangeline Barefoot, RN, MA, BSN, SANE-A, SANE-P, CEN
Forensic Nurse Examiner
Emergency Department, St. David's Round
  Rock Medical Center
Round Rock, Texas

Polly Campbell, RN, BS, BA (IAFN Board President, 2013)
Director, Sexual Assault Forensic Examiner
  Program
Office of Violence Prevention
Department of Health and Human Services
Augusta, Maine

Eileen Caraker, MSN, RN, FN-CSA, SANE-A, SANE-P
Coordinator, SART and Forensic Nursing
  Services
Gloucester County Prosecutor Office
Woodbury, New Jersey

Kim Day, RN, SANE-A, SANE-P
SAFEta Project Director
International Association of Forensic Nurses
Elkridge, Maryland

Stacy A. Drake, PhD, MPH, RN, AFN-BC, D-ABMDI
Assistant Professor of Nursing, Track Director,
  Forensic Nursing Science Post-Graduate
  Program
The University of Texas Health Science Center
Houston, Texas

Sheila Early, RN, BScN (IAFN Board President, 2014)
Forensic Nursing Consultant, Program
  Coordinator/Instructor, Forensic Health
  Sciences Option
British Columbia Institute of Technology
  (BCIT) Forensic Science and Technology,
  BCIT
Burnaby, British Columbia, Canada

Carolyn Porta Garcia, PhD, MPH, RN, SANE-A (IAFN Board Member, 2015)
Associate Professor, School of Nursing
University of Minnesota
Minneapolis, Minnesota

Stephen Goux, MSN, RN, AFN-BC, SANE-A, SANE-P (IAFN Board Treasurer, 2015)
Sexual Assault Nurse Examiner
Gwinnett Sexual Assault and Child Advocacy
  Center
Duluth, Georgia

Rachel Jacquet, MSN, RN-BC, CA-SANE, CP-SANE, SANE-A, SANE-P, CMI-IV, CFN, CEN, CFRN, CTRN
Forensic Nurse, Forensic Nurse Examiner
  Program
Christus Hospital—St. Elizabeth
Beaumont, Texas

Sara B. Jennings, MSN, RN, SANE-A, SANE-P, AFN-BC (IAFN Board Secretary, 2014-2015)
Clinical Care Leader, RN 4, Bon Secours
  Richmond Forensic Nursing Services
Bon Secours Richmond Health System
Richmond, Virginia

Elizabeth (Liz) Louden, RN, BN, MSN, SANE-A (IAFN Board Member, 2014)
Adjunct Professor
School of Nursing/Forensic Science and Law
Duquesne University
Welland, Ontario, Canada

Virginia A. Lynch, MSN, RN, FAAS, FAAN
Forensic Clinical Nurse Specialist
Divide, Colorado

Jennifer McConnell, BSN, RN, SANE-A (IAFN Board Member, 2014-2015)
Forensic Nurse Examiner Program Coordinator
St. Anthony Summit Medical Center
Frisco, Colorado

Susan McDonald, BA, MSN, RN, CCRN, CEN, SANE-A, SANE-P
CNII MSICU/Forensic Nurse Examiner
MSICU/Emergency Department, York Hospital
York, Pennsylvania

Stacey A. Mitchell, DNP, MBA, RN, SANE-A, SANE-P
Administrative Director
Risk Management and Patient Safety
    Department, Forensic Nursing Services,
    Harris Health System
Houston, Texas

Jennifer Pierce-Weeks, RN, SANE-A, SANE-P
Education Director
International Association of Forensic Nurses
Elkridge, Maryland

C. Jill Poarch, BSN, RN, SANE-A, SANE-P
Registered Nurse, Sexual Assault Nurse
    Examiner
Emergency Department, Sauk Prairie
    Healthcare
Prairie du Sac, Wisconsin

L. Kathleen Sekula, PhD, APRN-BC, FAAN
Professor, Director of Graduate Forensic
    Programs
School of Nursing, Duquesne University
Pittsburgh, Pennsylvania

Sharon W. Stark, PhD, RN, APRN-BC, CFN, CPG
Associate Dean, Coordinator Nurse
    Practitioner and Forensic Nursing Programs
MK Unterberg School of Nursing and Health
    Studies, Monmouth University
West Long Branch, New Jersey

Pamela D. Tabor, DNP-Forensics, AFN-BC (IAFN Board Member, 2014-2016)
Director of Arkansas Infant and Child Death
    Review Program
Injury Prevention Center, Arkansas Children's
    Hospital; University of Arkansas for
    Medical Sciences
Little Rock, Arkansas

Kimberly A. Womack, DHSc, ARNP-BC, SANE-A (IAFN Board President, 2015)
Director
Emerald Coast Forensic Services
Gulf Breeze, Florida

Carolyn E. Ziminski Pickering, PhD, RN
Assistant Professor
College of Nursing, Michigan State University
East Lansing, Michigan

Preface

In 1992, a dedicated group of nurses established a new professional organization – the International Association of Forensic Nurses, the leading professional organization for forensic nurses. Forensic nursing professionals practice in areas where the healthcare system and the law intersect. The forensic nurse provides care for both victims of intentional and unintentional injuries and for suspects and perpetrators of crime in a variety of settings, such as clinical, psychiatric, correctional, and death investigation.

In 1995, the American Nurses Association (ANA) recognized forensic nursing as a unique nursing specialty. This milestone ushered in another: the ANA and the Association's joint publication of the *Scope and Standards of Forensic Nursing Practice* (now entitled *Forensic Nursing: Scope and Standards of Practice*). The International Association of Forensic Nurses has since developed other foundational documents, including education guidelines for the sexual assault nurse examiner, the forensic nurse death investigator, the nurse who addresses elder abuse, and the nurse who cares for those who have experienced intimate partner violence. These resources have been instrumental in guiding the growth and progress of forensic nursing and are merely the beginning for this robust and rapidly evolving specialty.

In January 2010, the Board of Directors of the International Association of Forensic Nurses identified the need to develop and implement a comprehensive forensic nursing core curriculum, one that is designed to enhance the basic, core knowledge of the entry-level forensic nurse. For the purpose of this curriculum, an entry-level forensic nurse is defined as a registered nurse who has completed a diploma, associate degree, or baccalaureate nursing program and will be caring for patients who have been victims, suspects, or perpetrators of violence or trauma. The *Core Curriculum for Forensic Nursing* has been designed to address the knowledge, skills, and scope of practice of this entry-level forensic nurse.

The *Core Curriculum* is the first of its kind to be endorsed and offered by the International Association of Forensic Nurses; its goal is to standardize the educational preparation of the entry-level generalist forensic nurse by establishing a core foundation of knowledge and ensuring consistent content delivery. The *Core Curriculum* will be an invaluable resource for those seeking professional development and continuing education in the specialty of forensic nursing. A foreseeable aspiration is that the *Core Curriculum for Forensic Nursing* will serve as a comprehensive, standardized base of knowledge upon which the International Association of Forensic Nurses will develop a certification for the generalist forensic nurse.

The future beckons and, as is their tradition, forensic nurses are inspired to respond.

The Core Curriculum for Forensic Nursing *is dedicated to forensic nurses around the world who give of themselves every day to care for others.*

Bonnie Price and Kathleen Maguire

Contents

CHAPTER   7A

Overarching Issues: Testifying   221

Judy Malmgren

Cyndi Leahy

CHAPTER   7B

Overarching Issues: Vicarious Trauma   231

Cyndi Leahy

CHAPTER **1**

Introduction

Judy Waldman
Karen S. Neill

OBJECTIVES

At the completion of this chapter, the learner will be able to:

- Describe the social, political, and public health issues that have contributed to the evolution of forensic nursing as a nursing specialty.
- Apply nursing ethics to forensic nursing practice.
- Describe the domains of knowledge from which forensic nursing derives its theoretical framework, and the concepts of caring, holism, person-centered approach, and collaboration.
- Identify the four components of the metaparadigm of forensic nursing.
- Discuss the various roles and settings in which a forensic nurse may practice.
- Describe key concepts related to the scope and standards of forensic nursing practice.
- Identify current trends for the future of forensic nursing.

KEY TERMS

Competency: "An expected and measurable level of nursing performance that integrates knowledge, skills, abilities and judgment based on established scientific knowledge and expectations for nursing practice" (Mariano, 2013; p. 11).

Forensic: Pertaining or related to the law.

Forensic nurse examiner (FNE): A registered nurse qualified by education, experience, and specialized training; provides comprehensive nursing care to forensic patients in healthcare and community settings; includes clinical forensic assessment, investigation, and analysis regarding victims, suspects, or perpetrators of intentional or unintentional physical and/or psychological violence or trauma (i.e., child/elder abuse, intimate partner violence, sexual assault, natural disasters, etc.) and/or death; "appropriate [term] for any of the subspecialties of forensic nursing where forensic examinations are performed" (Lynch & Duval, 2011; pp. 199–200).

Forensic nursing: "The practice of nursing globally where health and legal systems intersect" (IAFN & ANA, 2009).

The icons represent various aspects of forensic nursing: death investigation, legal/criminal justice, intimate partner violence, administrative, correctional/psychiatric-mental health.

Forensic science: "The application of science to the law"; encompasses a number of discrete disciplines that promote the application of science to the legal system (Lynch & Duval, 2011; p. 10).

Holism: Integration, harmony, and balance of the mind, body, and spirit; a focus on the individual as a whole person with an emphasis on the process of self-healing; the view of illness as an opportunity for growth and self-awareness; and the reciprocal nurse–patient relationship with an emphasis on self-responsibility, health promotion, and lifestyle (Boschma, 1994; Povlsen & Borup, 2011).

Human rights: "Human rights are basic rights and freedoms that all people are entitled to regardless of nationality, sex, national or ethnic origin, race, religion, language, or other status"; "includ[ing] civil and political rights, such as the right to life, liberty and freedom of expression; and social, cultural and economic rights including the right to participate in culture, the right to food, and the right to work and receive an education . . . are protected and upheld by international and national laws and treaties" (Amnesty International, 2015).

Nursing: "The protection, promotion, and optimization of health and abilities, prevention of illness and injury, alleviation of suffering through the diagnosis and treatment of human response, and advocacy in the care of individuals, families, communities, and populations" (ANA, 2010; p. 66).

Nursing process: "A critical thinking model used by nurses that comprises the integration of the singular, concurrent actions of these six components: assessment, diagnosis, identification of outcomes, planning, implementation, and evaluation" (ANA, 2010; p. 66; Lynch, 2006).

Patient: "The recipient of forensic nursing practice, whether an individual, family, community, or population. The recipient may also be called client, resident, group, or system" (ANA, 2004).

- When the patient is an *individual,* the focus is on the health state, problems, or needs of a single person.
- When the patient is a *family* or a group, the focus is on the health state of that unit as a whole or the reciprocal effects of any individual's health state on any other members of the unit.
- When the patient is a *community* or *population,* the focus is on personal and environmental health and the health risks of the community or entire population" (IAFN & ANA, 2009; p. 51).

Public health: "[R]efers to all organized measures (whether public or private) to prevent disease, promote health, and prolong life among the population as a whole"; "aim [is] to provide conditions in which people can be healthy and focus on entire populations, not on individual patients or diseases"; "concerned with the total system and not only the eradication of a particular disease" (WHO, 2015).

Standards of practice/Standards of professional performance: Authoritative statements by which nurses practicing within the role, population, and specialty are governed, given the unique body of knowledge of forensic nursing.

Suspect/Accused/Offender or Perpetrator: One who is suspected of and/or formally charged with the commission of a criminal act or "who commits, executes, or performs a criminal act of any kind" (IAFN & ANA, 2009; p. 51).

Trauma: When an individual is exposed "to actual or threatened death, serious injury, or sexual violence" (American Psychiatric Association, 2013; p. 271); "trauma results from an event, series of events, or set of circumstances that is experienced by an individual as physically or emotionally harmful or threatening and that has lasting adverse effects on the individual's functioning and physical, social, emotional, or spiritual well-being" (SAMHSA, 2012; p. 2; SAMHSA, 2014b; p. 7); "sometimes . . . defined in reference to circumstances that are outside the realm of normal human experience" (Briere & Scott, 2006; Center for Nonviolence and Social Justice, 2014).

Victim: One who is harmed or killed by another; harmed by or made to suffer by an act, agency, or condition; suffers injury, loss, or death as a result of an involuntary undertaking; or who is tricked, swindled, or taken advantage of (Hammer, Moynihan, & Pagliaro, 2013).

Violence: "The intentional use of physical force or power, threatened or actual, against oneself, another person, or against a group or community, that either results in or has a high likelihood of resulting in injury, death, psychological harm, maldevelopment or deprivation" (WHO, 2002; p. 5).

Vulnerable populations: Groups that are at risk for poor psychological, physical, or social health, and thus, have greater health needs (Nyamathi, Koniak-Griffin, & Greengold, 2007).

EVOLUTION OF FORENSIC NURSING

History of Forensic Sciences/Medicine

Similar to the practice of nursing, the practice of forensic medicine predates any formal recognition of the discipline in Europe and Asia. Evidence exists of medical practitioners involved in the primitive justice systems during the Roman Empire and in thirteenth-century China (Smith, 1951). The role of coroner existed in Britain as early as the twelfth century and ample evidence exists of medical testimony in the courts of sixteenth-century Great Britain (Mant, 1987; Smith, 1951). In 1887, Britain formalized the role of coroner by enacting the Coroner's Act (Mant, 1987). It is the Coroner system of Great Britain upon which the structure of the United States and the countries of the British Empire (e.g., Canada, Australia) are based.

In the United States, the term "forensic" typically conjures an association with the deceased. The term actually refers to debate in courts of law. More specifically, "forensic science" is defined as relating to the "application of biochemical and other scientific techniques to the investigation of crime" (Barber, 2004; p. 582). Most people are familiar with the role of forensic examiners in death investigation, such as coroners and medical examiners (MEs). In 1983, the first two articles specifically addressing forensic medicine and the care of patients in the emergency department (ED) were published in the medical literature in the United States (Mittleman, Goldberg, & Waksman, 1983; Smialek, 1983). Both articles emphasized the need for recognition and preservation of evidence for patients presenting to the ED; the focus was on patients who were treated, but who subsequently died in the hospital.

Until the 1980s, the issues of the living forensic patient had been largely neglected in the United States. In contrast, this medical practice had existed in Europe and Great Britain for more than two centuries (McLay, 1990). With the publication of *Forensic Sciences: The Clinical or Living Aspects*, however, William Eckert brought the living forensic patient to the forefront of contemporary medicine in the United States (Eckert, 1990; Lynch, 2006). Eckert's work is the basis for the concept of applying forensic techniques to living patients. In 1986, the American Academy of Forensic Sciences published its first article dedicated to living – or clinical – forensic medicine. This new interest opened the door for other medical professionals, including emergency nurses.

History of Forensic Nursing

The history of forensic nursing may date as far back as the Crimean War. Clements and Sekula (2005) suggest that Florence Nightingale's practice demonstrated an early example of forensic nursing by using research, theory, and practice with victims and offenders (soldiers) during the Crimean War.

More than a century later, around the time that clinicians were identifying weaknesses in the practice of forensic medicine, Virginia Lynch was studying as her master's thesis the role of ED nurses working with trauma patients and the lack of forensic care. She subsequently published the first literature on forensic nursing, entitled *Clinical Forensic Nursing: A Descriptive Study in Role Development* (Lynch, 1990). This work clearly identified the gaps in practice, and the value of the role of the forensic nurse and of a multidisciplinary approach in caring for the forensic patient. Lynch provided strong support and acceptance of forensic nursing practices, which according to Smock, set the stage for ongoing development of this new discipline; and challenged clinicians, nurses, and hospital administrators to meet the responsibilities of the needs and demands of society (Smock, 2006). Virginia Lynch also strongly advocated for forensic nursing education to be incorporated into nursing school curricula. In 1991, the American Academy of Forensic Sciences formally recognized forensic nursing as a unique scientific discipline, and in 1995, the American Nurses Association officially recognized forensic nursing as a specialty area of nursing. The Canadian Nurses Association (2007) subsequently recognized forensic nursing as an emerging subspecialty of nursing with the formation of the Forensic Nurses' Society of Canada. Within the specialty area of forensic nursing, subspecialties have developed, each with their own history and influences.

Early Roles

Sexual Assault Nurse Examiner (SANE). This was the first well-established, formal role of a clinical forensic nurse. Nurses began volunteering at rape crisis centers in the 1970s (See Table 1.1). From practice in this setting as volunteers, nurses developed scientific knowledge, expertise, and critical thinking about the legal issues surrounding patient care (Burgess, Berger, & Boersma, 2004). Even before the movement toward forensic nursing in the ED, clinical forensic nurses were addressing the gaps in care and the inadequate response in hospitals to patients who had been sexually assaulted. Patients who were victims of sexual assault presented to EDs, where they were subjected to long waits, examined by untrained clinicians, and underwent inadequate collection of evidence. This often resulted in retraumatization of the patient, poor coordination between hospital staff and law enforcement personnel, and the lack of ability to fully prosecute the sexual assault case (Campbell, Wasco, Ahrens, Sefl, & Barnes, 2001; Hutson, 2002).

Psychiatric or Mental Health Forensic Nurse. This involves caring for victims or perpetrators of crime who have a mental illness. Paralleling the evolution of forensic nurses in the ED and sexual assault programs, psychiatric nurses were practicing in forensic psychiatric settings long before the concept of forensic nursing existed. According to Kent-Wilkinson (2010), the roots of forensic psychiatric nursing were established in the United Kingdom (UK); the role began in other developed countries in the 1970s and 1980s. This is attributed to the human rights legislation and reforms of the criminal justice system that demanded taking responsibility for the health of inmates (Kent-Wilkinson, 2010).

Death Investigation. The role of the nurse in death investigation was established in North America after the Chief Medical Examiner in Alberta, Canada, conducted a study concluding that nurses had the qualities essential for the investigation of death (Lynch & Duval, 2011). Thus, Canadian nurses began working in the area of death investigation in 1975 under Dr. John Butt, a forensic pathologist in Calgary, Alberta (Anderson, 2007). In the United States, this forensic nursing role began in the 1980s first in New Jersey and then Texas (Lynch, personal communication, 2015).

International Association of Forensic Nurses

The International Association of Forensic Nurses (IAFN) was established in 1992 when 72 registered nurses from Canada and the United States met for the first time in Minneapolis, Minnesota (IAFN, 2015b; Ledray, 1999). They sought to share their experiences and knowledge base of what was, at the time, a narrow field. Although most of the attendees specialized as SANEs, these nurses had a vision of developing an organization that included a wide and diverse body of nurses working in concert with any arena of the law (Hammer, Moynihan, & Pagliaro, 2013). In 1996, the Canadian Forensic Nurses' Society formed and became affiliated with the IAFN in 2012 (Forensic Nurses' Society of Canada, 2015).

Forensic nursing practice encompasses the nurse who applies concepts and principles of forensic science while providing nursing care. Since its founding, the IAFN has grown to include more than 3,000 members from 19 different countries and territories (IAFN, 2013b). As of 2015, 184 members were from countries outside the United States, including Australia, Barbados, Bermuda, Brazil, Canada, England, Germany, Guam, Israel, Japan, Kenya, Lebanon, the Netherlands, New Zealand, Puerto Rico, Singapore, South Africa, and Sweden (IAFN, 2015a). The IAFN promotes forensic nursing

TABLE 1.1 Forensic Nursing Timeline

Timeline

1970s	First programs established to provide care for patients who had been sexually assaulted (Kansas City, Missouri; Memphis, Tennessee; Honolulu, Hawaii; Minneapolis, Minnesota; and Amarillo, Texas) (National Sexual Violence Resource Center, 2015; Ledray, 2001)
1975	John Butt, MD, Chief Medical Examiner in Alberta, Canada, recognizes the registered nurse as a valuable resource to the field of death investigation (Lynch & Duval, 2011)
1986	Lynch develops formal curricula for forensic nursing with focus on death investigation (University of Texas at Arlington) (Lynch & Duval, 2011)
1988	Lynch expands curricula to include clinical forensic nursing (Lynch & Duval, 2011)
1989	Lynch introduces forensic nursing as a scientific discipline (Lynch & Duval, 2011)
1991	American Academy of Forensic Sciences (AAFS) recognizes forensic nursing as a scientific discipline (Lynch & Duval, 2011)
1992	First meeting of forensic nurses, most of whom were sexual assault nurse examiners; the International Association of Forensic Nurses (IAFN) is established as the first professional nursing organization for forensic nurses (IAFN, 2015b)
1994	Violence Against Women Act is enacted (US)
1995	American Nurses Association's Congress of Nursing Practice recognizes forensic nursing as a specialty (ANA & IAFN, 1997)
1996	*Sexual Assault Nurse Examiner Standards of Practice* are issued (IAFN, 1996)
1997	*Scope and Standards of Forensic Nursing* (1st ed.) is published (IAFN & ANA, 1997)
1999	*Sexual Assault Nurse Examiner (SANE) Development and Operation Guide* is published (Ledray, 1999)
2002	IAFN offers first certification for SANE - Adult/Adolescent (SANE-A®) Forensic Nursing Certification Board (FNCB) is established
2004	*National Protocol for Sexual Assault Medical Forensic Examinations, Adult/Adolescent* (1st ed.) is published (U.S. Department of Justice, 2004)
2005	*Journal of Forensic Nursing* publishes its first issue
2007	IAFN offers first certification for SANE - Pediatric (SANE-P®)
2009	*Forensic Nurse Death Investigator Education Guidelines* are published (IAFN, 2009a)
2012	Commission for Forensic Nursing Certification (CFNC) is established *Intimate Partner Violence Education Guidelines* are published (IAFN, 2012)
2013	*Sexual Assault Nurse Examiner Education Guidelines, Adult/Adolescent and Pediatric* are published (IAFN, 2013a)

roles worldwide and advocates for forensic nursing education globally. The IAFN publishes guidelines and scopes of practice for forensic nursing roles and hosts an annual International Conference on Forensic Nursing Science and Practice to promote the dissemination of knowledge and expertise to members and nonmembers alike from around the world.

Mission: To promote leadership in forensic nursing practice by developing, promoting, and disseminating information internationally about forensic nursing science.

Values:

- Access to forensic nursing care
- A world without violence
- Fidelity to patients
- Responsibility to the public
- Obligation to science
- Respect for colleagues
- Commitment to social justice

Vision: Forensic nurses will be universally recognized as the essential component of health care's response to violence and trauma.

Forensic Nursing Pioneers

The following pioneers deserve particular recognition for their contribution to forensic nursing.

Virginia A. Lynch, MSN, RN, FAAFS, FAAN. In 1982, Virginia Lynch, an ED nurse, embarked on a mission to determine how nurses could assist in preventing the loss and destruction of evidence. Lynch evaluated a crime laboratory that year where she learned that healthcare professionals often destroyed key evidence when providing care to victims. This knowledge sparked her interest in the preservation of evidence and documentation of injuries (Waszak, 2013). Lynch recognized that nurses possessed the ideal combination of medical and psychological skills to formulate a unique body of knowledge and discipline of nursing. She began her forensic career in 1984 as a death investigator in Fort Worth, Texas, and was the first woman and nurse to hold the position in that region, covering a 960-square-mile area (Waszak, 2013). Virginia Lynch, the founding president of IAFN, has been recognized as the founder of forensic nursing as a scientific discipline. Her research and master's thesis, *Clinical Forensic Nursing: A Descriptive Study in Role Development*, launched the emerging specialty of forensic nursing. Lynch went on to publish numerous articles and books on forensic nursing, including the first forensic nursing textbook, *Forensic Nursing* (2006), and *Forensic Nursing Science* (2011). Lynch has also contributed significantly to the education of forensic nurses. In 1986, she designed and developed a forensic nursing graduate program at the University of Texas. She was the first to complete a Master of Science in Nursing in forensic nursing and the first to receive an advanced practice nursing credential as a clinical nurse specialist in this new discipline. In her name, the IAFN awards the Virginia A. Lynch Pioneer Award in Forensic Nursing as the highest honor for exceptional contributions to the field of forensic nursing (IAFN, 2015a).

Ann Wolbert Burgess, DNSc, RN, FAAN. Ann Burgess is renowned as a practitioner, researcher, educator, and pioneer in the study of sexual assault. Well known for her research on the psychological impact of sexual assault, she has expanded her work to many areas of forensic practice and psychiatric nursing. Cofounding one of the first hospital-based crisis intervention services at the Boston City Hospital, she laid the groundwork for her subsequent research on victims and trauma. In 1974, she and Lynda Lytle Holmstrom first described the physical and psychological effects of rape as "rape trauma syndrome" (Burgess & Holmstrom, 1974). Burgess was one of the first nurses to demonstrate that nurses could be clinicians and researchers (Ann Burgess, 1991). Studying both victims and perpetrators, and the links between the two, she has contributed greatly to the understanding and appreciation of the mental health connections; her work remains influential today (O'Donohue, Carlson, Benuto, & Bennett, 2014). She has published prolifically and has authored numerous textbooks on psychiatric nursing and crisis intervention, and books on assessment and treatment of victims and offenders.

Comprehensive Roles of Forensic Nursing

- Forensic nursing is multidimensional, addressing issues related to both health care and the law.
- The role incorporates the diagnosis and treatment of human responses to actual and potential health problems among patients (individuals, families, groups, communities) who are victims, suspects, or perpetrators of crime, violence, or trauma (Hammer, Moynihan, & Pagliaro, 2013).
- A forensic nurse must use general and specialized nursing skills from varied settings or areas of practice, such as emergency care, critical care, women's health, psychiatry, geriatrics, pediatrics, and community health, as well as from areas outside traditional nursing practice, such as knowledge of forensic sciences and the criminal justice system, and the scientific investigation of death.
- Through the application of these specialty skills in practice, forensic nurses promote and enhance the use of assessment and interventions that are most appropriate to the individual, family, and community experiencing violence.
- Models of forensic nursing care apply to victims, suspects, and perpetrators of crime; the phenomenon of violence affects each and tends to present common issues and problems.

- Above all, forensic nurses remain unbiased and objective in their approach to all patients.
- Understanding psychological trauma is a key component in the forensic nursing assessment and treatment of victims, suspects, and offenders.
- The forensic nurse uses the nursing process to assess the needs of the public related to significant public health issues, such as sexual assault, communicable diseases, child maltreatment, suicide, interpersonal violence (domestic, elder abuse, homicide), gun violence, and human trafficking.

FUNDAMENTALS OF FORENSIC NURSING SCIENCE

The science of nursing, when merged with the forensic sciences and the justice system, creates a distinct discipline: Forensic nursing science. This scientific discipline offers the registered nurse unique opportunities at all levels of practice, ranging from the basic or generalist nursing role to advanced practice in forensic nursing.

- The IAFN defines "forensic nursing" as "the practice of nursing globally when health and legal systems intersect" (IAFN & ANA, 2009; p. 3).
- The foundation of forensic nursing practice is the bio-psycho-social-spiritual education of registered nurses who use the nursing process and research evidence to diagnose and treat victims, suspects, and perpetrators of trauma, and their families, communities, and the systems that respond to them (Lynch, 2006). Forensic nursing focuses on the identification, management, and prevention of intentional and unintentional injuries in a global community, collaborating with agents in the healthcare, social, and legal systems to investigate and interpret clinical presentations and pathologies. This is done by evaluating physical and psychological injury, describing the injury and evidence, as well as interpreting the associated influencing factors.
- Forensic nurses integrate forensic and nursing sciences in their assessment and care of victims, suspects, and perpetrators of physical, psychological, or social trauma.
- Forensic nurses provide care throughout the domains of nursing practice, including education, research, and consultation, and practice independently and collaboratively as needed in various settings whenever and wherever health and legal issues intersect.
- Forensic nurses share a unique body of knowledge related to the identification, assessment, and analysis of forensic patient data rooted in nursing science, forensic science, and public health to care for individuals, families, and communities.

Nursing Process

The nursing process is a "critical thinking model used by nurses that comprises the integration of the singular, concurrent actions of these six components: assessment, diagnosis, identification of outcomes, planning, implementation, and evaluation" (ANA, 2010, p. 66; Lynch, 2006). The specialty of forensic nursing was developed around the core criteria of the nursing process (Lynch, 2006). This concept is applied to the specific processes involved in the clinical investigation of trauma or death of the forensic patient.

The structure of the entire forensic nursing process is predicated on maintaining a certain state of mind—an investigative, interpretive, dogmatic search for the facts and the truth. Indeed, all healthcare personnel must be able to use interview skills and physical assessment indicators to detect abuse and neglect.

The forensic nurse may develop diagnoses based on the criteria of the North American Nursing Diagnosis Association (NANDA), now known as NANDA, International. Diagnoses may include a syndrome or cluster of diagnoses as recognized by NANDA, such as rape trauma syndrome (Herdman & Kamitsuru, 2014). The forensic nurse uses the nursing process as a framework to support appropriate intervention and reevaluation of care as necessary. Lynch (2006) identifies the following concepts related to the nursing process:

- Assessment: Identification of the forensic situation, identification of actual and potential victims, and patient assessment using subjective and objective data.

TABLE 1.7 Principles of the Criminal Justice System

Presumption of innocence	The accused is innocent until it is proven beyond a reasonable doubt that the accused committed the crime.
Due process	Involves a thorough examination of the facts of the case and the importance of protecting the legal rights of those charged with offences.
Independent judiciary	The accused has the right to have his or her case decided by a fair and impartial judge, without interference or influence of any kind.
Openness and accessibility of court	Through an open and public process, the public can have confidence in the justice system that all parties are treated fairly.
Equality before the law	All people are equal under the law.

Adapted from Justice BC. (n.d.). *Goals, basic principles and sources of criminal law*. Retrieved from. http://www.justicebc.ca/en/cjis/understanding/basic_principles.html

cope or integrate the emotions involved with the experience (SAMHSA, 2014a). Trauma may involve a single incident, such as a sexual assault, or an accumulation of traumas over time, as with child sexual abuse. Typical reactions may include, but are not limited to, emotional lability or difficulty with affect regulation, intrusive thoughts or memories, hypervigilance, avoidance, dissociation, difficulties with impulse control, and interpersonal difficulties (Briere & Spinazzola, 2005; Herman, 1992a, 1992b). These symptoms may occur immediately or over a period of time. The forensic nurse understands the psychological impact of trauma and how to evaluate the behaviors and experiences of victimization.

Criminal Justice. The forensic nurse is familiar with the domains of the criminal justice system in the jurisdiction in which he or she practices. In the United States, Canada, and many other countries, the criminal justice system is derived from the common law system, which descended from the British legal system. The common law criminal justice systems around the world share the principles outlined in Table 1.7.

Public Health

Violence. Violence is a healthcare issue (IAFN, 2009b). In the past, violence was primarily viewed as a criminal justice problem. Today, as a result of the work of many healthcare workers, public health figures, organizations, and agencies, including forensic nurses, violence has been constructed as a public health problem.

Notably, US Surgeon General C. Everett Koop (1916–2013) was instrumental in the effort to address the growing concern of violence in the United States. In 1985, he led the *Workshop on Violence and Public Health*, recommending a multidisciplinary healthcare approach to violence as a public health issue (Burgess, Berger, & Boersma, 2004; US Public Health Service, Office of the Surgeon General, US Department of Justice, Office of Juvenile Justice and Delinquency Prevention, 1986). In 1988, Koop criticized the response of the social and legal systems to forensic victims, characterizing it as late and inadequate (Hammer, Moynihan, & Pagliaro, 2013). He advised that medical and healthcare services should be included as resources for victims and recommended that healthcare professionals have a high index of suspicion in protection of victim rights (Arias, 2008; Hammer, Moynihan, & Pagliaro, 2013; Watts, 2013).

Effects of Violence. Approaching violence as a healthcare issue allows for applying epidemiological tools to investigate the phenomenon and its effect on society. Violence costs society in many ways: economically, socially, and regarding health and well-being.

- Rivara and colleagues (2007) demonstrated that the healthcare costs for women as a result of interpersonal violence (IPV) is 19% higher and the annual healthcare costs for their children are 11% higher. In addition, the researchers found that the higher healthcare costs existed for the children even if the abuse stopped before the child was born.

- According to Corso, Mercy, Simon, Finkelstein, and Miller (2007), violence is a leading cause of mortality and morbidity in the United States; violence-related injuries result in $5.6 billion in medical costs and a further $64.8 billion in productivity losses.
- The phenomenon of intergenerational trauma is particularly evident in Aboriginal or First Nations people. North American First Nations people experience higher levels of adverse childhood experiences, such as abuse, neglect, and household substance abuse (Blackstock, Trocmé, & Bennett, 2004; Duran, Malcoe, Sanders, Waitzkin, Skipper, & Yager, 2004) and are more likely to experience stressful events in adulthood, including poverty, unemployment, violence, homicide, assault, and witnessing traumatic events (Bombay, Matheson, & Anisman, 2009).

Recognizing the magnitude of the problem of violence and abuse on population health, several nursing organizations have issued position statements concerning various aspects of violence, including but not limited to the American Nurses Association, *Violence Against Women* (2000); the American Association of Colleges of Nursing, *Violence as a Public Health Problem* (1999); and the Emergency Nurses Association and the International Association of Forensic Nurses, *Intimate Partner Violence* (2013).

The IAFN position statement *Violence Is a Public Health and Healthcare Issue* (2009b) describes seven tenets:

1. Forensic nurses have a professional and ethical responsibility to serve, advocate for and empower patients, families, and their communities.
2. Forensic nurses organize and participate in facilitating the development of policies and procedures that foster the implementation of prevention and intervention programs in response to violence.
3. Recognition of violence as a global, healthcare problem is the first step towards solving this critical issue.
4. Forensic nurses have the opportunity to improve the ultimate health outcomes that result from violence as forensic nurses are uniquely positioned in intersecting systems such as healthcare, community and legal environments for early identification of patients at risk of victimization or perpetration of violence.
5. Increased awareness and education for all healthcare providers and attention to the effects of violence is needed in an effort to reduce immediate, intermediate, and long-term physical and psychological injuries that are associated with violence.
6. Forensic nurses are able to establish and promote identification, intervention and prevention programs, with the recognition that sustained societal change requires action that includes support of research, development of public policy and passage of legislation to effectively reduce and eliminate the causes, consequences and costs of violence.
7. Public and private institutions that regulate or provide accreditation for healthcare facilities must promote the development of a coordinated and culturally sensitive response and care for patients who have experienced violence or abuse to include the intervention of forensic nursing.

US Department of Justice: Office on Violence Against Women. The Office on Violence Against Women (OVW) is a part of the US Department of Justice, whose mission is to provide federal leadership in developing the nation's capacity to reduce VAW, strengthen services, and administer justice for victims of domestic or dating violence, sexual assault, and stalking (OVW, 2014). The OVW was created in 1995 to provide assistance to communities establishing programs, policies, and practices for DV, sexual assault, and stalking (OVW, 2014). Although services for victims had been established in the 1970s and 1980s, the services were not standard across the country. The efforts of advocates and survivors, including forensic nurses, informed the work of the government on these issues and served as the impetus for addressing violence toward women. The Violence Against Women Act (VAWA) was passed in 1994 following extensive efforts from advocates and professionals working with victims of domestic and sexual violence. The VAWA was reauthorized in 2013. The VAWA funds services for victims (men, women, and children) and has since expanded to include dating violence and stalking. The Act also supports training on these issues and ensures consistent responses to these victims across the country by emphasizing a coordinated community response (National Network to End Domestic Violence, 2015). The VAWA also supports community-based agencies working toward ending VAW, particularly those that are culturally specific, including Native American women.

Violence Prevention. Forensic nurses recognize their role in the prevention of violence by examining and understanding the societal influences and social injustices that promote violence or contribute to the cycle of violence, such as racism, oppression, poverty, and social inequities (IAFN, 2008). Forensic nurses work to improve the lives and health outcomes of their patients and society through their interactions within the legal system, healthcare system, and community agencies (Trujillo, Delapp, & Hendrix, 2014). Prevention programs must be driven by policy, be evidence-based, involve and meet the needs of the community, and be sustainable (Baum, Blakeslee, Lloyd, & Petrosino, 2013).

Public health prevention models target the population as a whole and consider prevention at three levels: primary, secondary, and tertiary.

- Primary prevention: Focuses on the promotion of change through knowledge, attitudes, and behaviors. The goal of primary prevention is to stop victimization and perpetration before it happens, which must take place through changes to the root causes of violence (Trujillo, Delapp, & Hendrix, 2014). For instance, forensic nurses can increase public awareness of issues of gender-based violence, such as domestic abuse and sexual assault.

  The IAFN has developed the Primary Sexual Violence Prevention Project to integrate primary prevention of sexual violence into forensic nursing practice through the use of evidence-based practices. The Project provides a roadmap for integrating primary prevention strategies, which includes five opportunities:
  - Develop individual prevention skills.
  - Seek opportunities to promote sexual violence prevention in all communities.
  - Incorporate primary sexual violence prevention strategies into healthcare provider education.
  - Collaborate with individuals and organizations to strengthen and promote community-wide sexual violence prevention.
  - Identify areas within your healthcare institution or organization that can integrate primary sexual violence prevention principles.
  - Advocate for public policy changes to prioritize sexual violence prevention and support efforts to create a world without violence (IAFN, n.d.a).

- Secondary prevention: This type is most familiar to forensic nurses as they care for victims, suspects, and perpetrators following an event or events with the goals of preventing injury, sequelae, or further violence. Forensic nurses promote prevention activities with populations at risk, such as children or women who are pregnant. For example, although still a controversial issue, screening women for DV or interpersonal violence has been recommended and implemented in many EDs. In a review, Anglin and Sachs (2003) found that insufficient outcome evaluation research exists to support a recommendation for or against universal screening in the ED. The researchers, however, concluded that, based on the impact of DV on women and children and the burden of suffering, mortality, morbidity, and the societal costs, screening for DV should be implemented in a private, nonjudgmental manner, and should include evaluation of effectiveness and outcomes (Anglin & Sachs, 2003). The CDC guideline, *Intimate Partner Violence and Sexual Violence Victimization Assessment Instruments for Use in Healthcare Settings* (Basille, Hertz, & Back, 2007), provides a compilation of assessment instruments, including evaluation of the psychometric properties of the instruments. However, "[t]hese assessment instruments should only be used if there are resources available to distribute to clients for primary prevention purposes (preventing violence before it starts); and if there are mechanisms in place to refer clients exposed to IPV [intimate partner violence] or SV [sexual violence] for a comprehensive assessment and appropriate victim services" (Basille, Hertz, & Back, 2007; p. 9).

- Tertiary prevention: Like secondary interventions, this type of prevention occurs after an event but seeks to prevent long-term harm to the individual; this includes policy and legislation development, public education, and prevention program development and evaluation. Forensic nurses promote prevention by assisting victims and perpetrators directly with behavior-changing strategies, using culturally competent means for teaching effective coping techniques (IAFN, 2009b).

Prevention begins with knowledge and recognition of the phenomenon of violence. Forensic nurses should assess for lifetime exposure to violence, hidden risk behaviors, such as substance abuse and self-harm, long-term sequelae of trauma, and safety. Forensic nurses provide interventions that promote prevention of violence at all levels. Examples include providing education to individuals, families, and communities about risk factors or intervening in high-risk groups to build awareness of issues that target that group (e.g., financial fraud of the older adult). According to Ferguson and Speck (2010), the framework for addressing violence as a public health issue requires a holistic approach that includes all stakeholders, including forensic nurses, and involves nursing community assessment, epidemiology, and forensic investigations.

Core Competencies of Public Health Nursing. Forensic nursing education includes public health nursing competencies that support increased knowledge of the role of prevention in improving the health of individuals, families, and communities.

The competencies were developed by the Quad Council for Public Health Nursing Organizations, which is an alliance of the four national nursing organizations that address public health nursing issues: the Association of Community Health Nurse Educators (ACHNE), the American Nurses Association's Congress on Nursing Practice and Economics (ANA), the American Public Health Association-PHN Section (APHA), and the Association of State and Territorial Directors of Nursing (ASTDN).

Last revised in 2011 and adopted in 2014, the competencies contain eight domains:

- Analytic and Assessment Skills
- Policy Development/Program Planning Skills
- Communications Skills
- Cultural Competencies Skills
- Community Dimensions of Practice
- Public Health Science Skills
- Financial Planning and Management Skills
- Leadership and Systems Thinking Skills (Quad Council of Public Health Nursing Organizations, 2011).

PRACTICE SETTINGS

Paralleling the diverse roles of forensic nurses are the practice settings in which forensic nurses function. These include but are not limited to hospital or healthcare settings; legal, correctional, or educational settings; governmental or nongovernmental organizations (NGOs); and commercial or industrial enterprises. The following is a summary of possible practice sites in which forensic nurses may work.

Hospital/Pre-Hospital/Clinics

- Emergency Department (ED): SANEs and forensic nurse examiners (FNEs) may work out of hospital EDs. Sexual assault nurse examiners work with victims of sexual assault and, in some settings, with victims of DV. Forensic nurse examiners tend to have a broader scope of practice, responding to different forensic populations that may include sexual assault and DV victims; child maltreatment; elder abuse; and victims of interpersonal violence, crime, and death.
- Sexual Assault Response Teams (SART)/Sexual Assault Treatment Centers (SATC): Sexual assault nurse examiners may work on SARTs/SATCs in EDs, in a hospital clinic setting, or in a free-standing clinic, providing medical and forensic interventions for victims of sexual assault. Many SARTs/SATCs have expanded their role to respond to and provide care for victims of DV.

- Child Maltreatment Clinics: Sexual assault nurse examiners and FNEs who specialize in pediatrics may work in a hospital-based outpatient clinic, responding to EDs, or in a child advocacy center, providing care for victims of child maltreatment, including physical and sexual abuse or emotional abuse and neglect.
- Child Advocacy Center (CAC)/Child and Youth Advocacy Center (CYAC): A CAC/CYAC is a child-focused facility in a neutral setting used for the multidisciplinary approach to the investigation of child maltreatment. These centers emphasize a coordinated, collaborative effort of multidisciplinary professionals and agencies for investigation (law enforcement, child protection) and intervention (medical, social, psychological) and seek to create a child-focused approach and a safe, secure, child-friendly environment. The CAC model was developed by the National Children's Alliance (NCA), which is the national association and accrediting body for CACs.

Legal/Investigative Settings

- Crime Laboratory: Requires additional specialized training in the forensic sciences and technology; roles include analysis of trace evidence involving forensic biology, forensic chemistry, forensic toxicology, questioned documents, and firearms and tool mark examination.
- Crime Scene Investigator (CSI): Requires additional specialized training in crime scene evidence collection techniques and analysis; may work directly at the scene of crimes conducting forensic photography, fingerprinting, collecting DNA, and performing blood spatter pattern analysis. However, not all jurisdictions allow forensic nurses to perform these roles; in many locales, CSIs must be sworn law enforcement officers.
- Legal Nurse Consultant (LNC): Works directly with the legal system in private practice or legal settings, such as attorney's offices. The American Association of Legal Nurse Consultants (2013) describes legal nurse consulting as "the application of knowledge acquired during the course of professional nursing education, training, and clinical experience to the evaluation of standards of care, causation, damages and other medically related issues in medical-legal cases or claims."
- Nurse Attorney: Requires the additional education of a law degree; involves practicing law in a variety of settings, such as private practice, legal aid, or within a prosecutor's office, a healthcare setting, or with an advocacy or nongovernmental agency or organization, such as the Innocence Project.
- Law Enforcement Agencies: Works as a consultant for the police department or another law enforcement agency or as a forensic specialist who provides a connection between law enforcement and healthcare agencies; may assume other specialist roles, such as a trainer or educator. In the United Kingdom, for example, forensic nurses are employed within local police stations, where they provide medical, forensic, and mental health assessments (Collins, personal communication, 2014; Cowley, Walsh, & Horrocks, 2014).
- Victim Services: Works with victims through the criminal justice system by providing nursing care at a scene following a violent crime or through partnerships for care delivery, such as in a women's shelter or within an advocacy agency.

Governmental Institutions/Organizations

- Politics: Works at any level of local, regional, or national politics in roles such as education, advocacy, and policy development.
- Boards of Health: Works within public health or community boards of health; roles include investigation, risk management, health prevention and promotion, and education and policy development using an epidemiological approach to forensic issues, such as violence.
- Violence Prevention and Response Teams: Is often employed within governmental or community violence prevention programs; applies knowledge of violence epidemiology and public health forensic content expertise to raise awareness, educate, advocate, and provide community assessment and program development.
- National Health Organizations: Works within federal institutions, such as the Centers for Disease Control and Prevention (CDC) and the Federal Emergency Management Agency (FEMA), in various capacities, including emergency response.

Nongovernmental/Not-for-Profit Organizations

- Advocacy Groups: Work involves VAW or other groups that advocate for violence prevention and intervention or investigation, such as Rape Abuse Incest National Network (RAINN).
- Human Rights Organizations: Works with enterprises such as Amnesty International, Physicians for Human Rights (PHR), and the International Rescue Committee (IRC), applying forensic knowledge to human rights issues locally or globally.
- Community-Based Organizations: Involves work with advocacy groups or service agencies that provide investigative, advocacy, research, education, health promotion, and prevention or support services.
- International Organizations: Includes positions with the WHO or the UN in roles such as investigation, health promotion and prevention, education, advocacy, research, and policy development. Forensic nurses have contributed to WHO position statements and clinical and policy guideline publications (e.g., *Guidelines for Medico-Legal Care for Victims of Sexual Violence* (WHO, 2003) and *Responding to Intimate Partner Violence and Sexual Violence Against Women* (WHO, 2013)).

Commercial Enterprises

- Technology Development and Sales: With knowledge of forensic sciences and technology, forensic nurses may work in a variety of technological settings, including research and development or on a consultative basis for companies that support the advancement of forensic science and technology.

Industrial

- Workplace Safety: Works within healthcare settings or external workplace safety settings in risk management, accident prevention/safety, or in an investigative role, such as evaluating workplace accidents, injuries, and deaths. Harris (2013) reports that the forensic nurse is ideally poised to evaluate workplace injuries/accidents/fatalities as he or she has "the ability to evaluate both medical and physical injuries, describing the scientific relationship between injury and evidence and interpreting the factors that influence them" (p. 198). Harris (2013) advocates for forensic nursing expertise to be used in consultation or as an applied role in occupational injury and workplace fatality investigations.
- Occupational Health: Interprets physical and psychological trauma by determining the mechanism of injury, perhaps by accident reconstruction and conducting trauma assessment. Forensic nurses may also provide psychological services through employee assistance programs.
- Risk Management: Proactively applies forensic knowledge to prevent unsafe environments or practices and promote safety and quality improvement. The clinical risk manager is a new forensic nursing role with a strong educational component in preventing error; other roles include but are not limited to record review, complaint/claim investigations, and as a legal resource for staff (Benak, 2005).

Custodial Institutions

- Jails, Detention Centers, and Prisons: Work occurs at any level of the correctional system, including medical or psychological services, providing care to perpetrators of crime, violence, and abuse.
- Psychiatric Facilities: Work setting involves various types of mental health facilities, hospital units, clinics, or group homes.
- Psychiatric Correctional Facilities: Works within an interprofessional team on a forensic psychiatric unit, caring for perpetrators and helping assess these patients for the criminal justice system. Forensic nurses may work on forensic units of large regional hospitals, such as a provincial or state mental health hospital, or on a unit within a general hospital or a forensic psychiatric facility.

Educational

- Colleges/Universities: Teaches forensic sciences or forensic nursing curricula at the undergraduate, graduate, and doctoral level.

- Public Health Offices: Works directly with the public or other professionals in the education and prevention of violence and trauma, or at a policy development or research level.
- Public Health Department: Involves work at a larger, regional public health setting, such as at the state or provincial level as an educator, clinician, or statistician; may work in the clinical, epidemiology, outreach, or prevention arms of the public health services.
- Conferences/Scientific Assemblies/Trainings: Works in the education field as a presenter or indirectly through an employer by translating knowledge in local, national, and international settings. The IAFN, for instance, holds an annual International Conference on Forensic Nursing Science and Practice where hundreds of forensic nurses gather to learn from not only experts, but also from their colleagues.

Death Investigation

- Medical examiner (ME)/Coroner's Office: Works as a death investigator or a nurse coroner; may also work in the records, research, or administrative offices of the ME or coroner.

ROLES OF THE FORENSIC NURSE

Table 1.8 outlines the various roles of the forensic nurse.

Levels of Practice

The two levels of forensic nursing practice are basic and advanced.

Basic Forensic Nursing Practice. Forensic nursing is practiced by registered nurses who have the requisite knowledge and skills, based on the scope and standards of practice (IAFN & ANA, 2009). Basic forensic nursing practice is considered generalist and is guided by forensic nursing protocols for specific forensic patient populations. Forensic nurses at the basic level achieve specialized knowledge through training programs, continuing education, and certification programs, among other avenues. Most generalists who practice basic forensic nursing are prepared for their nursing career at the diploma, associate degree, and bachelor's degree level.

Forensic Nursing in an Advanced Role. Forensic nursing in an advanced role incorporates expanded and specialized knowledge and skills, and is characterized by the integration and application of a range of theoretical and evidence-based knowledge that is acquired as a part of graduate-level academic preparation. Forensic nurses prepared to function in an advanced role and in advanced practice hold an academic master's or doctoral degree from an accredited institution.

Educational Preparation

In 1986, Virginia Lynch introduced the first master's program for a forensic clinical nurse specialist at the University of Texas, Arlington (Lynch, 2011a). In Canada in 1996, Arlene Kent-Wilkinson established the first two online forensic nursing courses for Mount Royal University in Calgary, Alberta. In 1998, Catherine Carter-Snell developed this into a six-course certificate program. Originally designed only for nurses, the course was expanded to include police officers, paramedics, and social workers per their request. Many countries now offer forensic nursing programs, such as a Master of Forensic Nursing in Italy and a forensic nursing course in India (Lynch, 2011b). In 2000, Bangkok introduced a forensic nursing program; in 2001, Zimbabwe introduced an FNE program for victims of torture (Lynch, 2011b). Educational opportunities continue to expand, ranging from continuing education courses and certificate programs to graduate programs.

Nurses can obtain an academic degree at the master's level in the forensic nursing specialty, or complete a graduate degree at the master's or doctoral level with some emphasis in forensics/forensic nursing, such as completion of a master's degree program in the option of forensic nursing or completion of a master's degree program with a thesis or capstone on a forensic topic area; completion of a Ph.D. with a dissertation devoted to a forensics/forensic nursing topic area; or a Doctor of Nursing Practice (DNP) degree with the completion of a scholarly project in a forensics/

TABLE 1.8 Roles of the Forensic Nurse

	Role Definition	Reference
Medical clinical	Gather and document physical and nonphysical evidence. Improve patient care management with clinical service, legal order, and forensic procedure.	PubMed.gov. Retrieved from: http://www.ncbi.nlm.nih.gov/pubmed/10646459
Legal	Analyze medical portions of legal documents. Inform attorneys of medical issues. Attend medical examinations and report evidence at trial. Assist in preparation for trial.	American Association of Legal Nurse Consultants. Retrieved from: http://www.aalnc.org/?page=WhatisanLNC http://www.theforensicnurse.com/ http://www.americannursetoday.com/assets/0/434/436/440/8364/8366/8378/8428/326dcefb-22dd-440a-a9fe-d15c36cb8ba1.pdf
Correctional	Provide health care to those in the criminal justice system. The forensic nurse is often the first to see an inmate about a medical problem. Provide medical care while maintaining security and public safety.	International Association of Forensic Nurses. Retrieved from: http://www.iafn.org/displaycommon.cfm?an=1&subarticlenbr=762
Geriatric	Care for elderly patients in cases of abuse or neglect. Assist patients who are vulnerable to abuse. Help law enforcement involved with the case.	Nursing School Degrees. Retrieved from: http://www.nursing-school-degrees.com/Nursing-Careers/forensic-geriatric-nurse.html
Psychiatric	Provide care to individuals with mental disorders who are at risk to commit crimes or cause injury. Apply principles of forensic psychiatry and nursing to assess and treat individuals with crime-related mental disorders.	*Forensic Nursing: Scope and Standards of Practice*, 2009; p. 9
Pediatric	Help children who are victims of abuse or other crimes. Conduct physical, psychological, and social evaluations and document evidence. Help child work through trauma from both physical and emotional harm. Find forensic evidence and provide expertise in prosecution.	Nursing School Degrees. Retrieved from: http://www.nursing-school-degrees.com/Nursing-Careers/pediatric-forensic-nurse.html
Forensic nurse examiner (FNE)	Provide care for patients who have experienced or perpetrated physical and/or psychological violence or trauma and/or death.	Lynch & Duval, 2011
Nurse death investigator/ Nurse coroner	Conduct medicolegal death investigation. Establish a death, identify individual, and notify kin. Provide expertise in assisting medical examiners in determining cause of death.	Medscape Multispecialty. Retrieved from: http://www.medscape.com/viewarticle/571555_4
Sexual assault nurse examiner (SANE)	Care for victims of sexual assault and abuse. Conduct physical assessments. Provide emotional and social support resources. Testify at legal proceedings related to the examination. Ensure that patient is treated with compassion and provide potential evidence to criminal justice.	International Association of Forensic Nurses. Retrieved from: http://www.iafn.org/displaycommon.cfm?an=1&subarticlenbr=546
Nurse attorney	Must be an RN and earn a law degree. Practice law with a specialization in health law. Provide medical knowledge for cases.	Nursing School Degrees. Retrieved from: http://www.nursing-school-degrees.com/Nursing-Careers/nurse-attorney.html

(continued)

TABLE 1.8 Roles of the Forensic Nurse (continued)

	Role Definition	Reference
Risk management	Develop a plan for data collection and responses to patient or staff risk in the healthcare setting. Collaborate to provide data that support solutions to risk.	*Forensic Nursing: Scope and Standards of Practice,* 2009; p. 8
Community	Maintain patient confidentiality. Prevent violence in the community. Conduct unbiased research that is based on science.	International Association of Forensic Nurses. Retrieved from: http://www.iafn.org/displaycommon.cfm?an=1&subarticlenbr=56
Systems	Form connections between the medical, healthcare, and human, social, and criminal justice systems.	
International	Form networks and share best practice methods. Build alliances to promote the exchange of ideas or expansion of educational programs. Share knowledge, skills, and expertise across the globe.	International Association of Forensic Nurses. Retrieved from: http://www.iafn.org/associations/8556/files/IAFN%20Going%20Intl%20White%20Pape.pdf
Forensic nurse researcher	Participate in the development of original research, which builds the knowledge base for forensic nursing. Work collaboratively with forensic and other nurses to translate research evidence into practice to improve outcomes for individuals, families, and communities.	

forensic nursing practice area. Multiple avenues exist for obtaining academic degrees that provide for practice in the forensic nursing specialty (See Appendix B).

Credentialing

Sexual Assault Nurse Examiner Certification (SANE-A®, SANE-P®). The Commission for Forensic Nursing Certification offers certification as SANE-Adult/Adolescent and SANE-Pediatric. Certification is achieved through meeting eligibility requirements for education and successful completion of a certification examination. Certification renewal is required every 3 years and is accomplished through demonstration of a requisite amount of continuing education or achievement of a passing score on the certification examination.

Portfolio. In collaboration with the American Nurses Credentialing Center, the IAFN offers certification in Advanced Forensic Nursing (AFN-BC) through portfolio review. This is an alternative assessment process for any forensic nurse in a specialty area and is an important option for forensic nurses who hold an advanced nursing degree.

SCOPE AND STANDARDS OF FORENSIC NURSING PRACTICE

Function of the Scope of Practice Statement

First published in 1997, the *Scope and Standards of Forensic Nursing Practice* defines forensic nursing practice as a unique specialty in all settings and across varied roles. In 2009, the IAFN and the American Nurses Association revised the original document, and released *Forensic Nursing: Scope and Standards of Practice.* As of this printing, the second edition is forthcoming.

A primary function of the scope and standards of practice is to define and comprehensively describe forensic nursing, and provide direction for further development and recognition nationally and internationally. The scope of forensic nursing practice is recognized as having flexible boundaries across diverse settings and populations, intersecting varied healthcare settings and educational, legal, legislative, and scientific systems. The body of knowledge and practice identified as unique to forensic nursing continues to emerge, with the scope and standards of practice intended to serve as a foundation for legislation, policy, and professional regulation of forensic nursing. This document serves to inform forensic nurses, the nursing profession, other healthcare providers, employers, legislators, and the public of the unique scope of professional forensic nursing practice and priorities.

Function of the Standards

The *standards of practice* and the *standards of professional performance* are authoritative statements by which nurses practicing within the role, population, and specialty are governed, given the unique body of knowledge of the nursing specialty. During the Crimean War, Florence Nightingale conducted the first nursing research by collecting healthcare data and applying knowledge of statistics to patient care, thus creating the first standards of care (Finkelman & Kenner, 2013).

- All forensic nurses in practice, regardless of the role, population, or specialty are expected to perform competently. Competency is defined as "an expected and measurable level of nursing performance that integrates knowledge, skills, abilities and judgment based on established scientific knowledge and expectations for nursing practice" (Mariano, 2013; p. 11).
- The standards reflect the current state of knowledge, values, and priorities of forensic nursing practice.
- The standards of forensic nursing practice are specific to the multifaceted and complex specialty characterized by responsibilities, functions, roles, and skills that are derived from professional nursing practice and expected of all registered nurses, yet adapted in accordance with the distinctive practice environments and populations of forensic nursing.
- The standards provide guidance in the professional role comprised of knowledge, skills, attitudes, and behaviors that are relevant from novice to advanced levels of forensic nursing practice.
- The standards can be used as evidence of the legal standard of care for practicing within the role, population, and specialty of forensic nursing, recognizing that as the knowledge base unique to forensic nursing expands, so does the practice of forensic nursing.

FUTURE ISSUES

Although forensic nursing is a well-established specialty, forensic nursing concepts and roles will expand into additional settings as more nurses become interested, educated, and expert in forensic nursing practice and application. The future of forensic nursing depends on strong leadership, education, advocacy, and research. The elements that will spark the specialty's growth are (1) standardization of practice and competencies and (2) research and publication to build the knowledge base, professional status, identity, and recognition of forensic nurses (Jackson, 2011).

Presently, forensic nursing education is limited in nursing school and undergraduate curricula (Freedberg, 2008).

- Freedberg (2008) recommends forensic education and awareness-building in the nursing school curriculum and promotes using the nursing process to assess and plan care for persons affected by violence.
- The WHO report, *Preventing Violence* (WHO, 2004), highlights the need for trained forensic professionals who are qualified to conduct forensic examinations and are educated in the standards of evidence collection (Henderson, Harada, & Amar, 2012).

As forensic nursing grows and increases its recognition as a specialty practice across traditional and nontraditional nursing practice settings – and as more nurses pursue forensic nursing education – continued efforts are needed to gain professional recognition that will enhance the responsibilities and competencies of the forensic nurse (Jackson, 2011).

The forensic nurse must recognize and understand the broader role of public health intervention in providing care in a changing global environment. Advocacy and activism are essential to influencing the issues of violence, crime, and trauma in societies worldwide. Initiatives at the forefront of forensic nursing practice include:

- Advancing forensic education globally
- Developing and standardizing forensic nursing curricula
- Combating sexual assault as a weapon of war
- Preventing gender-based violence
- Engaging in political advocacy
- Promoting human rights
- Preventing interpersonal violence and child maltreatment
- Addressing transcultural violence issues
- Promoting forensic nursing roles globally
- Developing policy
- Addressing violence as a healthcare issue
- Advancing public health

Human Rights

A critical aspect of the future of forensic nursing is the issue of human rights. Forensic nurses worldwide must come together to address the cultural and religious practices that violate human rights and threaten the most vulnerable members of society—women, children, older adults, persons with disabilities, and the poor. Forensic nurses must have a comprehensive understanding of transcultural issues when working with people from socioculturally diverse populations (Hammer, Moynihan, & Pagliaro, 2013).

Hammer, Moynihan, and Pagliaro (2013) state that "we must strive to include issues that the WHO has identified as having the highest priority, not limiting our concerns to state or national agendas" (p. 13). In addition, forensic nurses must have knowledge of diverse cultural healthcare practices and be familiar with legislation at all levels of government.

Global Education

Education and advancement of forensic nursing worldwide are critical to addressing these priority issues. The IAFN is dedicated to promoting forensic nursing worldwide and has developed several initiatives based on the identified needs, which are presented in the document entitled *White Paper: Summary of IAFN's International Initiatives and Next Steps for Moving Forward Internationally* (Lugbil, 2007).

- The IAFN and the ANA published the *Forensic Nursing: Scope and Standards of Practice* (2009) to standardize forensic nursing practice nationally and internationally.
- The IAFN has developed education guidelines to provide specific standards for educational preparation of forensic nurses in focused areas of practice. These areas include the *Sexual Assault Nurse Examiner Education Guidelines: Adult/Adolescent and Pediatric* (IAFN, 2013a); *Forensic Nurse Death Investigator Education Guidelines* (IAFN, 2009a); and the *Intimate Partner Violence Education Guidelines* (IAFN, 2012).
- The forensic nurse is situated as a critical member in a multidisciplinary and multisectorial team approach to global education.

Global Influence

Forensic nurses possess the ability to influence policy development and legislation, and to promote governmental awareness of issues such as poverty, crime, and violence on a global level. Lynch (2007) has stated that the role of the forensic nurse has evolved toward a commitment to address the global agenda on poverty and human development through education, research, and early intervention to reduce the consequences associated with violence. Changing the world will require a collective action of which forensic nurses will be an integral part.

- The IAFN Governmental Affairs Committee provides documents to enable IAFN members to assert professional ideas and opinions aimed at influencing health policy issues worldwide (McDonald, 2012).
- Forensic nurses with specialized expertise in globally exploited populations, such as sex trafficking victims or torture victims, are well poised to influence policy formation for the prevention of these human rights violations (McDonald, 2012).

Research

Although recognized as a nursing specialty in the United States for more than 20 years, forensic nursing science is still a nascent science. It is imperative that forensic nurses conduct the research necessary to support evidence-based practice (Clements & Sekula, 2005).

- Stokowski (2008) has suggested that "research into the primary prevention of violence, the effects of violence, and the outcomes of forensic nursing practice is also needed, both in the United States and on a global scale" (p. 5).
- According to Koehler (2005), the role of the forensic nurse is a critical component of database development, as the information that is collected and documented can be incorporated into data-driven research in the specialty.

CASE STUDY

A forensic nurse is working in a medium-security correctional psychiatric facility. Over the last 2 days, a 30-year-old male patient has demonstrated increasingly agitated and violent behavior. The patient has been nonadherent with his prescribed medication for the same time. He now assaults a co-patient and has threatened a staff member.

- How does the nurse balance the respect for patient autonomy with the need for safety?
- What ethical justifications or principles guide the nurse's clinical decisions regarding the care of the patient/prisoner?

REVIEW QUESTIONS

1. A forensic nurse is a nurse who:
   a. applies forensic science concepts while providing nursing care.
   b. has specialized training in crime scene investigation.
   c. is skilled in collecting forensic evidence.
   d. works as a sexual assault nurse examiner (SANE).

2. Which of the following actions demonstrates the assessment phase of the nursing process for a forensic client?
   a. Interprofessional team peer review of child sexual abuse cases
   b. Providing a patient with information about psychological trauma
   c. Recognition of a patterned injury; bruising consistent with a belt mark on a child
   d. Reporting concerns of child maltreatment to a child protection service

3. A conceptual model is defined as:
   a. a connection of concepts based on values and beliefs.
   b. a general description of a phenomenon.
   c. a pattern of viewing the world.
   d. an organized representation of complex concepts.

4. Three ethical values of forensic nurses are:
   a. autonomy, maleficence, and equality.
   b. caring, advocacy, and justice.
   c. liberty, freedom, and beneficence.
   d. objectivity, confidentiality, and boundaries.

5. Match the forensic nursing role with the setting.
   a. Evaluates causes of accidents and injuries
   b. Provides education on violence prevention
   c. Collects evidence from the deceased
   d. Writes policy briefs and recommendations
   e. Collects epidemiological research data
   f. Consults legally on forensic issues

   1. Attorney's office
   2. Coroner's office
   3. Board of health
   4. Workers' compensation office
   5. City council
   6. Public health department

REFERENCES

Ali, A., & Lees, K. E. (2013). The therapist as advocate: Anti-oppression advocacy in psychological practice. *Journal of Clinical Psychology, 69*(2), 162–171.

American Association of Colleges of Nursing. (1999). *Position statement: Violence as a public health problem.* Retrieved from http://www.aacn.nche.edu/publications/position/violence-problem

American Association of Legal Nurse Consultants. (2013). *What is an LNC?* Retrieved from http://www.aalnc.org/?page=WhatisanLNC

American Nurses Association (ANA). (2000). *Position statement: Violence against women.* Retrieved from http://www.nursingworld.org/MainMenuCategories/Policy-Advocacy/Positions-and-Resolutions/ANAPositionStatements/Position-Statements-Alphabetically/Violence-Against-Women.html

American Nurses Association (ANA). (2004). *Nursing: Scope and standards of practice.* Silver Spring, MD: Nursesbooks.org.

American Nurses Association (ANA). (2010). *Nursing: Scope and standards of practice* (2nd ed.). Silver Spring, MD: Nursesbooks.org.

American Nurses Association (ANA) & International Association of Forensic Nurses (IAFN). (1997). *Scope and standards of forensic nursing practice.* Washington, DC: ANA.

American Psychiatric Association. (2013). *Diagnostic and statistical manual of mental health disorders (DSM-V).* Washington, DC: American Psychiatric Publishing.

Amnesty International. (2015). *Human rights basics.* Retrieved February 16, 2015, from http://www.amnestyusa.org/research/human-rights-basics

Anderson, G. S. (2007). *All you ever wanted to know about forensic science in Canada but didn't know who to ask.* Ottawa, Ontario, Canada: Canadian Society of Forensic Sciences. Retrieved from http://www.bcit.ca/files/cas/forensics/pdf/forensic_science_anderson.pdf

Anglin, D., & Sachs, C. (2003). Preventive care in the emergency department: Screening for domestic violence in the emergency department. *Academic Emergency Medicine, 10*(10), 1118–1127.

Ann Burgess: Psychosocial nurse of the year. (1991). *Journal of Psychosocial Nursing and Mental Health Services, 29*(12), 38.

Arias, C. D. (2008). C. Everett Koop: The nation's health conscience. *American Journal of Public Health, 98*(3), 396–399.

Barber, K. (Ed.). (2004). *Canadian Oxford dictionary* (2nd ed.). Ontario, Canada: Oxford University Press.

Basille, K. C., Hertz, M. F., & Back, S. E. (2007). *Intimate partner violence and sexual violence victimization assessment instruments for use in healthcare settings.* Atlanta, GA: Centers for Disease Control and Prevention, National Center for Injury Prevention and Control.

Baum, K., Blakeslee, K. M., Lloyd, J., & Petrosino, A. (2013). *Violence prevention: Moving from evidence to implementation.* Washington, DC: National Academy of Sciences. Retrieved from https://www.iom.edu/Global/Perspectives/2013/~/media/Files/Perspectives-Files/2013/Discussion-Papers/BGH-ViolencePreventionEvidenceImplementation.pdf

Beauchamp, T. L., & Childress, J. F. (2009). *Principles of biomedical ethics* (6th ed.). New York, NY: Oxford University Press.

Benak, L. (2005). Risk management-the forensic nursing responses "ability." *Journal of Forensic Nursing, 1*(2), 86–88.

Blackstock, C., Trocmé, N., & Bennett, M. (2004). Child maltreatment investigations among Aboriginal and non-Aboriginal families in Canada: A comparative analysis. *Violence Against Women, 10*(8), 901–916.

Bombay, A., Matheson, K., & Anisman, H. (2009). Intergenerational trauma: Convergence of multiple processes among First Nations peoples in Canada. *Journal of Aboriginal Health, 5*(3), 6–47.

Boschma, G. (1994). The meaning of holism in nursing: Historical shifts in holistic ideas. *Public Health Journal, 11*(5), 324–330.

Briere, J., & Scott, C. (2006). *Principles of trauma therapy: A guide to symptoms, evaluation, and treatment.* Thousand Oaks, CA: Sage Publications, Inc.

Briere, J., & Spinazzola, J. (2005). Phenomenology and psychological assessment of complex posttraumatic states. *Journal of Traumatic Stress, 18*(5), 401–412.

Burgess, A. W., Berger, A. D., & Boersma, R. R. (2004). Forensic nursing: Investigating the career potential in this emerging graduate specialty. *American Journal of Nursing, 104*(3), 58–64.

Burgess, A. W., & Holmstrom, L. L. (1974). Rape trauma syndrome. *American Journal of Psychiatry, 131*(9), 981–986.

Campbell, D. B. (2011). Oppression of the different: Impact and treatment. *International Journal of Applied Psychoanalytic Studies, 8*(1), 28–47.

Campbell, R., Greeson, M., Bybee, D., & Kennedy, A. (2013). *Adolescent sexual assault victims' experiences with SANE-SARTs and the criminal justice system, 1998–2007.* ICPSR - Interuniversity Consortium for Political and Social Research. Retrieved from http://www.icpsr.umich.edu/icpsrweb/NACJD/studies/29721/version/1

Campbell, R., Greeson, M., & Patterson, D. (2011). Defining the boundaries: How sexual assault nurse examiners (SANEs) balance patient care and law enforcement collaboration. *Journal of Forensic Nursing, 7*(1), 17–26.

Campbell, R., Wasco, S. M., Ahrens, C. E., Sefl, T., & Barnes, H. E. (2001). Preventing the "second rape": Rape survivors' experiences with community service providers. *Journal of Interpersonal Violence, 16*(12), 1239–1259.

Canadian Nurses Association. (2007). *Canadian regulatory framework for registered nurses. Position statement.* Ottawa, Canada: Canadian Nurses Association.

Center for Nonviolence and Social Justice. (2014). *What is trauma?* Retrieved from http://www.nonviolenceandsocialjustice.org/FAQs/What-is-Trauma/41/

Clements, P., & Sekula, K. (2005). Toward advancement and evolution of forensic nursing: The interface and interplay of research, theory, and practice. *Journal of Forensic Nursing, 1*(1), 35–38.

Collins, S. E., & Halpern, K. J. (2005). Forensic nursing: A collaborative practice paradigm. *Journal of Nursing and Law, 10*(1), 11–19.

Corso, P. S., Mercy, J. A., Simon, T. R., Finkelstein, E. A., & Miller, T. R. (2007). Medical costs and productivity losses due to interpersonal and self-directed violence in the United States. *American Journal of Preventative Medicine, 32*(6), 474–482.

Cowley, R., Walsh, E., & Horrocks, J. (2014). The role of the sexual assault nurse examiner in England: Nurse experiences and perspectives. *Journal of Forensic Nursing, 10*(2), 77–83.

Crane, P. (2005). Cultural competence and the advanced practice forensic nurse. *Topics in Emergency Medicine, 27*(2), 157–162.

Cunneen, C. (2006). Racism, discrimination and the over-representation of indigenous people in the criminal justice system: Some conceptual and explanatory issues. *Current Issues in Criminal Justice, 17*(3), 329–346.

Downing, N. R., & Mackin, M. L. (2012). The perception of role conflict in sexual assault nursing and its effects on care delivery. *Journal of Forensic Nursing, 8*(2), 53–60.

DuMont, J., MacDonald, S., White, M., Turner, L., White, D., Kaplan, S., & Smith, T. (2014). Client satisfaction with nursing-led sexual assault and domestic violence services in Ontario. *Journal of Forensic Nursing, 10*(3), 122–134.

DuMont, J., White, D., & McGregor, M. J. (2009). Investigating the medical forensic examination from the perspectives of sexually assaulted women. *Social Sciences and Medicine, 68*(4), 774–780.

Duran, B., Malcoe, L. H., Sanders, M., Waitzkin, H., Skipper, B., & Yager, J. (2004). Child maltreatment prevalence and mental disorders outcomes among American Indian women in primary care. *Child Abuse and Neglect, 28,* 131–145.

Eckert, W. (1990). Forensic sciences: The clinical or living aspects. *American Journal for Forensic Medicine and Pathology, 11*(4), 336–341.

Eisler, R. L., & Silverman, J. S. (2014). Criminal injustice. *Psychiatric Annals, 44*(3), 156–160.

Emergency Nurses Association, International Association of Forensic Nurses (IAFN). (2013). *Joint position statement: Intimate partner violence.* Retrieved from https://www.ena.org/SiteCollectionDocuments/Position%20Statements/IPV.pdf

Ericksen, J., Dudley, C., McIntosh, G., Ritch, L., Shumay, S., & Simpson, M. (2002). Client's experiences with a specialized sexual assault service. *Journal of Emergency Nursing, 28*(1), 86–90.

Evans, S. (2005). Beyond gender: Class, poverty and domestic violence. *Australian Social Work, 58*(1), 36–43.

Fehler-Cabral, G., Campbell, R., & Patterson, D. (2011). Adult sexual assault survivors' experiences with sexual assault nurse examiners (SANEs). *Journal of Interpersonal Violence, 26*(18), 3618–3639.

Ferguson, C. T., & Speck, P. (2010). The forensic nurse and violence prevention and response in public health. *Journal of Forensic Nursing, 6*(3), 151–156.

Finkelman, A., & Kenner, C. (2013). *Professional nursing concepts: Competencies for quality leadership* (2nd ed.). Sudbury, MA: Jones & Bartlett Learning.

Forensic Nurses' Society of Canada. (FNSC). (2015). *About: History.* Retrieved March 8, 2015, from http://forensicnurse.ca/about/

Fox, S., & Hoelscher, K. (2012). Political order, development and social violence. *Journal of Peace Research, 49*(3), 431–444.

Freedberg, P. (2008). Integrating forensic nursing into the undergraduate nursing curriculum: A solution for a disconnect. *Journal of Nursing Education, 47*(5), 201–208.

Gustafsson, L. K., Wigerblad, A., & Lindwall, L. (2013). Respecting dignity in forensic care: The challenge faced by nurses of maintaining patient dignity in clinical caring situations. *Journal of Psychiatric and Mental Health Nursing, 20*(1), 1–8.

Hammer, R. (2000). Caring in forensic nursing. Expanding the holistic model. *Journal of Psychosocial Nursing and Mental Health Services, 38*(11), 18–24.

Hammer, R. M., Moynihan, B., & Pagliaro, E. M. (2013). *Forensic nursing: A handbook for practice.* Sudbury, MA: Jones & Bartlett Learning.

Harris, C. (2013). Occupational injury and fatality investigations: The application of forensic nursing science. *Journal of Forensic Nursing, 9*(4), 193–199.

Henderson, E., Harada, N., & Amar, A. (2012). Caring for the forensic population: Recognizing the educational needs of emergency department nurses and physicians. *Journal of Forensic Nursing, 8*(4), 170–177.

Herdman, T. H., & Kamitsuru, S. (Eds.). (2014). *NANDA International nursing diagnoses: Definitions and classification 2015–2017.* Oxford, England: Wiley Blackwell.

Herman, J. L. (1992a). Complex PTSD: A syndrome in survivors of prolonged and repeated trauma. *Journal of Traumatic Stress, 5*(3), 377–391.

Herman, J. L. (1992b). *Trauma and recovery: The aftermath of violence – from domestic abuse to political terror.* New York, NY: Basic Books.

Hutson, L. A. (2002). Development of sexual assault nurse examiner programs. *Nursing Clinics of North America, 37*(1), 79–88.

International Association of Forensic Nurses (IAFN). (1996). *Sexual assault nurse examiner standards of practice.* Elkridge, MD: IAFN.

International Association of Forensic Nurses (IAFN). (2008). *Vision of ethical practice.* Elkridge, MD: IAFN. Retrieved from http://www.forensicnurses.org/?page=visionethicalpract

International Association of Forensic Nurses (IAFN). (2009a). *Forensic nurse death investigator education guidelines.* Elkridge, MD: IAFN. Retrieved from http://c.ymcdn.com/sites/www.forensicnurses.org/resource/resmgr/Education/Nurse_Death_Investigator_Edu.pdf

International Association of Forensic Nurses (IAFN). (2009b). *Position statement: Violence is a public health and health care issue.* Elkridge, MD: IAFN. Retrieved from http://c.ymcdn.com/sites/www.forensicnurses.org/resource/resmgr/Position_Papers/IAFN_Position_Statement-Viol.pdf

International Association of Forensic Nurses (IAFN). (2012). *Intimate partner violence education guidelines.* Elkridge, MD: IAFN. Retrieved from https://c.ymcdn.com/sites/iafn.site-ym.com/resource/resmgr/Education/Intimate_Partner_Violence_Nu.pdf

International Association of Forensic Nurses (IAFN). (2013a). *Sexual assault nurse examiner guidelines: Adult/adolescent and pediatric.* Elkridge, MD: IAFN. Retrieved March 10, 2015, from http://c.ymcdn.com/sites/www.forensicnurses.org/resource/resmgr/Education/Sexual_Assault_Nurse_Educati.pdf

International Association of Forensic Nurses (IAFN). (2013b). *2013 annual report.* Retrieved from http://www.forensicnurses.org/?page=2013Annual&hhSearchTerms=%222013+and+annual+and+report%22

International Association of Forensic Nurses (IAFN). (2015a). *A global organization.* Retrieved from http://www.forensicnurses.org/?page=IntlInitiative&hhSearchTerms=%22global+and+organization%22

International Association of Forensic Nurses (IAFN). (2015b). *History of the association.* Retrieved March 10, 2015, from http://www.forensicnurses.org/?page = AboutUS

International Association of Forensic Nurses (IAFN). (n.d.a). *Primary sexual assault prevention project.* Retrieved from http://c.ymcdn.com/sites/www.forensicnurses.org/resource/resmgr/imported/Primary%20Prevention%20Brochure.pdf

International Association of Forensic Nurses (IAFN) & American Nurses Association (ANA). (2009). *Forensic nursing: Scope and standards of practice.* Silver Spring, MD: Nursesbooks.org. (2nd ed. In press)

International Council of Nurses. (2012). *The ICN code of ethics for nurses.* Geneva, Switzerland: International Council of Nurses. Retrieved from http://www.icn.ch/images/stories/documents/about/icncode_english.pdf

International Council of Nurses. (2013). *Code of ethics for nurses.* Retrieved from http://www.icn.ch/who-we-are/code-of-ethics-for-nurses/

Itaborahy, L. P., Zhu, J., & International Lesbian Gay Bisexual Trans and Intersex Association. (2014). *State-sponsored homophobia: A world survey of laws: Criminalisation, protection and recognition of same-sex love* (9th ed.). Geneva, Switzerland: International Lesbian Gay Bisexual Trans and Intersex Association. Retrieved from http://old.ilga.org/Statehomophobia/ILGA_SSHR_2014_Eng.pdf

Jackson, J. (2011). The evolving role of the forensic nurse. *American Nurse Today, 6*(11), 42–43.

Kent-Wilkinson, A. (2010). Forensic psychiatric/mental health nursing: Responsive to social need. *Issues in Mental Health Nursing, 31*(6), 425–431.

Koehler, S. A. (2005). The use of coroners'/medical examiners' data by forensic nurses. *Journal of Forensic Nursing, 1*(1), 37–38.

Lawson, L. (2008). Person-centered forensic nursing. *Journal of Forensic Nursing, 4*(3), 101–103.

Ledray, L. (1999). *Sexual assault nurse examiner development and operation guide.* Washington, DC: Office for Victims of Crime, U.S. Department of Justice.

Ledray, L. E. (2001). *Evidence collection and care of the sexual assault survivor: The SANE-SART response.* Enola, PA: National Sexual Violence Resource Center. Retrieved from http://www.nsvrc.org/publications/guides/evidence-collection-and-care-sexual-assault-survivor-sane-sart-response

Leininger, M. (2002). Culture care theory: A major contribution to advance transcultural nursing knowledge and practices. *Journal of Transcultural Nursing, 13*(3), 189–192.

Leininger, M., & McFarland, M. R. (2002). *Transcultural nursing: Concepts, theories, research and practices* (3rd ed.). New York, NY: McGraw Hill.

Luce, H., Schrager, S., & Gilchrist, V. (2010). Sexual assault of women. *American Family Physician, 81*(4), 489–495.

Lugbil, C. A. (2007). *White paper: Summary of IAFN's international initiatives and next steps for moving forward internationally.* Elkridge, MD: International Association of Forensic Nurses. Retrieved from https://c.ymcdn.com/sites/iafn.site-ym.com/resource/resmgr/imported/IAFN%20Going%20Intl%20White%20Pape.pdf

Lynch, V. (1990). *Clinical forensic nursing: A descriptive study in role development* (Unpublished master's thesis). Arlington, VA: University of Texas Health Science Center.

Lynch, V. A. (2006). *Forensic nursing.* St. Louis, MO: Elsevier/Mosby.

Lynch, V. A. (2007). Forensic nursing science and the global agenda. *Journal of Forensic Nursing, 3*(3), 101–111.

Lynch, V. A. (2011a). Evolution of forensic nursing science. In V. A. Lynch, & J. B. Duval (Eds.), *Forensic nursing science* (2nd ed.) (pp. 1–9). St. Louis, MO: Elsevier/Mosby.

Lynch, V. A. (2011b). Global expansion and future perspectives. In V. A. Lynch, & J. B. Duval (Eds.), *Forensic nursing science* (2nd ed.) (pp. 617–629). St. Louis, MO: Elsevier/Mosby.

Lynch, V. A. (2014). Enrichment of theory through critique restructuring, and application. *Journal of Forensic Nursing, 10*(3), 120–121.

Lynch, V. A., & Duval, J. B. (2011). *Forensic nursing science* (2nd ed.). St. Louis, MO: Elsevier/Mosby.

Mant, A. K. (1987). Forensic medicine in Great Britain: The origins of the British medicolegal system and some historic cases. *American Journal of Forensic Medicine and Pathology, 8*(4), 354–361.

Mariano, C. (2013). Holistic nursing: Scope and standards of practice. In M. Helming, C. C. Barrere, K. Avino, & D. Shields (Eds.), *Core curriculum for holistic nursing* (pp. 11–20). Sudbury, MA: Jones & Bartlett Learning.

Markowitz, J. R., Steer, S., & Garland, M. (2005). Hospital-based intervention for intimate partner violence victims: A forensic nursing model. *Journal of Emergency Nursing, 31*(2), 166–170.

Masters, K. (2011). *Nursing theories: A framework for professional practice.* Sudbury, MA: Jones & Bartlett Learning.

McDonald, S. (2012). The first twenty years: Celebrating the anniversary of the International Association of Forensic Nurses. *On The Edge, 18*(2), 1.

McKenna, B., Furness, T., Dhital, D., Park, M., & Connally, F. (2014). Recovery-oriented care in a secure mental health setting: "Striving for a good life." *Journal of Forensic Nursing, 10*(2), 63–69.

McLay, W. D. S. (1990). *Clinical forensic medicine.* London, England: Pinter Publishers for the Association of Police Surgeons.

Mikkonen, J., & Raphael, D. (2010). *The social determinants of health: The Canadian facts.* Toronto, Canada: York University School of Health Policy and Management.

Mittleman, R., Goldberg, H., & Waksman, D. (1983). Preserving evidence in the emergency department. *American Journal of Nursing, 83*(12), 1652–1656.

National Network to End Domestic Violence. (2015). *Violence Against Women Act.* Retrieved from http://nnedv.org/policy/issues/vawa.html

National Sexual Violence Resource Center. (2015). *SART history.* Retrieved from http://www.nsvrc.org/projects/sart-history

Nyamathi, A., Koniak-Griffin, D., & Greengold, B. A. (2007). Development of nursing theory and science in vulnerable populations research. *Annual Review of Nursing Research, 25*, 3–25.

Office on Violence Against Women (OVW), U.S. Department of Justice. (2014). *About the office.* Retrieved from http://www.ovw.usdoj.gov/overview.htm

O'Donohue, W., Carlson, G. C., Benuto, L. T., & Bennett, N. M. (2014). Examining the scientific validity of rape trauma syndrome. *Psychiatry, Psychology and Law, 21*(6), 858–876.

Pietrantonio, A. M., Wright, E., Gibson, K. N., Alldred, T., Jacobson, D., & Niec, A. (2013). Mandatory reporting of child abuse and neglect: crafting a positive process for health professionals and caregivers. *Child Abuse and Neglect, 37*(2/3), 102–109.

Porter, J. E. (2012). Nursing professional ethics, law, and boundaries. *Journal of Nursing and Law, 15*(2), 61–63.

Povlsen, L., & Borup, I. (2011). Holism in nursing and health promotion. *Scandinavian Journal of Caring Sciences, 25*(4), 798–805.

Quad Council of Public Health Nursing Organizations. (2011). *Quad Council competencies for public health nurses.* Retrieved July 19, 2015, from http://www.achne.org/files/Quad%20Council/QuadCouncilCompetenciesforPublicHealthNurses.pdf

Rivara, F. R., Anderson, M. L., Fishman, P., Bonomi, A. E., Reid, R. J., Carrell, D., & Thompson, R. S. (2007). Intimate partner violence and health care costs and utilization for children living in the home. *Pediatrics, 120*(6), 1270–1277.

Sankar, P., Mora, S., Metz, J. F., & Jones, N. L. (2003). Patient perspectives of medical confidentiality: A review of the literature. *Journal of General Internal Medicine, 18*(8), 659–669.

Sedlak, A., Mettenberg, J., Baesna, M., Petta, I., McPherson, K., Green, A., & Li, S. (2010). *Fourth national incidence study of child abuse and neglect (NIS-4): Report to Congress.* Washington, DC: U.S. Department of Health and Human Services.

Shattell, M. (2004). Nurse-patient interaction: A review of the literature. *Journal of Clinical Nursing, 13*(6), 714–722.

Smialek, J. (1983). Forensic medicine in the emergency department. *Emergency Medicine Clinics of North America, 1*(3), 1685–1691.

Smith, S. (1951). The history and development of forensic medicine. *British Medical Journal, 1*(4707), 599–607.

Smock, W. S. (2006). Genesis and development. In V. A. Lynch, *Forensic nursing* (pp. 13–18). St. Louis, MO: Elsevier/ Mosby.

Stanhope, M. & Lancaster, J. (2014). *Public health nursing: Population-centered health care in the community.* Philadelphia, PA: Elsevier/Mosby.

Stokowski, L. A. (2008). Forensic nursing: Part 2. Inside forensic nursing. *Medscape.* Retrieved July 15, 2014, from http://www.medscape.com/viewarticle/571555

Substance Abuse and Mental Health Services Administration (SAMHSA). (2012). *Trauma and justice strategic initiative,* Rockville, MD: SAMHSA.

Substance Abuse and Mental Health Services Administration (SAMHSA). (2014a). Key terms: Definitions. *SAMHSA News, 22*(2). Retrieved July 30, 2014, from http://www.samhsa.gov/samhsaNewsLetter/Volume_22_Number_2/ trauma_tip/key_terms.html

Substance Abuse and Mental Health Services Administration (SAMHSA). (2014b). *Trauma-informed care in behavioral health services.* Treatment improvement protocol (TIP) series 57. Rockville, MD: SAMHSA. Retrieved from http:// store.samhsa.gov/shin/content/SMA14-4816/SMA14-4816.pdf

Trocmé, N., Fallon, B., MacLaurin, B., Sinha, V., Black, T., Fast, E., Felstiner, C., Hélie, S., Turcotte, D., Weightman, P., Douglas, J., & Holroyd, J. (2010). Canadian incidence study of reported child abuse and neglect – 2008: Major findings. Ottawa, Canada: *Public Health Agency of Canada.* Retrieved July 19, 2015, from http://www.phac-aspc. gc.ca/ncfv-cnivf//pdfs/nfnts-cis-2008-rprt-eng.pdf

Trujillo, A. C., Delapp, T. D., & Hendrix, T. J. (2014). A practical guide to prevention for forensic nursing. *Journal of Forensic Nursing, 10*(1), 20–26.

United Nations (UN). (1948). *Universal declaration of human rights.* Geneva, Switzerland: UN. Retrieved from http:// www.un.org/en/documents/udhr

United Nations (UN). (2008). *Making the law work for everyone, Volume 1: Report of the Commission on Legal Empowerment of the Poor.* New York, NY: UN Development Programme. Retrieved from http://www.unrol.org/files/Making_the_Law_Work_for_Everyone.pdf

United Nations (UN). (2015). *Millennium development goals.* Geneva, Switzerland: UN. Retrieved from http://www. un.org/millenniumgoals/

U.S. Department of Justice, Office on Violence Against Women. (2004). *A national protocol for sexual assault medical forensic examinations: Adults/adolescents* (1st ed.). Washington, DC: US Department of Justice, Office on Violence Against Women.

U.S. Public Health Service, Office of the Surgeon General, U.S. Department of Justice, Office of Juvenile Justice and Delinquency Prevention. (1986). *Report: Surgeon General's workshop on violence and public health.* Washington, DC: U.S. Department of Health and Human Services. Retrieved from http://profiles.nlm.nih.gov/ps/access/NNBCFX. pdf

Waszak, D. (2013). The birth of forensic nursing: How Virginia A. Lynch's determination to stop clinicians from unintentionally obstructing justice inspired a new nursing specialty. *Advance Healthcare Network for Nurse.* Retrieved from http://nursing.advanceweb.com/Features/Articles/The-Birth-of-Forensic-Nursing.aspx

Watts, G. (2013). Charles Everett Koop. *Lancet, 381*(9871), 990.

Wilkinson, R., & Marmot, M. (2003). *Social determinants of health: The solid facts* (2nd ed.). Geneva, Switzerland: World Health Organization.

Williams, D. (2006). Forensic nurses: A proliferation of experts? *Journal of Forensic Nursing, 2*(1), 44–45.

World Health Organization (WHO). (1948). *Constitution of the World Health Organization.* Geneva, Switzerland: WHO. Retrieved from http://whqlibdoc.who.int/hist/official_records/constitution.pdf

World Health Organization (WHO). (2002). *World report on violence and health.* Geneva, Switzerland: WHO. Retrieved from http://www.who.int/violence_injury_prevention/violence/world_report/en/

World Health Organization (WHO). (2003). *Guidelines for medico-legal care for victims of sexual violence.* Geneva, Switzerland: WHO. Retrieved from http://whqlibdoc.who.int/publications/2004/924154628X.pdf?ua = 1

World Health Organization (WHO). (2004). *Preventing violence: A guide to implementing the recommendations of the world report on violence and health.* Geneva, Switzerland: WHO. Retrieved from http://whqlibdoc.who.int/publications/2004/9241592079.pdf?ua = 1&ua = 1

World Health Organization (WHO). (2013). *Responding to intimate partner violence and sexual violence against women: WHO clinical and policy guidelines.* Geneva, Switzerland: WHO. Retrieved from http://apps.who.int/iris/bitstream/10665/85240/1/9789241548595_eng.pdf

World Health Organization (WHO). (2015). *Trade, foreign policy, diplomacy and health: Public health.* Retrieved on February 16, 2015, from http://www.who.int/trade/glossary/story076/en/

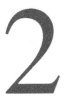

CHAPTER 2

Forensic Nursing in the Healthcare Setting

Catherine J. Carter-Snell
Annie Lewis-O'Connor

OBJECTIVES

At the completion of this chapter, the learner will be able to:

- Discuss key events in the development of forensic nursing in clinical settings.
- Describe the theoretical foundations of forensic nursing in healthcare settings.
- Compare and contrast individual and overlapping roles for key systems involving forensic clinical nurses.
- Describe forensic considerations in each phase of the nursing process.
- Identify key characteristics of injuries, including mechanism of force, patterns, patterned injury, and healing.
- Define "rules of evidence."
- Discuss basic principles of evidence collection, chain of custody, and documentation.
- Define "gender-based violence."
- Describe the health consequences of violence.
- Discuss strategies for preventing violence.

KEY TERMS

Acute stress reactions (ASR): Include responses such as distress, anxiety, sleep problems, avoidance, reexperiencing, substance abuse, guilt, anger, and shame (Bryant, Friedman, Spiegel, Ursano, & Strain, 2010). If symptoms are present at least 1 month posttrauma, then the person may have posttraumatic stress disorder (PTSD).

Alternate light sources: Ultraviolet lights used to aid in the collection of potential evidence.

Comprehensive care: Involves a focus on the individual patient and his or her significant others with consideration of physical, psychological, and social factors.

Drug-facilitated assault: The use of drugs and/or alcohol to incapacitate or render an individual unable to consent to sexual activity.

Focus of care: To prevent violence or intervene effectively to mitigate the effects of violence; for some patients, these interventions can include preservation and collection of evidence.

Forensic nursing science: Involves the "application of the forensic aspects of health care combined with the bio/psycho/social/spiritual education of the registered nurse in the scientific investigation and treatment of the trauma or death of victims and perpetrators of violence, criminal activity and traumatic accidents" (Lynch, 2011a; p. 5). The forensic nurse provides case management for victims of crime or the accused in a variety of settings with a goal to improve health outcomes and prevent violence (Lynch, 2014). This care may include recovery of clinical evidence and provision of legal testimony.

Informed consent: Consent in which the patient is able to communicate his or her choices, has the ability to understand the choices, appreciates the situation in the context of these values, and has the ability to weigh the values to reach a decision (Dhai & Payne-James, 2013).

Intimate partner violence (IPV): Physical, sexual, or psychological harm by a current or former partner or spouse; violence may occur among heterosexual or same-sex couples and sexual intimacy is not a requirement (CDC, 2014).

Mechanism of injury: Circumstances around how an injury occurred; injuries occur when an object contacts the body (or vice versa), and a transfer of energy takes place.

Patient-centered care (PCC): Focuses on the patient and family members as an integral part of the healthcare team.

Patterned injuries: Occur when an injury resembles the object that caused it.

Toluidine dye: Nuclear counterstain that aids in the detection of possible injury to the skin.

Trauma-informed approach (TIA): Recognizes that trauma results from an event, a series of events, or circumstances that an individual experiences (SAMHSA, 2011; TIP Project Team, 2013).

HISTORY AND THEORY

Forensic nursing in healthcare settings has evolved from the incorporation of forensic principles from a variety of disciplines. Nurses recognized a need to improve healthcare services for patients who experienced trauma and violence, and to address violence prevention. Trauma and violence exact significant health consequences, both short- and long-term. These deleterious effects, the perpetuation of violence across the lifespan, and the need for trauma-informed approaches (TIAs) to care provide the underlying theory for forensic nursing practice.

Health Consequences of Violence

Violence affects millions worldwide (WHO, 2014a). The health consequences are substantial and long-lasting, affecting individuals, relationships, and the community. In the United States (US), the Centers for Disease Control and Prevention (CDC) in collaboration with Kaiser Permanente conducted the Adverse Childhood Experiences (ACE) study (CDC, 2012). During the initial phase of the study, approximately 17,000 adults were enrolled to examine the relationship between exposure to adverse events during childhood and health and well-being later in life. The findings indicate that the more that a child is exposed to abuse, neglect, and other traumatic stressors, the more at risk the child is for a host of health problems, including but not limited to depression, illicit drug use, chronic obstructive pulmonary disease, ischemic heart disease, liver disease, and risk for intimate partner violence (IPV). The events measured included self-reported personal childhood emotional and physical abuse and neglect, such as childhood sexual abuse, history of household illicit drug use, maternal abuse, parental separation or divorce, family member mental illness, incarceration, or attempted suicide (Felitti, Anda, Nordenberg, Williamson, Spitz,

Edwards, Koss, & Marks, 1998). Similar negative health consequences in adults with histories of childhood abuse have been found in other countries and populations (Bellis, Hughes, Leckenby et al., 2014a, 2014b; Raposo, Mackenzie, Henriksen & Affifi, 2014). The link between the trauma experience and the physical and psychological health consequences is in large part due to the neurobiological stress response.

Stress, the Neurobiology of Trauma, and Health Consequences

Patients' responses to trauma vary substantially. The public and even some professionals expect victims of assault or trauma to be distraught and emotional, but no one "typical" presentation exists. Emotional responses can range from silence, dissociation, or immobility to visible fear, anxiety, or hysteria. By the time health professionals see the patient, calmness may be the most common response, as demonstrated by a study of 817 women who sought health care within 5 days after a sexual assault (Carter-Snell, 2007). The vast majority appeared conversational, calm, and cooperative (67%), while only 2.2% were extremely agitated. The patient's response is individual and depends upon factors such as the time between the assault and seeking assistance, support systems, lifetime exposure to trauma, and current health status. Prior trauma and severity of the current trauma influence the neurobiological response to trauma and subsequent development of stress disorders or other health challenges.

Neurobiology of Stress. The physiologic response to stress involves a number of key neuroendocrine systems. The stress response relies on the actions of the locus caeruleus/norepinephrine (LC/NE) system, the limbic system (amygdala and hippocampus), the hypothalamic-pituitary-adrenal (HPA) axis, and the autonomic nervous system (Charmandari, Tsigos, & Chrousos, 2005; Olson, Marc, Grude, McManus, & Kellerman, 2011). When a fearful situation occurs, the LC/NE system releases norepinephrine, which in turn activates the limbic system, the HPA axis, and the sympathetic nervous system (See Figure 2.1). The limbic system causes arousal and primitive fear responses. The hypothalamus releases corticotropin releasing factor (CRF) to the pituitary, which releases adrenocorticotropic hormone, which in turn leads to the release of cortisol and catecholamines from the adrenal glands. The sympathetic system releases mainly epinephrine and some norepinephrine. The combined actions of these hormones and their effector organs result in increases in blood sugar, respiration, blood pressure and heart rate, increased focus, and decreased activity of nonessential organs (e.g., the digestive system).

The result of the neuroendocrine response is preparation for the "fight or flight" responses first described by Cannon (1929) and later included in the General Adaptation Syndrome by Selye (1976). A third response has also been identified: the "freeze" response (Bracha, 2004) or "tonic immobility." This freezing response results in an involuntary immobilization of the victim. Professionals can misinterpret this lack of resistance or attempts to escape the situation as the victim having consented.

The stress response is meant to be self-limiting, with acute stress responses generally resolving within two to three days posttrauma (Bryant, 2011, 2013). Normally, the increased cortisol levels are detected by glucocorticoid receptors in the brain, which reduces the CRF and ACTH production. The parasympathetic nervous system antagonizes the stress response as does the prefrontal cortex (Charmandari, Tsigos, & Chrousos, 2005). The oxytocin released with ACTH from the pituitary also helps to create a calming response and a need for connection with others (Uvnas-Moberg, Arn, & Magnusson, 2005).

Negative Effects of the Acute Stress Response. Three key functional changes that affect nursing assessment include the freeze response and the effects of stress on memory and potentially speech. The freeze response to stress may have negative repercussions for victims of violence, as police and healthcare professionals might not understand why the victim did not fight back or flee the assault. The freezing or immobility response is perhaps more common than previously realized, especially with sexual assault. Previous victims of sexual assault reported rates of freezing as high as 89% (Moor, Ben-Meir, Golan-Shapira, & Farchi, 2013), particularly if victims felt dehumanized or humiliated. Although a Danish study of bank employees who experienced a robbery

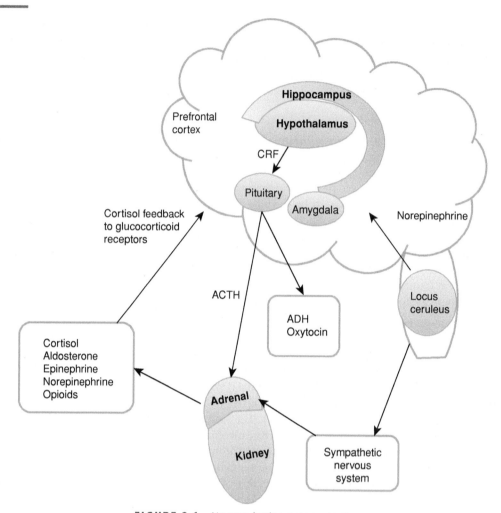

FIGURE 2.1   Neuroendocrine response to stress.

found that women experienced significantly more tonic immobility or freezing than men (Christiansen & Hansen, 2015), the response may vary with the type of trauma. Freezing responses were found across all forms of stressors in the studies, although sexual assault victims had higher levels of all forms of traumatic responses. High rates of tonic immobility are also found across the research on adult male victims of sexual assault, both heterosexual and homosexual (Coxell & King, 2010). In addition, tonic immobility responses during childhood sexual abuse have been linked to posttraumatic stress disorder (PTSD) symptoms in adulthood (Humphreys, Sauder, Martin, & Marx, 2010). Although more research is emerging in these areas, the findings highlight the need for the nurse to understand the patient's reactions at the time of the trauma and the implications for followup treatment.

The stress hormones negatively affect some aspects of memory, which may create gaps or inconsistencies in the recall of events, especially in the acute phase. Memory and speed of information processing are also significantly affected with the development of stress disorders such as PTSD (Scott, Matt, Wrocklage, Crnich, Jordan, Southwick, Krystal, & Schweinsburg, 2014). The hippocampus and amygdala are responsible for encoding and consolidating memories. The interaction of catecholamines and cortisol in some circumstances can impair memory encoding and retrieval (Campbell, 2012; Schwabe & Wolf, 2014; Tiller & Baker, 2014). High stress levels, especially with high cortisol, have been found to impair conscious memory retrieval (Finsterwald & Alberini, 2014; Van Stegeren, 2009).

Stress may also affect speech and the ability to modulate the stress response. Diagnostic imaging studies of veterans with PTSD who were subjected to subsequent stressors have demonstrated changes in blood flow (Pitman, Shin, & Rauch, 2001). In particular, flow was increased to the limbic (fear) centers, and decreased to the prefrontal and left temporal (speech) centers. Although this has not been tested on other populations, it offers possible support for the difficulty patients may experience when asked to relate the details of their assault, and the importance of providing a relaxed atmosphere to limit stress.

Altered Stress Responses and Syndromes. Sustained or severe acute stress responses are linked to mental health, behavioral, and neurologic changes. Sustained or significant stress alters the ability of the stress system to self-regulate and physiologic changes occur. The result may include the development of stress disorders, such as acute stress disorder (ASD), PTSD, major depressive disorder (MDD), and anxiety disorders.

Acute stress reactions (ASR) include responses such as distress, anxiety, sleep problems, avoidance, reexperiencing, substance abuse, guilt, anger, and shame (Bryant, Friedman, Spiegel, Ursano, & Strain, 2010). Acute stress disorder is considered to be present if acute stress responses persist for days or weeks after the trauma. Symptoms of ASD typically include intrusion (e.g., nightmares, unexpected reminders of the event), avoidance of reminders, and hyperarousal (WHO, 2013). The revised diagnostic definition of ASD requires 9 of 14 these possible stress reactions to be present, of which some form of reexperiencing and/or avoidance behaviors must be present (American Psychiatric Association, 2013). If symptoms are present at least a month posttrauma, then the person may have PTSD.

Posttraumatic stress disorder is one of the most common responses after victimization, and is commonly associated with secondary disorders, such as depression, substance abuse, and panic (Burgess, Roberts, & Regehr, 2010; Jakubec, Carter-Snell, Ofrim, & Skanderup, 2013). Victims of sexual assault and IPV as well as victims of war and disaster commonly develop PTSD (Burri & Maercker, 2014; Kilpatrick, Resnick, Milanak, Miller, Keyes, & Friedman, 2013; Norris & Slone, 2013). Studies of both adolescent and adult females have demonstrated rates of PTSD two to three times higher than in males (Kilpatrick, Resnick, Milanak, Miller, Keyes, & Friedman, 2013; McLaughlin, Koenen, Hill, Petukhova, Sampson, Zaslavsky, & Kessler, 2013). Presence of dissociation during and immediately after the trauma indicates a greater risk for PTSD after sexual assault (Ozer, Best, Lipsey, & Weiss, 2003) as does the presence of initial anxiety or panic (Bracha, 2004). The presence of freezing responses is even more predictive than peritraumatic panic or dissociation (Bovin, Jager Hyman, Gold, Marx, & Sloan, 2008). The forensic nurse's role is not to diagnose ASD or PTSD, but the nurse must be aware of the symptoms and document them as risks for stress disorders. While in the clinical setting, the patient may require a referral to psychiatry or need to be educated about potential symptoms of PTSD and community resources for discharge. The criteria for PTSD include having experienced or witnessed a trauma involving death, serious injury, or sexual violation as well as impairment of function or distress and evidence of symptoms from each of four groups or clusters of symptoms shown in Table 2.1 (American Psychiatric Association, 2013).

TABLE 2.1 Symptom Clusters of PTSD

Cluster	Symptoms
Reexperiencing	Spontaneous memories, recurrent dreams, intrusive thoughts, or prolonged distress or "flashbacks"
Avoidance	Attempts to avoid memories, feelings, thoughts, or reminders of the trauma, including use of alcohol or substances
Negative cognitions or mood	Distorted sense of blame (of self or others), decreased interest in activities, inability to remember key portions of trauma, withdrawing from others
Arousal	Sleep difficulties, hypervigilance, fight or flight reactions, self-destructive or high-risk behavior

Specific nursing diagnoses relate to stress reactions. One of the first was "rape trauma syndrome" (Burgess & Holmstrom, 1974). At the time this term was proposed, the *Diagnostic and Statistical Manual of Mental Disorders* (*DSM*) diagnosis of PTSD referred only to ASR that persisted for four weeks or began four weeks posttrauma. Until the fourth edition of the *DSM* was developed in 1994, no diagnosis described the acute disorganization and reactions that patients experience in the initial weeks posttrauma. Rape trauma syndrome encompasses the symptoms seen in PTSD, but symptoms may begin prior to the assault, during, or postassault (Burgess, 1983; Burgess & Holmstrom, 1974). Examples include guilt, self-blame, and anxiety symptoms. Rape trauma syndrome is now described as part of the posttrauma syndrome nursing diagnosis, which is described as a sustained, maladaptive response to an overwhelming event (Carpenito, 2013).

"Battered woman syndrome" (BWS) emerged in 1978; psychologists used the term to describe the psychological effects of IPV (Walker, 1984, 2006). Battered woman syndrome has been described as a subset of PTSD within the context of IPV (Walker, 2006). Intimate partner violence is typified by power and control imbalances, learned helplessness, and psychological dependency. In addition to the PTSD symptoms of numbing, reexperiencing, and hyperarousal, Walker describes those with BWS as demonstrating disruptions in their relationships and body image, and experiencing somatic complaints and problems with sexuality.

Stress Disorders and Long-Term Health. Clear links have been made between the psychological impacts of stress, such as PTSD and other disorders such as MDD (Kilpatrick, Ruggiero, Acierno, Saunders, Resnick, & Best, 2003), and chronic diseases such as cancer, autoimmune disorders, and heart disease (Sledjeski, Speisman, & Dierker, 2008). Healthcare utilization and costs for victims of violence are significantly higher than for nonabused patients (Bonomi, Anderson, Rivara, & Thompson, 2009; CDC, 2014; Fishman, Bonomi, Anderson, Reid, & Rivara, 2010). A patient who arrives at the emergency department may have experienced violence but appear to have a seemingly unrelated health problem. For instance, a patient with a substance abuse problem may be referred to a rehabilitation clinic, whereas a patient with vague abdominal pain may be labeled as "drug seeking." The underlying issue for both could be avoidance of prior trauma, each requiring different referrals. This underscores the need for a trauma-informed approach to care.

Despite the toll that violence can have on one's health, much research has found the significant role that resiliency has for victims. The forensic nurse can help promote resiliency through the initial response to a victim of trauma or violence.

Resiliency to Trauma. Resiliency to trauma is the ability to rebound from the event. The normal process of recovery after trauma involves alternating between avoidance of trauma memories and awareness of events (Davis & Reich, 2014). The patient may not be ready to discuss the effects of trauma with his or her healthcare provider. The speed of this process is individual and must be respected. The response of healthcare professionals and police to victims impacts their recovery. Some researchers have found that victims experience disbelief, stigmatization, or blaming when they disclose (Campbell, 2006; Maier, 2008). These negative responses are linked to greater risks of poor psychological outcomes, such as PTSD (Ullman & Peter-Hagene, 2014). Presence of supportive responses from both professionals and informal support people, such as comfort, provision of choice, and believing the patient, are linked to lower levels of stress disorders or PTSD symptoms (Ozbay, Johnson, Dimoulas, Morgan, Charney, & Southwick, 2007; Ullman & Peter-Hagene, 2014).

Violence Perpetuation Across the Lifespan

Established associations exist between past and present experiences of violence and lifetime exposures. The following are examples of consequences to violent exposures:

- Girls who have experienced sexual abuse are more likely to become victims of subsequent physical abuse and repeated sexual assault, and experience self-harm and IPV (Silverman, Raj, Mucci, & Hathaway, 2001; Trickett, Noll, & Putnam, 2011).

- Children who have been abused or neglected are more likely to experience bullying and teen dating violence (Duke, Pettingell, McMorris, & Borowsky, 2010).
- Both men and women who experienced childhood sexual abuse are more likely to be victims of sexual assault as adults (Classen, Palesh, & Aggarwal, 2005; Coxell, King, Mezey, & Gordon, 1999).
- Those who have experienced physical dating violence have likely been victims of child abuse, sexual assault, or have witnessed family violence in their home (Hamby, Finkelhor, & Turner, 2012).
- Men exposed to IPV as children were found to be more likely to bully (Espelage, Low, Rao, Hong, & Little, 2014). Men who were school bullies were found to be more likely to later abuse intimate partners (Falb, McCauley, Decker, Gupta, Raj, & Silverman, 2011).
- Adults who abuse partners are more likely to abuse their children (Duffy, Hughes, Asnes, & Leventhal, 2014).

Researchers have found that childhood exposures to violence have a cyclical effect on violent experiences and revictimization. Nurses are in key positions to assess for exposures to violence and identify risks for perpetrating violence. Recognizing that a patient may have a trauma history provides an opportunity to identify victims and perpetrators.

Trauma-Informed and Patient-Centered Care

The correlation between trauma and health and between past and present violence exposure has led to a focus on a trauma-informed approach to health care. As noted, a patient in a healthcare setting may present with one problem when the underlying problem is actually a history of a traumatic event that has not been identified or resolved. Examples include patients who seek care for substance abuse problems, report somatic abdominal pain or depression, exhibit high-risk behaviors, or experience repeat assaults. Understanding the impact of trauma on health allows the nurse to focus more broadly on the needs of the patient and reduces the risk of misdiagnosis (TIP Project Team, 2013).

A TIA recognizes that trauma results from an event, series of events, or circumstances that an individual experiences (SAMHSA, 2011; TIP Project Team, 2013). When a person struggles with the effects of trauma, the healthcare provider should be cognizant of the signs and symptoms of trauma exposure and the short- and long-term impact on health. A TIA refers to how a program, agency, organization, or community thinks about and responds to those who have experienced or may be at risk for experiencing trauma. To truly embrace TIA means to change the organizational culture. All components of the organization must incorporate a thorough understanding of the prevalence and impact of trauma and the complex and varied paths in which people recover and heal from trauma. Finally, a TIA is designed to avoid retraumatizing those who seek assistance, to focus on "safety first" and a commitment to "do no harm," and to facilitate participation and meaningful involvement of consumers, families, and trauma survivors in the planning of services and programs. A TIA incorporates three key elements:

- Realizing the prevalence of trauma
- Recognizing how trauma affects all individuals involved with the program, organization, or system, including the workforce
- Responding by putting this knowledge into practice (SAMSHA, 2011).

Patient-centered care (PCC) is another approach that can be used along with trauma-informed care. Patient-centered care has been identified as a core competency in education of health professionals who work with victims of violence (Ambuel, Trent, Lenehan, et al., 2011). In a PCC approach, the patient and family members are part of the healthcare team. Instead of providing care "to" the patient or "for" the patient, a patient-centered approach would be to do "with" the patient. A qualitative analysis of PCC revealed five key domains: biopsychosocial perspective, patient as person, shared power, shared responsibility, and therapeutic alliance (Slatore, Hansen, Ganzini, Press, Osborne, Chesnutt, & Mularski, 2012). The Institute for Patient- and Family-Centered Care (2010) cites the following core concepts of PCC:

- Respect and dignity – Listening to and honoring patient and family choices, and incorporating these and the patient's and family's beliefs and culture into care planning

TABLE 2.2 Traditional Versus Trauma- and Patient-Informed Services

Philosophical Organizational Changes

Traditional	Trauma- and Patient-Informed
Deficits focus	Strengths focus
Expert model	Partnership
Control	Collaboration
Gatekeeping	Sharing
System-structured (business model)	Patient-centric (not system-driven)
Prescribed	Choices
Dependence	Empowerment

- Information-sharing – Providing unbiased information to patients and families in a manner that is affirming, useful, timely, and accurate so they may participate in care
- Participation – Encouraging patients and families to participate in care and decisions at whatever level they choose
- Collaboration – Involving patients and families in institutional planning, design, evaluation, and professional education

These concepts resonate with the needs of patients who have experienced violence and trauma; restoration of control, empowerment, and choice are key components of care when a patient has little control over the events experienced. Changes are needed to move traditional organizations of care to patient- and trauma-informed organizations changes (See Table 2.2).

Forensic Nursing Foundations and Theories

Nurses with forensic expertise provide sound, ethical nursing care while incorporating forensic science principles. As such, they are governed by nursing professional practice regulations and codes of ethics in their region and/or country (e.g., practice standards, ethics, and licensure requirements). Examples include standards of practice and the code of ethics from provincial or state organizations, national organizations (e.g., American Nurses Association, Canadian Nurses' Association), and international sources (e.g., International Council of Nurses, International Association of Forensic Nurses). The primary objective of forensic nursing is comprehensive physical and psychosocial nursing care for the patient (victim suspect, or perpetrator of violence). Provision of care using a trauma-informed and patient-centered framework benefits patients.

Research on theories of forensic nursing is emerging. One of the first theories for forensic nursing practice is the Integrated Practice Model of Forensic Nursing Science (Lynch & Duval, 2006; Valentine, 2014). The model depicts justice, medicine, and nursing as intersecting circles. It emphasizes a need to understand scope and standards of practice, evidence-based practice, and the clinical investigation of trauma. The model also emphasizes the importance of fields of expertise (nursing science, criminal justice, and forensic science), the societal impacts on forensic nursing (social sanctions, rule of law, and human violence), and the healthcare system (forensic nursing, public health, and human rights).

Forensic nursing relies upon knowledge from and interaction with many disciplines. Examples include criminal justice, biological and forensic sciences, psychology, sociology, medicine, and ethics. The diversity of knowledge, disciplines, and clinical practice settings all contribute to the complexity of developing a theory for forensic clinical nursing. Regardless of the framework or theory used, it is important that it be responsive and adapt to changes in practice (Lynch, 2014).

Timeline for Clinical Forensic Nursing

A number of key events have shaped the current practice of forensic nursing in the healthcare setting. Many of the initial clinical forensic initiatives related to services for victims of sexual assault. Records indicate that as early as the 14th century, midwives testified in court related to virginity and rape (Lynch, 2011b). In 1972, Ann Burgess, a psychiatric nurse, and Lynda Lytle Holmstrom, a sociology professor, began taking "call" to counsel women who sought care at Boston City Hospital emergency department in the United States following sexual assault (Office for Victims of Crime, 2011). Their work and research led to the development of the nursing diagnosis of "rape trauma syndrome." The first programs to care for patients who had been sexually assaulted began in the United States in the 1970s in Kansas City, Missouri; Memphis, Tennessee; Honolulu, Hawaii; Minneapolis, Minnesota; and Amarillo, Texas (Ledray, 2001; National Sexual Violence Resource Center, 2015). By the 1990s, programs began to develop in Canada and were introduced in the United Kingdom (UK) in 2001 (Rutty, 2006). In 2004, the US military's *Task Force Report on Care for Victims of Sexual Assault* recommended integration of sexual assault nurse examiners (SANEs) across the Department of Defense (DOD), 2004. In 2008, SANE programs were introduced in Peru (Lynch, 2011b). Having been introduced in a variety of clinical settings worldwide, SANE programs continue to expand.

Clinical services for victims of IPV began to appear in the 1980s. Dr. Jacquelyn Campbell (1981) introduced the danger assessment (DA) scale to identify women at risk for femicide in intimate partner relationships. Daniel Sheridan introduced the Family Violence Program for victims of family violence and sexual assault at Chicago Rush-Presbyterian-St. Luke's Medical Center (Primeau & Sheridan, 2013). In 1996, South Africa adopted a National Crime Prevention Strategy, which led to the development of forensic nurse examiners (FNEs) to address homicide, rape, IPV, and alcohol abuse (Lynch, 2011b). Combined services for victims of either IPV and/or sexual assault are now found in a number of clinical settings.

INTERSECTING SYSTEMS AND SERVICES

People affected by violence and trauma require an inter-collaborative response between professionals. Nurses trained in forensic concepts offer a unique and complimentary component.

Health Care

Nurses and physicians in the healthcare setting are often the first to identify a victim of violence. Patients can present to a variety of settings including primary care, emergency services, obstetrics/gynecology, and pediatrics, as well as in schools and universities. Some clinical settings also employ forensic specialists or have access to them for consultation. An example is a SANE or FNE who works with victims of sexual assault; some also work with victims of IPV. Over the past two decades, nurses have been recognized as experts in domestic violence, human trafficking, elder abuse, child maltreatment, corrections (prison) health, death investigation, and teen dating violence.

Emergency Medical Services

Often the "first responders" to victims of violence are emergency medical technicians (EMTs)/paramedics, police officers, and firefighters. First responders are often familiar with evidence preservation at the scene and chain of custody issues when transporting patients to clinical sites. Subjective and objective documentation is critical to both the medical and legal teams. For example, EMTs who responded to a home of an unresponsive 3-month-old child note that the home appears to have no crib. This observation may lead both the medical and legal teams to consider co-sleeping and possible sudden infant death syndrome.

Legal System and Mandatory Reporting

When law enforcement officials are involved at the scene of a violent episode, they will typically come to the hospital where the victim/suspect/offender is taken. The police officers may ask to interview the patient and determine the type of injuries sustained, which often informs the police in their role. In cases of mandatory reporting, police officers must speak with the patient once he or she is medically cleared by medical staff. Health professionals are often mandated to report injuries such as gunshot wounds, significant injuries from stabbing, or burns.

Some types of violence require health professionals to report to police or child protective services (i.e., mandatory reporting). Worldwide variation exists on mandatory reporting laws. Some examples of mandatory reporting are as follows:

- Suspected child abuse/sexual assault of minors – Reporting is mandatory across North America. It is also typical to require reporting of assaults that occur in publicly funded institutions (e.g., prisons, hospitals, care facilities).
- Disabled persons – Abuse of a physically or mentally impaired person.
- Elder abuse – Reporting is mandatory across the United States, although compliance among physicians is inconsistent (Rodriguez, Wallace, Woolf, & Mangione, 2006). In Canada, all abuse that occurs in publicly funded facilities and abuse of elders who lack capacity must be reported. However, an older adult who is abused, but does not lack capacity, is not reportable in all provinces (Canadian Centre for Elder Law, 2011). Less than half of the countries studied by the World Health Organization (WHO) have plans for elder abuse policy; elder abuse is considered the most neglected form of abuse (WHO, 2014b).
- Generally, IPV is only reported to the police with patient consent unless an immediate threat to life or safety to the individual exists, or the incident involves a minor.
- Gunshot wounds are almost universally required to be reported in North America and some regions require stabbings (nonaccidental) and burns to be reported. Many victim advocates have argued against mandatory reporting out of concern that victims will refrain from seeking help if they know it will be reported to police (Renke, 2005). Reporting of gunshot wounds was overturned due to concerns about public safety, but in some countries, arguments continue related to elder abuse and IPV.

Patient Counseling and Advocacy

Some commentators have argued that nurses cannot advocate for their patients as this may be construed as bias by the courts (Gorham & Brown, 2008). Although nurses must remain objective, they have an ethical obligation to advocate for the healthcare needs of their patient. Both the American Nurses Association's *Code of Ethics for Nurses* (ANA, 2015) and the International Congress of Nurses' *Code of Ethics for Nurses* (ICN, 2012) require that nurses act compassionately and advocate for the healthcare needs of their patients.

Other disciplines or groups also provide advocacy services. Social workers advocate and bring additional knowledge in assessment risk and safety, counseling, crisis support, and referrals to community agencies. Many police departments in the United States have victim services units whose goal is to support the victim throughout the reporting and legal process. Victim services personnel provide support, information, and can serve as the liaison with community agencies. In some settings, victim or family advocates are available to provide further support or advocacy through volunteer groups. The advocate's role is to provide both individual and system supports (Lonsway & Archambault, 2013). One study indicated that victims of sexual assault who had an advocate received higher rates of medical care and experienced less shame, self-blame, or distress than those without an advocate (Campbell, 2006). The forensic nurse and advocate collaborate to ensure that the patient is supported and receives comprehensive care.

Protective Services and Agencies

Protective services exist for some at-risk populations, such as children, persons with disabilities, and older adults, although this varies greatly by country. Many industrialized countries have robust laws similar to North America. In developing countries, international organizations such as the WHO, UNICEF, and USAID continue to advocate and strive to ensure human rights for all.

Community Support Agencies

Community agencies are important allies in violence intervention and prevention efforts. The forensic nurse must know the available community agencies. Examples include counseling centers, shelters, pastoral services, and public health agencies. Effective prevention and intervention requires multidisciplinary and intersectoral collaboration (Carnochan, Butchart, Feucht, Mikton, & Shepherd, 2010). The WHO (2014a) has noted that some of the highest risk countries for violence (e.g., in Africa) have the least resources and services in place.

Medical Examiner/Coroners in the Clinical Setting

Legislation requires that some types of deaths in healthcare settings are reported to either the medical examiner or the coroner. Examples include suspicious or unexpected deaths, or those in which a police investigation is ongoing. In some jurisdictions, nurse death investigators work with the medical examiner's office and may be required to investigate in-hospital deaths under certain circumstances.

POPULATIONS AT RISK

Women

Women are extremely vulnerable to violence (i.e., "gender-based violence"). Population-level surveys provide the most accurate estimates of the prevalence of gender-based violence in non-conflict settings. In 2005, the WHO published the *WHO Multi-Country Study on Women's Health and Domestic Violence Against Women*. Some 24,000 women from 10 developing countries were interviewed. The findings among women aged 15 to 49 years revealed:

- Fifteen percent of women in Japan and 71% of women in Ethiopia reported physical and/or sexual violence by an intimate partner in their lifetime.
- Between 0.3% and 11.5% of women reported experiencing sexual violence by a nonpartner since the age of 15 years.
- Many women reported their first sexual experience as forced – 17% in rural Tanzania, 24% in rural Peru, and 30% in rural Bangladesh (WHO, 2005).

North American studies have shown that almost half of all women surveyed have been sexually assaulted by age 16 (Johnson, 2006) or 18 years (Black, Basile, Brieding, Smith, Walters, Merrick, Chen, & Stevens, 2011). The true extent of violence is difficult to determine as population surveys have shown that as many as 60% of women tell no one about the violence they experience (WHO, 2005). Repeated Canadian surveys show that only 10% of women report sexual assaults to police officials although 30% seek health care (Johnson, 2006). Findings are similar across many countries worldwide, with only 36% of injured women seeking health care after sexual assault or domestic violence (WHO, 2005).

Experiencing one form of abuse poses a risk for revictimization. For instance, a child who has been a victim of child abuse is at higher risk of becoming a victim of dating violence (Felitti, Anda, Nordenberg, Williamson, Spitz, Edwards, Koss, & Marks, 1998; Martsolf & Draucker, 2008). A person who has been sexually assaulted is at higher risk of being sexually assaulted again, particularly if he or she has PTSD and struggles with alcohol use (Messman-Moore, Ward, & Brown, 2009). Increasingly, collaborative prevention programs across violence types are being developed due to the recognition of overlapping risk and protective factors and interrelationships across the lifespan (Foshee, Reyes, Ennett, Suchindran, Mathias, Karriker-Jaffe, Bauman, & Benefield, 2011).

Women are particularly vulnerable following natural disasters. The most compelling data on gender-based violence after natural disasters shows that women and children are disproportionately affected. This increased incidence of violence has been evidenced following hurricanes (Anastario, Shehab, & Lawry, 2009; Curtis, Miller, & Berry, 2000), the earthquake in Haiti (Kolbe, Hutson, Shannon, et al., 2010), and the tsunami in Thailand (Pittaway, Bartolomei, & Rees, 2007). Violent acts include sexual assault and physical abuse of women and children, forced prostitution or marriage, and genital mutilation (WHO, 2005).

Infants and Children

Physical and sexual assaults against children are generally committed by someone close to the child, rather than a stranger (Sinha, 2012). Childhood physical abuse, emotional abuse, and neglect are similar for both boys and girls internationally (Stoltenborgh, Bakermans-Kranenburg, & van Ijzendoom, 2012; Stoltenborgh, Bakermans-Kranenburg, van Ijzendoom, & Alink, 2013). At least one third of an international sample of adults reported three or more adverse childhood experiences (Cohen, Paul, Stroud, et al., 2006). The experiences were similar and some were significantly associated with adult distress and anxiety, including emotional abuse, neglect, and family conflict, violence, or breakup.

Gender differences exist for sexual assault: 18% of girls experience childhood sexual abuse compared to 7.6% of boys (Stoltenborgh, van Ijzendoom, Euser, & Bakermans-Kranenburg, 2011). The WHO data (2014a) indicate that between 1 in 3 and 1 in 5 female children have been sexually abused in childhood.

Bullying and cyberbullying are common in children of all ages, but this type of violence is particularly common between grades six and ten (Craig & McCuaig, 2012). Almost half of children have been in both the bully and victim roles. Screening tools for violence may help detect bullying issues for younger patients. Given the significant impact of bullying on health, the WHO has called for countries to implement public health policies aimed at prevention and intervention (Srabstein & Leventhal, 2010). The United States (AAP, n.d.) and Canada (Government of Canada, 2012) have developed national protocols, policies, and resources for screening and intervention. Screening for bullying with adolescents and children is an important aspect of forensic clinical practice. The injuries or symptoms with which these patients present may be rooted in violence.

Adolescents and young adults are at particular risk for dating violence and sexual assault. A US study revealed that 2.7% of 12- to 17-year-old girls experienced dating violence, compared to 0.6% of male teens (Wolitzky-Taylor, Ruggiero, Danielson, Resnick, Hanson, Smith, Saunders, & Kilpatrick, 2008). At least 20% to 30% of college students in various countries have experienced dating violence (Krebs, Lindquist, Warner, Fisher, & Martin, 2007; Lehrer, Lehrer, & Zhao, 2010; Straus, 2004). By the age of 16 years, at least half of Canadian girls reported experiencing at least one unwanted sexual experience (Johnson, 2006).

Early preventive work for sexual assault focused on "stranger danger." Although assaults by strangers occur, they comprise the minority of sexual assaults. A national survey in the United States revealed that for adolescents and adults, the assailant is most often a friend or someone the victim has met recently in a social setting (Catalano, 2011). The assailant may also be an intimate partner, but not as frequently as a friend or acquaintance. A 2013 survey showed that the rates of stranger assaults had decreased further (Truman & Langton, 2014). For females under 12 years old, the assailant is more often a family member, according to Canadian national data (Sinha, 2013). These findings should be considered when developing an adolescent patient's safety plan predischarge or when assessing the family members in the history of the event.

Elderly

Older adults are at risk for physical, emotional, or financial abuse or neglect. A paucity of data exists, but one global study estimates that 6% of elderly reported significant abuse (Cooper, Selwood, & Livingston, 2008). This rate does not account, however, for those older adults who do not report abuse. National variation seems to exist; rates range from as low as 0.8% in Spain to 32% in Belgium (WHO, 2014b). Abuse that occurs outside of care institutions is typically perpetrated by a family member – most often a spouse or adult child (Walsh & Yon, 2012). Elders most at risk are those who have health problems and functional decline (Eulitt, Tomberg, Cunningham, Counselman, & Palmer, 2014), are financially dependent, and have poor social support (Cohen, 2013; Reis, 2000; Wangmo, Teaster, Grace, Wong, Mendiondo, Blandford, Fisher, & Fardo, 2014). Rates are consistently higher, at approximately 25%, if older adults suffer from dementia or live in residential institutions.

Caregivers may be either institutional staff or family members, and most often have drug, alcohol, or psychiatric problems (Cohen, 2013; Wangmo, Teaster, Grace, Wong, Mendiondo, Blandford, Fisher, & Fardo, 2014), share living accommodations (Wangmo, Teaster, Grace, Wong, Mendiondo, Blandford, Fisher, & Fardo, 2014), or have poor social networks (Cohen, 2013). Factors most often associated with elder abuse are caregivers who do not interact well with others and an elderly person who was abused in the past and who has inadequate social support (Reis, 2000).

Minorities

Sexual Minorities. Sexual minorities such as lesbian, gay, transgender, or bisexual are at higher risk of both physical and sexual assault. These assaults may result from sexism, classism, and hate crimes. The forensic nurse should ensure that questioning of these patients is gender-neutral (using "partner" vs. "boyfriend") and nonjudgmental. For instance, one must not assume that an assault was perpetrated by a person of the opposite sex.

Aboriginal/Native People. Aboriginal women face significantly higher rates of physical and sexual assault than Caucasian women in North America (NCAI Policy Research Center, 2013; Sinha, 2013). Furthermore, when they are assaulted, Aboriginal women face greater rates of injury, hospitalization, and death (Department of Justice, 2015; Lloyd, 2014). The women may be unable to disclose the specifics of their assault due to shame or cultural beliefs/practices. The forensic nurse must understand the cultural factors impacting minority groups in his or her practice area and take every effort to create a culturally safe environment.

Persons with Disabilities

Mental or physical disabilities may be either acute or chronic. People of any age with disabilities are four times more likely to experience violence than persons without disabilities (WHO, 2014b). In Canada and most states in the United States, laws mandate reporting if a belief exists that a person with a disability is being harmed.

Drugs and Alcohol

Drugs and/or alcohol can render a person unable to resist or consent and, thus, vulnerable to harm. Alcohol is associated with increased risks of violence across all cultures and countries (Cherpitel, Ye, Bond, Borges, & Monteiro, 2015; WHO, 2009). Victims become more vulnerable and perpetrators become more aggressive. Alcohol has also been shown to decrease awareness of risk (Abbey, Saenz, & Buck, 2005). The amount required to incapacitate someone varies by factors such as gender, age, and body size. Therefore, the capacity to consent is not directly tied to blood alcohol or drug levels. Although the amount consumed and the time period of ingestion are relevant to determining one's ability to consent, it is also important to know the patient's level of consciousness and awareness at the time of the assault.

Homelessness

Individuals who are homeless may feel stigmatized when seeking health care, potentially worsening their mental health through secondary victimization. It is extremely common for persons who are homeless to have histories of prior abuse, as well as resulting mental health and addictions issues, school dropouts, poverty, or isolation (Wong, Clark, & Marlotte, 2014). They live in unsafe and unstable conditions. Once people become homeless, they are at significant risk of being reassaulted, lured into prostitution, or becoming victims of human trafficking. At least half of such people experience violence while homeless, especially if they are older or female (Meinbresse, Brinkley-Rubinstein, Grassette, Benson, Hall, Hamilton, Malott, & Henkins, 2014).

PRACTICE AND PREVENTION

Forensic nursing care involves the application of the nursing process in caring for patients with an added focus on forensic-legal implications. These processes include screening for violence; responding to disclosures with sensitivity; obtaining informed consent and a patient history; completing a physical and psychosocial assessment; performing a complete head-to-toe physical examination; collecting evidence; testing; and providing treatment, referral, and followup care.

Screening for Violence

A number of professional organizations (Allen, Larsen, Javdani, & Lehrner, 2012) and governmental agencies (U.S. Preventive Services Task Force, 2013; WHO, 2014a) have recommended that healthcare providers screen for violence; yet this is not widely implemented, even in North America. Only 13.6% of 191 Canadian emergency departments studied routinely screened their patients for IPV (McClennan, Worster, & Macmillan, 2008). Even when screening protocols are in place, issues arise with noncompliance among staff due to lack of knowledge or discomfort with resources (Hussain, Sprague, Madden, Hussain, Pindiprolu, & Bhandari, 2013). Electronic health records help ensure that providers are reminded to screen their patients by including questions in the health history; however, ongoing education and knowledge about available resources are critical.

The definition and practices of universal screening differ across regions and countries. Sufficient evidence exists to recommend that all women of childbearing age be screened for violence (U.S. Preventive Services Task Force, 2013), making it universal to this group. A review of 33 studies indicated that the benefits of screening include reduced episodes of violence and improved health outcomes in various populations (Nelson, Bougatsos, & Blazina, 2012). The extent and significance of the improvements varied by population, but outcomes were consistently positive (Joubert & Posenelli, 2009; Stark, 2012; Touza, Prado, & Segura, 2012). One Canadian city has extended universal screening to all patients, both male and female of any age who seek care in emergency departments across the city (Snell, McCracken, & Lind, 2012). The WHO (2014a) suggests that perhaps not all women in all settings should be asked about violence; immediate care, and available support and resources must be in place to meet their needs. The way in which patients are asked about violence is also important.

How Should Patients Be Asked About Violence?

Although the nurse can sometimes have an index of suspicion, identifying a victim of violence is not always obvious or predictable, and highlights the need for universal screening. Patients should be asked privately with no family or friend present, and should be informed that all patients are asked. The use of professional interpreters is the standard of practice; a family member or friend should never be used to screen. Although a lack of agreement exists as to frequency of inquiry and in which settings, a consensus exists around screening any women with concerns, pregnant women each trimester, women who are postpartum, and women at their annual primary care visits.

Assessment for IPV and Risk

If a patient discloses violence during screening, then the patient's safety and that of the family (including pets) should be determined prior to discharge. Studies indicate that asking women about the likelihood of their partner reabusing them is a relatively accurate predictor of revictimization (Bennett Cattaneo & Goodman, 2003; Hanson, Helmus, & Bourgon, 2007). A number of tools or scales are available to screen for IPV or to assess lethality risk (See Table 2.3). The DA was one of the earliest tools and was intended to predict risk of lethality for women (Campbell, 1981). A combination of asking the victim and using a risk or screening tool has been found to more accurately determine risk compared to either one alone (Connor-Smith, Henning, Moore, & Holdford,

TABLE 2.3 Victim-Focused IPV Screening and Risk Assessment Tools

Instrument	Description	Authors
Abuse Assessment Screen (AAS)	• Three items (five in original), clinically administered • Severity and frequency of abuse in pregnancy • Initial screen for IPV	McFarlane, Parker, Soeken, & Bullock, 1992
Index of Spouse Abuse (ISA)	• Thirty-item self-report • Changes in severity or degree of abuse	Hudson, Walter, & Rau, 1981
Partner Violence Screen (PVS)	• Three questions, clinician administered for emergency • Past and present abuse and perceived safety	Feldhaus et al., 1997
Danger Assessment (DA)	• Fifteen-item danger assessment self-report • Risk factors for lethality	Campbell, 1981
Hurt, Insult, Threat, Scream (HITS)	• Four-item self-report • Frequency of abuse	Sherin et al., 1998
Woman Abuse Screening Tool (WAST)	• Seven-item self-report • Initial screening for abuse behaviors	Brown et al., 1996
HARASS Tool	• Twelve-item self-report • Frequency of forms of harassment in relationship, for use with domestic abuse scale	Primeau & Sheridan, 2011, 2013; Sheridan, 1998

2011). Nurses are advised to choose a method of screening that suits their clinical setting, patient population, length of contact time, and type of patients. Victim-based tools have received some validation in different settings with different languages (Gerth, Rossegger, Urbaniok, & Endrass, 2014) and cultures (McWhinney-Delaney, 2006), and for different populations of women, such as immigrants (Messing, Amanor-Boadu, Cavanaugh, Glass, & Campbell, 2013). A continued need exists to establish validity and reliability for these tools (Hanson, Helmus, & Bourgon, 2007) and to develop assessment strategies for male victims of IPV.

Another key consideration is the format or location of the screening (Lewis-O'Connor, 2007). For instance, victims may be placed at risk if they are questioned in front of the abuser. A meta-analysis of different methods of screening suggests that the odds of women disclosing IPV increased by 37% if they used a computer-assisted, self-administered format rather than face-to-face or written screening tools (Hussain, Sprague, Madden, Hussain, Pindiprolu, & Bhandari, 2013). A comparison of self-administered questionnaires and face-to-face screening among women seen in primary care demonstrated higher rates of disclosure of IPV with the self-administered scales; no differences were found for males who reported (Kapur & Windish, 2011).

The majority of victim-focused scales are designed for younger adult women. Elder abuse screening tools are also available, and vary in length and content. Cohen (2013) argues that since each elder's situation is unique, using multiple tools to screen may be more accurate; however, the length of these tools can provide challenges in the context of busy healthcare settings. Some elder abuse tools include:

- Indicators of abuse (IOA) screen – A 29-item, professionally administered interview with 78% to 84% sensitivity and 99.2% specificity (Cohen, 2013; Reis, 2000)
- Elder Assessment Instrument – Designed to identify those who are at risk or need referral; consists of a 41-item questionnaire administered by the clinician, with a sensitivity of 71% and specificity of 93% (Fulmer, Guadagno, Dyer, & Connolly, 2004)
- Hwalek–Sengstock Elder Abuse Screening Test – A six-item self-report tool to differentiate abuse from nonabuse, reduced from the original 15-item scale (Neale, Hwalek, Scott, Sengstock, & Stahl, 1991)
- Caregiver abuse screen (CASE) – Is completed by the caregiver to assess abuse and neglect using nonblaming language (Reis & Nahmiash, 1995)

- Identification of Seniors at Risk (ISAR) – A six-item self-report tool that is based on functional impairment; to be used in emergency care settings (Eulitt, Tomberg, Cunningham, Counselman, & Palmer, 2014; McCusker, Bellevance, Cardin, Trepanier, Verdon, & Ardman, 1999)

Responding to Initial Disclosures

If a patient discloses abuse, the first priority is to ensure that the patient is safe, and that the nurse is also safe. The assailant may be present or searching for the victim in the healthcare setting. The next step is to gain an understanding of the violence: the perpetrator's behaviors (using the DA tool), the patient's current resources and available supports, and the patient's physical and emotional well-being. The goal is to determine how best to assist the patient.

A major tenet of providing trauma-informed care requires the avoidance of "secondary victimization" (Burgess, Roberts, & Regehr, 2010; Campbell, 2006). In Campbell's study of patients who had been sexually assaulted, the healthcare staff and police discouraged reporting, did not consider the assault serious enough to investigate, or blamed the victim for how he or she dressed or behaved to "provoke" the assault (Campbell, 2006). The victims reported feeling blamed, depressed, anxious, violated, and not wanting to seek help again. Self-blame and shame are closely linked to acute stress symptoms and the development of PTSD (La Bash & Papa, 2014; Moscardino, Scrimin, Capello, & Altoe, 2014). Suggestions to reduce victimization and promote resilience are to:

- Limit questions about trauma to what is needed and by whom – Asking a victim to recall an event too soon after it occurs or when the person is not ready to discuss the issue can impair resilience, increase the risk of ineffective coping strategies (Bicknell-Hentges & Lynch, 2009), and increase the risk of posttraumatic stress symptoms (Gittins, Paterson, & Sharpe, 2015). Strategies include limiting the history to those who will conduct the examination, allowing the patient time to respond, watching for signs of dissociation or distress, stopping the history if such signs occur, and restricting the questions to essential information (e.g., health care, prevention of complications).
- React positively to disclosures – Positive responses (e.g., emotional support, provision of information) promote coping, while negative reactions (e.g., blaming, taking control) are linked to avoidance behaviors, decreased perception of control over recovery, and posttraumatic stress symptoms (Ullman & Peter-Hagene, 2014).
- Promote patient strengths and self-worth – A Spanish study of adolescents found that self-esteem and feelings of worth moderated the effect of victimization on mental health symptoms in both boys and girls (Soler, Kirchner, Paretilla, & Forns, 2013).

Obtaining a History

Both a medical history and a history of the events are required. Starting with the medical history allows a gradual transition from least threatening to more threatening information for the patient, as well offering as an opportunity to build rapport.

Medical History. The medical history is critical to guiding the physical examination, interpreting the physical findings, and determining psychological risks. The medical history should move from general health to the specifics of the event. Items to include in the medical history are: past medical history, allergies, current medications, prior hospitalizations, past surgical history, mental health history (including self-harm), and social history. Physicians and advanced practice nurses should also include a review of systems prior to conducting the physical examination.

History of Events. An experienced healthcare provider (ideally with advanced training in caring for victims of violence) should obtain the history of the event/assault. The focus of the history is to determine a patient's physical and psychological risks, required treatment and referrals, and the potential for evidence collection during the examination. Examples of required information and the purpose are shown in Table 2.4, using sexual assault protocols (DOJ, 2013). Note that the purpose of the questions can be justified in relation to health care or interventions. The law enforcement official generally asks more detailed questions about the setting and suspect(s) than does the nurse as

TABLE 2.4 Examples of Sexual Assault Health History Questions

Focus	Information	Purpose
Events of assault	• Where touched or contacted and with what (e.g., object, hand, mouth, penis, use of restraints, strangulation) • Use of threats, weapons • Ejaculation • Loss of consciousness • Other symptoms (e.g., memory, dissociation, freezing)	• To identify areas of focus for injury or other physical findings, risks for other injury (e.g., head, hyoid); not all contact will hurt or cause injury so ask where touched • To determine potential psychological impact, safety, injuries (also affects level of charges in some countries)
Substance use	• Voluntary or involuntary use of drugs or alcohol and symptoms (e.g., toxidromes)	• To determine immediate risks to health, need for toxicology testing, ability to resist
Suspect	• Relationship to patient • Number of assailants • Markings left on assailants • Intravenous drug user, male who has sex with men, prison history	• Risks for injury and infection • Safety concerns if likely to reencounter • Transfer of evidence (e.g., under fingernails)
Setting	• Setting/surface (e.g., grass, in car)	• Aids in understanding injuries, evidence transfer
Postassault activities	• Showering, voiding • Time between assault and seeking help	• May affect likelihood of evidence recovery or presence of physical findings (e.g., body injuries may appear later than genital injuries)
Recent sexual activities	• Consensual activities within last week (vaginal penetration) or 3 days (anal/oral penetration)	• To determine potential for presence of other DNA • Assists in understanding injuries

the purpose of the former is investigation. Overlap between law enforcement and nursing histories are usually limited to avoid inconsistencies in the history. Although inconsistencies are typical of memory effects during acute stress, they can and do complicate later prosecution if not understood. The nurse uses open-ended questions as much as possible (e.g., What happened? Where were you touched?) rather than closed or leading questions (e.g., Did she grab you here?).

Response to Examination

Patients demonstrate a variety of responses to the examination, ranging from cooperation to dissociation. The examination may trigger intrusive recollections or physical responses that are distressing. The patient may exhibit a sudden change in behavior, such as agitation or anxiety, or signs of dissociation (e.g., detachment, gazing into space, being unaware of the surroundings, failing to react to pain, or a lack of engagement). As noted previously, dissociation in the peritraumatic period can indicate an increased risk for PTSD. Strategies to support the patient include:

- Suspending the examination or history-taking until the patient feels safe and is actively ready to resume the process. The nurse should validate that the patient's feelings are normal and offer reassurance to work with the patient at his or her pace.
- Using "grounding" techniques with reexperiencing symptoms such as flashbacks or dissociation (Haskell, 2003). The goal is to reconnect the patient to his or her body and senses. The care team may need to consult behavioral/psychiatric services.
- Being aware that touching the patient may provoke an exaggerated startle response or anxiety, the nurse should ask permission to touch the patient or to perform a procedure.
- Providing comfort measures and breaks as needed and allowing the patient autonomy, control over timing of the procedures, and choices.

Informed Consent. An informed consent is required before a patient undergoes a forensic examination. Because some components of the examination are not part of the health examination and are not emergently medically necessary, they should be treated as a special form of consent. This allows the patient to regain control over what he or she has experienced. Considerations include:

- The patient needs to understand the range of choices, be able to ask questions, and recognize that a forensic examination is a choice.
- An informed consent should include:
  - components of the examination and evidence collection
  - photography (if appropriate or available)
  - the option to release evidence collection kits and reports to law enforcement in reported cases
- A patient may choose to refuse any portion or all of the examination.
- A patient should have the capacity for informed consent, that is, the patient is able to communicate his or her choices, understand the choices, appreciate the situation in the context of his or her own values, and weigh values to reach a decision (Dhai & Payne-James, 2013). The patient may temporarily lose capacity, as with the influence of drugs or alcohol or illness. If the patient does not demonstrate capacity for consent, the examination cannot be conducted unless medically necessary (most are not). Local guidelines and regulations vary as to who may give consent on behalf of the incapacitated patient. A number of sexual assault centers have developed guidelines for unconscious or incapacitated victims, such as those of the provincial network in Ontario, Canada (Macdonald & Norris, 2007).
- Age of consent is also a consideration – In some regions or countries, parental consent is required for all patients under the age of majority unless emancipation laws exist for minors living on their own. In other countries, such as Canada, there is no minimum age for consent. Children can give their own consent at any age as long as they demonstrate capacity as previously described (Canadian Bar Association, 2012). The parents cannot overturn the child's decision nor can the nurse share the child's health information with the parents without the child's consent. The forensic nurse must be familiar with local consent and health information laws.

Physical Assessment

It is recommended that a complete medical examination be offered to all victims of violence. Some general IOA or interpersonal violence are injuries that are inconsistent with the history, multiple injuries in various stages of healing, unusual delays in seeking care, and patterned injuries (Darnell, 2011). A primary survey includes a physical assessment of any immediate threats to life or limb (airway, breathing, circulation, disability of neurological system). These threats should be managed immediately. Once resolved, a secondary survey (head-to-toe examination of the patient) is then completed, looking for any signs of the assault or physical findings that might be related to the assault. The examination should include both subjective and objective data, and include both inspection and palpation. A review of research on sexual assault patients with injuries revealed that a median of only 18% reported pain (subjective), while almost half were observed to have tenderness to palpation (Carter-Snell, 2007). A full assessment and documentation are recommended even if the patient chooses not to report to law enforcement officials.

Patterns of Injury

"Patterns of injury" should be noted while conducting the physical examination. These are combinations of injuries that occur with specific mechanisms or types of violence. (Note: A detailed description of injuries is included in the "Concepts" and Issues section of this chapter).

Self-Inflicted Injury. Self-inflicted injuries are generally nonfatal and have some key characteristics:

- Although multiple injuries may be present, they are often parallel, located in accessible areas, and are generally of similar severity and inflicted involving a single mechanism (e.g., incision or abrasion).

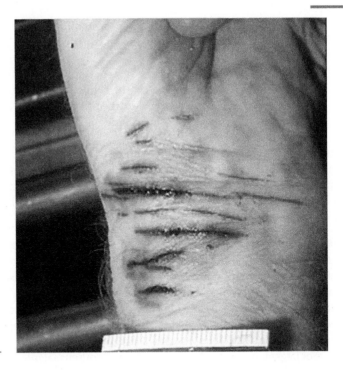

FIGURE 2.2 Hesitation wounds.

- Self-inflicted injuries may be nonsuicidal (e.g., cutting behaviors), indicate risk for completed suicide, or in some cases, be an attempt at false allegations.
- Suicidal incised wounds are typically at the throat or chest for men, or the wrists for men and women (Saukko & Knight, 2009). They often have "hesitation" incisions, which are more shallow incisions during the preliminary phases of attempted suicide (Gall, Goldney, & Payne-James, 2011) (See Figure 2.2).

Suffocation. Lack of oxygen, either from insufficient oxygen in the environment or due to blockage of the airway, is considered suffocation (Saukko & Knight, 2009). Suffocation can result from smothering or gagging, choking on a foreign body, arm-lock holds to the neck, or strangulation. Deaths due to hypoxic suffocation (e.g., fire victims, plastic bag suffocation) often lack visible signs or injuries. Smothering forms of suffocation may be from occlusion of the mouth and nose, which may be intentional or nonintentional. Patterns of injury with smothering, if present, may include pressure abrasions and/or bruises to the face, cheeks, or mouth; marks on the face; and sometimes lacerations of the inner lips from pressure of the teeth. A patient may also display defensive wounds from trying to protect him- or herself. Traumatic asphyxiation (e.g., crushing in a crowd, vehicle on top of a person's chest) results in discoloration above the level of compression. The entire sclera and conjunctivae can be engorged with blood. The face, lips, and scalp may be congested and have petechiae and ecchymoses. Bruising also may be present on the chest at the site of compression. Patterned injuries can include, for instance, the tire mark of a motor vehicle that has struck a pedestrian.

Strangulation. In the United States, strangulation is the fifth leading cause of homicide (Federal Bureau of Investigation, 2011). Patients who have been strangled are at significant risk for morbidity and mortality (Glass, Laughon, Campbell, Wolf, Block, Hanson, Sharps, & Taliaferro, 2008). Prior nonfatal strangulation is associated with more than six times the rate of becoming an attempted homicide, and seven times the odds of becoming a completed homicide. These statistics emphasize how critical it is for nurses in emergency department settings to screen for strangulation when assessing women who have been abused. Typical findings of strangulation include:

- Bruises or abrasions to the neck (intradermal injuries may be seen with alternate light sources)
- Localized pain

- Airway symptoms (voice changes, hoarseness, difficulty swallowing, coughing)
- Neurological symptoms (dizziness, loss of consciousness with/without incontinence, headache, memory loss)
- Vomiting
- Petechiae in the conjunctiva and on the skin above the strangulation, especially with jugular occlusion (carotid rupture is too sudden for petechiae to develop) (Faugno, Waszak, Strack, Brooks, & Gwinn, 2013; Primeau & Sheridan, 2013).

Head Injury. Blows to the head, with or without skull fractures, may be associated with concussions, loss of consciousness or confusion, memory impairment, hemotympanum, and nausea or vomiting. Basal skull fractures may also have associated indirect injuries, such as periorbital ecchymosis or Battle sign (bruising behind the ears). A complete examination of the head, nose, eyes, ear, and mouth is always warranted.

Sexual Assault. A systematic review of research on sexual assault injuries revealed that at least a third or more of women will not have any injuries after sexual assault, although wide variability occurred in rates of injury, nomenclature, and techniques used to visualize the injuries (Carter-Snell, 2007). When injuries are present, however, the patterns of injury are less clear than with some other forms of violence. The literature revealed significant variation in terms used to describe injuries, methods of documentation, skill of examiners in identifying injuries, and visualization techniques, such as toluidine dye or colposcopy. Despite these challenges, a pattern is emerging that suggests more or larger injuries may be present with nonconsensual intercourse versus consensual intercourse:

- Patients were more likely to be in the nonconsensual group if they exhibited two or more genital injuries or had genital bruising or abrasions (Anderson, McClain, & Riviello, 2006).
- Patients who had been sexually assaulted had larger surface areas of injury (Anderson, Parker, & Bourguignon, 2009) and more severe injuries than those who had consensual intercourse (Larkin, Cosby, Kelly, & Paolinetti, 2012).

Patterned Injury

Injuries are said to be "patterned" when the injury resembles the object that caused the injury. Bruises are less likely to be the same size or exact replications of the pattern due to extravasation of blood and compression of underlying tissue, while abrasions are usually more superficial and provide a more accurate reflection of the pattern (Saukko & Knight, 2009).

Fingertip Bruising. Tips of fingers typically leave oval or circular bruises approximately 0.5 cm to 1 cm, also described as dime-sized (Sheridan, 2007). The bruises may be single or multiple, and sometimes may be arranged in a full or partial fan shape consistent with the spread of some or all of the fingers on a hand.

Bite Marks. Bite marks may be a combination of blunt and penetrating injury. Blunt injuries include bruises, friction abrasions, redness, and in some cases, lacerations. A complete human bite mark consists of two facing arches, each with a set of aligned patterned bruises, abrasions, and/or lacerations (See Figure 2.3).

Tram Line Bruising. This is a pattern with two parallel lines of bruising and no central bruising (central clearing). This sparing of the central tissue is from the inward compression of the object on the skin, which drags the skin inward and tears the blood vessels on the margins (Saukko & Knight, 2009).

When documenting an injury, the forensic nurse should include a detailed description of the finding (i.e., measurements, shape, color). Suspected findings such as fingertip bruising and bite marks should not be labeled as such. If the patient is able to report what caused the finding, the response should be documented in quotes. For example, the patient stated, "Those bruises are where he grabbed me by the arm."

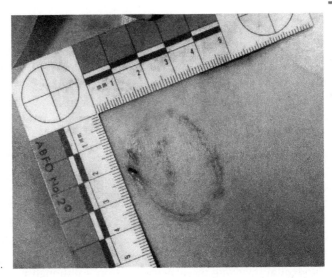

FIGURE 2.3 Bite mark.

Accidental Versus Nonaccidental Injuries in Children

Bruises. Accidental bruises are seen in children as they become mobile. These injuries occur on bony prominences (chin, elbows, etc.). In contrast, nonaccidental bruising is more likely to be located on the head, trunk, back, and genital area. The bruising may also be patterned, reflecting the object used to inflict the injury. A history is critically important in these cases.

Head Trauma. In one study, a large sample of children with head trauma was found to have more diffuse axonal injury and subdural hemorrhage if the trauma happened to be abusive; accidental injury was associated with higher rates of skull fractures and epidural hemorrhage (Roach, Acker, Bensard, Sirotnak, Karrer, & Partrick, 2014). Although some studies describe retinal hemorrhage associated with head trauma, a systematic review has found no retinal sign that would distinguish abusive versus accidental head trauma (Maguire, Watts, Shaw, Holden, Taylor, Watkins, Mann, Tempest, & Kemp, 2013). Small children who have been shaken may have sustained deficits and, in some cases, this injury may result in death.

Fractures. According to the American Academy of Pediatrics (AAP), "Fractures are a common childhood injury and account for between 8% and 12% of all pediatric injuries" (Flaherty, Perez-Rossello, Levine, Hennrikus, & American Academy of Pediatrics Committee on Child Abuse and Neglect, 2014; p. e477). Certain fractures are likely to be accidental; however, others are highly suspicious. The AAP uses three criteria for suspicion in infants and toddlers; high specificity; moderate specificity; and common, but low, specificity.

- High specificity:
  - Classic metaphyseal lesions
  - Rib fractures
  - Scapular fractures
  - Sternal fractures
- Moderate specificity:
  - Multiple fractures, especially bilateral
  - Fractures of different ages
  - Epiphyseal separations
  - Vertebral body fractures and subluxations
  - Digital fractures
  - Complex skull fractures
- Common, but low, specificity:
  - Subperiosteal new bone formation

- Clavicular fractures
- Long-bone shaft fractures
- Linear skull fractures (Flaherty, Perez-Rossello, Levine, Hennrikus, & American Academy of Pediatrics Committee on Child Abuse and Neglect, 2014; p. e478).

Followup skeletal surveys for suspected nonaccidental trauma should be performed within 2 weeks of the initial screening as "[f]ollow-up skeletal surveys have been shown to improve rate of fracture detection in suspected cases of nonaccidental trauma" (Sonik, Stein-Wexler, Rogers, Coulter, & Wootton-Gorges, 2010; p. 804).

Burns. Abusive burns have been found more often in younger children, cover larger surface areas, have immersion lines, use tap water, or are associated with delays in seeking care (Wibbenmeyer, Liao, Heard, Kealey, Kealey, & Oral, 2014). Many accidental burns can be attributed to neglect or poor supervision of the child. Nonaccidental burns were also found to be more likely symmetrical and lack splash marks or to be imprinted, such as cigarette burns (Mok, 2008).

Abdominal Trauma. A systematic review of research of abdominal injuries revealed that abused children are more likely to be younger (2 to 3 years of age) and incur injuries to the lower duodenum involving the pancreas or liver – although not exhibiting external bruising – compared to children with accidental abdominal injuries (Maguire, Upadhyaya, Evans, Mann, Haroon, Tempest, Lumb, & Kemp, 2013). The abused children also were more likely to exhibit other injuries, such as burns, head injuries, and fractures.

Sexual Trauma. Evaluation of children for sexual abuse is challenging and rarely straightforward. To add to this challenge, the majority of examinations for suspected sexual abuse will be normal. In a landmark paper, Adams and colleagues concluded that, in cases of confirmed sexual abuse, normal findings are typical (Adams, Harper, Knudson, & Revilla, 1994). Forensic nurses with specialized training in pediatric sexual abuse are filling a gap in providing care to this vulnerable population.

Tools to Aid Injury Visualization

Some physical findings, especially those to the genital area, are difficult to identify. Genital injuries may be subtle and less experienced examiners may not be able to reliably see them (Sachs, Benson, Schriger, & Wheeler, 2011). Tools are available that enhance visualization, such as alternate light sources, colposcopy, toluidine dye, and photography.

Alternate Light Sources. Light sources can be used on all areas of the body as a preliminary test to aid in the collection of potential evidence. Ultraviolet lights (<400 nm) are no longer used because they are nonspecific and cause many substances to fluoresce (Carter-Snell & Soltys, 2005). Newer lights use wavelengths >400 nm and are more specific to semen and other bodily fluids. However, other substances may react to alternate lights as well. Lights are held approximately 6 in to 8 in from the skin with the examiner wearing orange goggles; all surfaces of the skin are inspected for the presence of stains. If reactions to the light are identified, they should be swabbed, placed in the forensic kit, and documented.

Colposcopy. In the United States, colposcopy has been included as an addition to the sexual assault examination for many years to help visualize genital injuries and often to conduct photodocumentation (DOJ, 2013). The equipment can be expensive and may not be readily available in rural or remote health settings.

Toluidine Blue Dye. Genital injuries are often subtle and difficult to visualize. Toluidine dye can be applied to nonmucosal areas (e.g., external genitalia) to highlight and identify injuries. Breaks in the skin that extend into the dermis and expose nucleated mast cells will absorb the dye and appear as distinct dark purple/blue areas. The dye is applied and left in place for 60 seconds. It is then removed either with water-soluble lubricant on a gauze or with diluted (1%) acetic acid spray. Toluidine dye has been shown to be more effective than direct visualization or colposcopy in detecting external genital lacerations (Zink, Fargo, Baker, Bushur, Fisher, & Sommers, 2010).

Q-Tip/Catheter. Injuries to the hymen can be difficult to visualize, especially if the hymen is redundant (folded on itself). A balloon-tipped swab or a urinary catheter with a balloon can be used after the forensic samples are taken (White, 2013). The catheter is inserted into the vagina, the balloon is inflated, and the catheter is gently withdrawn to rest behind the hymen. This allows the examiner to assess the hymen for lacerations or bruising. The catheter balloon should only be used in postpubertal patients and by providers with an advanced education.

Photography. Photography is a valuable tool to preserve evidence that could be absent at a later time, such as injuries or trace evidence. Photography also provides a means for training, peer review, and quality assurance. A photographic image provides objective, reliable data.

- Consent to photograph – Consent to photograph is required (Pasqualone, 2011). Consents should include the types of photographs to be taken, who will have access to them, and how they will be used and stored (Ledray, 2008). Institutions must have policies and procedures in place for obtaining and storing photographs.
- Suitable equipment – The choice of camera is influenced by the training required for reliable photographs. The main requirement is that the photograph is a true and accurate representation of what was seen (Smock & Besant-Matthews, 2007).
- Secure storage and chain of custody – Photographic images (i.e., memory card, CD, DVD) should be labeled and stored in a secure location. Forensic nurses must be able to attest to the authenticity of the photographic image.
- Views to photograph – Three different views are typical with each injury. A full-body view gives perspective; a mid-range photograph conveys the image in context; and a close-up view with and without a ruler placed in the same plane as the injury conveys detail (Linden, Lewis-O'Connor, & Jackson, 2007; Pasqualone, 2011).
- Release of photographs – The consent form may include the release of photographs, along with health information to law enforcement personnel. In some regions, a separate consent is used for photography and release to law enforcement officials.

Injury Nomenclature and Classification Systems

Significant variability exists across the literature in the use and definitions of injuries. Recent efforts are underway to standardize the nomenclature and classification of injuries. The nomenclature and systems used to classify injuries are inconsistent, which confounds the identification of patterns of injury across settings and types of assault (Sommers, Brunner, Brown, Buschur, Fargo, Fisher, Hinkle, & Zink, 2012).

One of the original systems to standardize injury regarding sexual assault genital examination was the TEARS system developed by Laura Slaughter (Sommers, Brunner, Brown, Buschur, Fargo, Fisher, Hinkle, & Zink, 2012). The acronym "TEARS" stands for tears (T), ecchymosis (E), abrasions (A), redness (R), and swelling (S). Although it has not been consistently adopted, the system provides a guide for examiners to standardize terminology and injury documentation. However, some limitations exist. For example, the more accurate term for tears is "lacerations," and the term "ecchymosis" should not be used to mean "bruises."

The BALD STEP guide was subsequently developed to include a broad range of physical findings and to facilitate consistency and efficiency of documentation (Carter-Snell, 2011). The components of the guide are shown in Table 2.5. The BALD STEP guide is intended to prompt staff to look for these findings, promote consistent terminology, and aid in efficiency and clarity of documentation (See Figure 2.4; Table 2.5).

Systems for classifying severity of injury have also been developed, including the Penn Injury Typology (Sommers, Brunner, Brown, Buschur, Fargo, Fisher, Hinkle, & Zink, 2012), the nongenital injury severity score (Dunlap, Brazeau, Stermac, & Addison, 2004), and the genital injury score (Kelly, Larkin, Cosby, & Paolinetti, 2013). The use of more consistent terminology and methods for estimating severity improves understanding of injuries and patterns of injury with various types of violence.

Blood Testing and Toxicology

If testing services are available, blood and urine may be obtained for a variety of reasons. The patient's history of events will assist the forensic nurse in determining if potential drug and/or

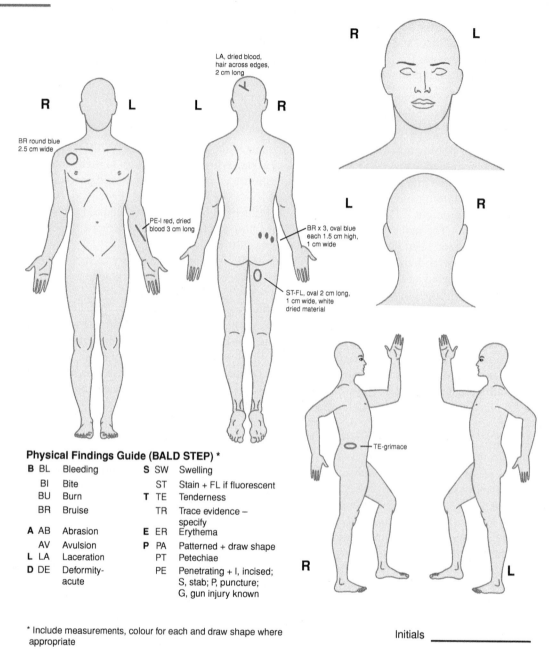

FIGURE 2.4   Documentation with BALD STEP.

alcohol testing should be conducted. When indicated, these specimens should be collected as soon as possible after receiving the patient. Some agents are quickly metabolized and may not be detectable hours after the event (Du Mont, Macdonald, Rotbard, Bainbridge, Asilani, Smith, & Cohen, 2010; UN, 2011). If the patient arrives more than 24 hours to 48 hours postevent, some laboratory protocols request only a urine sample as metabolites will be absent in the blood after that time. The UN guidelines (UN, 2011) for testing include the following recommendations:

- Blood – Use of blood tubes containing sodium fluoride–potassium oxalate are used (typically grey-top tubes) as they stop further degradation of agents and do not require refrigeration. Two tubes are collected: one for the defense and one for the prosecution.

TABLE 2.5 BALD STEP Guide for Physical Findings

B	Bruises (BR)	S	Stains (ST) + FL if fluorescent
	Bite marks (BI)		Swelling (SW)
	Bleeding (BL)	T	Tenderness (TE)
	Burns (BU)		Trace evidence (TR)-specify
A	Abrasions (AB)	E	Erythema (ER)
	Avulsions (AV)	P	Patterned injury (PA)
L	Lacerations (LA)		Petechiae (PT)
D	Deformities-acute		Penetrating Injury (PE)
	(DE)		Incised (PE-I)
			Stab (PE-S)
			Puncture (PE-P)
			Gun injury known (PE-G)

- Urine – The recommended collection is at least 50 mL of urine. Some laboratories request that, if the sample cannot be analyzed within hours, then the urine should be frozen or transferred into two additional sodium fluoride–potassium oxalate tubes.

Studies of drug-facilitated sexual assaults in multiple countries reveal that the most commonly used agent is alcohol (Du Mont, Macdonald, White, Turner, White, Kaplan, & Smith, 2014; El Sohly & Salamone, 1999). The next most commonly identified drugs are cocaine and marijuana, with only rare identification of traditionally described "date rape" drugs, such as flunitrazepam (Rohypnol) and gammahydroxybutyrate (GHB). Prior to the patient's arrival at the hospital, the drug may have metabolized, so the nurse should ask about possible signs of drug facilitation. These may include sudden loss of consciousness or intoxication beyond what would be expected for the amount of alcohol consumed, prolonged hangover-type symptoms, and memory loss (Du Mont, Macdonald, Rotbard, Bainbridge, Asilani, Smith, & Cohen, 2010). Groups of symptoms known as "toxidromes" may assist nurses in the clinical setting or the laboratory in determining the types of agents ingested (See Figure. 2.5). Toxidromes are assessed mainly by examining the pupils, vital signs, skin moisture and temperature, odors, and level of consciousness (Hack &

Type	Pupils	HR	RR	Consciousness	Skin/Gastrointestinal	Medications
Sympatho-mimetic	↑	↑	↑	Agitation, excess speech & motor activity, hyperreflexia, seizures	Sweaty, increased gut activity, anorexia	Cocaine, PCP, amphetamines
Withdrawal	↑	↑		Agitation, hallucinations	Sweaty, piloerection (goosebumps, diarrhea)	Narcotic or alcohol
Anticholinergic	↓	↑		Agitation, variable, visual disturbances, seizures	Dry mucous membranes, flushed hot skin, decreased gut activity, urinary retention	Antihistamines, antinauseants
Opioid	↓	↓	↓	Drowsy/unconscious, hyporeflexia, (meperidine may cause larger pupils)	Decreased gut, hypothermia	Morphine, oxycodone
Sedative/hypnotic	↓	↓		Drowsy, no respiratory depression, nystagmus, hallucinations, amnesia	Decreased gut activity	Benzodiazepines (Rohypnol, Valium), alcohol, antidepressants, anti-convulsants

FIGURE 2.5   Toxidromes.

TABLE 2.6 Evidence Persistence

Location	Possible Persistence*	References
Semen in mouth	<31 hrs	Allard, 1997
Saliva on skin	0–96 hrs	Kenna et al., 2011
Sperm in anus	<3 d	Allard, 1997
Semen in vagina	24 hrs to 6–7 d or more	Silverman & Silverman, 1978
Sperm on cervix	Up to 10 d or more	Mayntz-Press et al., 2008; Morgan, 2008; Perloff & Steinberger, 1964; Silverman & Silverman, 1978
DNA from fingers on neck	10 d	Rutty, 2002

*Based on estimates across the literature

Hoffman, 2011; Lam, Engebretsen, & Bauer, 2011). Some toxicology evidence kits include forms for the laboratory that require this information. Without knowing these symptoms, the toxicology samples may come back negative as only a few agents out of each major grouping are tested. Furthermore, some medications are not typically tested at all, such as prescription medications (e.g., Ambien, Benadryl, and narcotics) and can be precipitated by the effects of alcohol.

Evidence Considerations

Evidence collection in adults has typically been offered within the first 72 hours post sexual assault, but research suggests that the timeframe to examine and treat patients is longer (Archambault, 2005). From a healthcare perspective, emergency contraception may be provided as late as 5 days after sexual assault, compared to 3 days with older forms of contraception. Research indicates that DNA persists longest on the cervix (See Table 2.6). Although most DNA is retrieved within 72 hours (Joki-Erkkila, Tuomisto, Seppanen, Huhtala, Ahola, Raino, & Karhunen, 2014), studies have shown DNA retrieval postcoitus after 4 days (Hall & Ballantyne, 2003; Morgan, 2008), 6 days (Joki-Erkkila, Tuomisto, Seppanen, Huhtala, Ahola, Raino, & Karhunen, 2014), 7 days (Mayntz-Press, Sims, Hall, & Ballantyne, 2008), and even 10 days later (Silverman & Silverman, 1978). An expanded window for treatment and evidence collection is helpful, as patients often delay seeking health care for hours or even days after a sexual assault, especially if they know the assailant (Millar, Stermac, & Addison, 2002; Vertamatti, deAbreu, Otsuka, Costa, Ferreira, Tavares, Santos, & Barbosa, 2012).

The timing of evidence collection for adolescents is similar to adults (Christian, 2011). For prepubertal children, however, the window for evidence collection is somewhat narrower. Most positive body swabs are obtained within the first 24 hours postassault (Christian, 2011; Thackeray, Hornor, Benzinger, & Scribano, 2011). In addition, with children, DNA is often found on clothing and bed linens and DNA evidence has been found beyond 24 hours from both body swabs and clothing, with 23% of positive results recovered within 48 hours (Thackeray, Hornor, Benzinger, & Scribano, 2011). In three cases, the child's underwear tested positive for semen as long as 63 hours later. The importance of this evidence has now expanded recommendations for prepubertal evidence collection to at least 72 hours (Christian, 2011). Christian describes the potential for this timing to expand further with newer DNA analysis techniques, an example of which is Y-STR analysis.

Ultimately, the timing of treatment and evidence collection depends on the capacity of the clinical setting, the law enforcement resources, and the probability of persistence of evidence from a particular anatomical location. Examples of time ranges in which evidence may persist are shown in Table 2.6. It should be noted, however, that these are only averages; other variables affect persistence. Even if the victim has showered, DNA recovery from the skin in areas that has had saliva contact (e.g., the nipples) is possible, so attempts should be made (Williams, Panacek, Green, Kanthaswamy, Hopkins, & Calloway, 2014). Local police and forensic laboratory protocols and forensic nursing protocols should be consulted for timeframes involving evidence collection.

Crime Scene Preservation and Collection. Although the patient is being cared for in the health setting, the forensic nurse may provide relevant information to assist with the law enforcement investigation. The forensic nurse's actions to preserve and collect evidence are critical.

- For instance, the history of the assault may reveal a need for law enforcement officials to examine the scene of the violence for evidence ("She assaulted me in my car.").
- The type of injuries may direct the officers' search for specific items (e.g., a rod or bat if the patient exhibits linear, patterned bruises; a hangar if the patterned injury is in a loop shape). Alternatively, the police officials may find an object at the scene and ask the patient about it or ask the nurse for information regarding injuries that might be consistent with this object.
- The patient may bring evidence from the scene to the clinical setting (e.g., a condom, a piece of clothing). The forensic nurse should retain this evidence and give it to law enforcement officials (i.e., place it in a paper vs. a plastic bag).

Evidence Principles. The type of evidence and method of collection vary with the type of violence or trauma, but some key principles exist:

Gloving. Gloves must be worn at all times during the physical examination and the handling of evidence. Ideally, gloves should be changed between each item collected to prevent cross-contamination.

Chain of Custody. The nurse must be able to account for all persons who have had contact with the evidence. The evidence should remain with the nurse or delegate at all times or be locked in a secure area until it can be handed over to law enforcement officers.

Eating/Drinking. If oral penetration has occurred within the last 24 hours, the nurse should obtain oral swabs along the lower gum and behind the molars. Once the swab or oral rinse is obtained, the patient may eat or drink unless other medical contraindications direct otherwise.

Voiding. If a female patient has experienced vaginal penetration and needs to void before the examination, she should be instructed not to wipe after voiding to limit the loss of any potential biological evidence.

Undressing. Trace evidence may be present on the patient's clothing. Unless the patient has significant trauma that must be managed, the patient should remain dressed until ready to begin the examination. If a forensic kit is to be obtained, a drop-sheet is typically used in which the patient stands on top of two sheets of paper while disrobing, to catch potential trace evidence. Although respecting privacy, the nurse should remain in the room. The patient should be asked to remove only one piece of clothing at a time and hand each item to the nurse. The nurse will place each item in a separate paper bag to be sealed and labeled. The top drop-sheet is then folded, labeled, and placed with the kit as evidence. Staff should ensure that the patient has a change of underwear and clothing available.

Swabs. If the nurse suspects that the patient has had contact with bodily fluids from the assailant, the nurse swabs the area and places the specimen in the forensic kit. The method for swabbing depends on the history provided, the illumination using alternate light sources, and the area being sampled:

- Dry stains – A wet/dry technique is used for all dry stains and bite marks. This may be accomplished using the double-swab technique (i.e., using one swab moistened with water, then immediately rewiping the area with a dry swab) (Sweet, Lorente, Lorente, Valenzuela, & Villenueva, 1997) or by wetting one side of a swab, rubbing it over the area, turning it to the dry side, and reswabbing (RCMP Laboratory, 2014). The nurse moistens the swabs with water only; saline can degrade the specimen.
- Wet stains – The nurse uses dry swabs.

Paper Versus Plastic. DNA will degrade if it becomes moldy in storage. Whenever possible, samples should be placed into paper or cardboard containers. If the item is a hazard (e.g., jagged piece of glass) or is exceptionally wet (e.g., tampon), a plastic urine container can be used, but the sample may need to be refrigerated or frozen to prevent degradation. The forensic nurse should check with the local forensic laboratory regarding recommendations.

DNA Reference Samples. The patient's own DNA is required as a reference sample. The DNA reference sample is obtained with a buccal swab (i.e., a sample of the patient's blood or a vigorous swab of the inner cheek to obtain epithelial cells).

Labeling. The nurse should seal and label all samples as soon as possible and place them in the kit. The source of the sample and the examiner's initials should appear on the outside of the sample. The patient's initials or identifying numbers should also be documented on the sample as the samples will be removed from the kit during processing by law enforcement or laboratory personnel. Chain of custody must be maintained during this process; instructions are packaged in the forensic kits.

Types of Evidence to Collect. The type of evidence to collect varies with the situation. Below are some general practices for collection:

* Biological – Bodily fluids (e.g., semen, blood, saliva) that are recovered may be potential evidence. Swabs of the mouth, external genitals, vagina/cervix, and anus/rectum may be indicated and are based on the patient's history. In child sexual abuse cases, the areas swabbed and the collection method are somewhat modified.
* Trace evidence – Examples may include hair, makeup, glass, loose debris, or fibers. These items can be scraped into paper envelopes or bindles. A "bindle" is created by folding a piece of paper inward multiple times to prevent the loss of material. Pieces of tape or a sticky note can also be used to pick up smaller pieces of debris.
* Chemical – In cases of fire, poisoning, or metal exposure, much of the evidence may be at the scene. Clothing or swabs from the patient's body may be needed if contact occurred with the chemicals.
* Firearms – Whenever possible, a bullet or bullet fragment that has exited the body or has been removed in surgery should be retained in a paper envelope or a sterile cup. It should not be handled with anything metal (e.g., forceps) as contact with the metal could alter the markings on the bullet. In some locales, forensic nurses also use gunshot residue kits to collect possible firearm discharge residue from the patient's hands.

Evidence Storage for Patients Not Reporting to Law Enforcement. Some clinical settings have made provisions for evidence storage for those patients who wish to have evidence collected, but have not yet decided to report to law enforcement officials. In some regions, these are called "anonymous" or "third party" kits. The kit is securely stored and chain of custody is maintained for a specified period of time, either in the clinical unit or with law enforcement personnel, using only an identification number. After a specified period of time, the kit is destroyed.

Documentation

Documentation of nursing interactions should occur throughout all phases of care. The documentation should be thorough and objective; and list assessment findings, interventions, and evaluation of interventions. Confidentiality of health information and secure storage of documentation (and any photographic images) is important. Arrangements should be in place for secure storage of these records and limiting access to health personnel unless necessary.

Nursing Diagnosis

The nursing diagnosis phase of the nursing process requires integration and analysis of the history and physical examination to determine the best plan of care, treatment, and followup services. Each assessment has recommended interventions (nursing and collaborative) (Carpenito, 2013). Some of the nursing diagnoses that may be used with patients who have experienced a violent or traumatic event are shown in Table 2.7.

Planning

Any threats to life or limb identified in the primary survey must be resolved before proceeding with further interventions. Subsequent issues identified in the assessment and diagnosis phase are prioritized, based on patient safety (physical or psychological) and need (Darnell, 2011). In the

TABLE 2.7 Possible Nursing Diagnoses Related to Violence, Stress, or Trauma

Patient Unit	Possible Nursing Diagnoses
Individual-psychological	Anxiety, death anxiety
	Impaired communication
	Acute confusion
	Ineffective coping
	Defensive coping
	Ineffective impulse control
	Decisional conflict
	Fatigue
	Fear
	Anticipatory grieving
	Delayed growth and development
	Risk-prone health behavior
	Hopelessness
	Risk for compromised human dignity
	Posttrauma syndrome
	Powerlessness
	Ineffective relationship
	Risk for compromised resilience
	Ineffective role performance
	Ineffective family processes
	Disturbed self-concept
	Risk for self-harm
	Social isolation
	Spiritual distress
	Stress overload
	Risk for other-directed violence
	Risk for self-directed violence/suicide
	Risk for bleeding
Individual-physical	Impaired comfort (acute or chronic pain)
	Risk for infection transmission
	Risk for injury
	Decreased intracranial adaptive capacity
	Impaired memory
Family/Community	Caregiver role strain
	Family coping
	Interrupted family processes
	Dysfunctional family processes
	Impaired parenting
	Contamination: community (e.g., related to disaster)
	Ineffective community coping
	Deficient community health
	Inefficient community self-health management

context of patient-centered and trauma-informed care, the patient needs to be included in planning to ensure that interventions are consistent with his or her wishes, abilities, resources, and lifestyle. The respective and unique roles of members of the healthcare team should be clear and concise to best meet the patient's needs. The patient's perspective should be central to the planning and prioritization. The patient's lifestyle, concerns, and unique situation may not support the implementation of some of the recommended strategies. Restoring control and choice, however, are critical to recovery and resilience.

Provision of holistic nursing care must include patient safety considerations, be focused on achieving outcomes to meet the needs or promote strengths in the areas identified, and be consistent with the care that the patient requests (Darnell, 2011). Some recommendations for the care of patients who have experienced violent or traumatic events include advocacy, crisis intervention, and safety and risk assessment. Patients are also provided care and treatment of injuries, prophylaxis for infection and pregnancy, and referral and discharge planning. In some instances, forensic nurses may be asked to consult on patients located in the inpatient clinical setting.

Crisis Intervention

Effective communication techniques and crisis interventions should be used throughout the healthcare interaction. The patient may initially appear calm, but when asked about the assault/trauma, may become more anxious and agitated. If the patient has PTSD or other mental health issues, his or her emotions/behaviors may escalate at various points during the examination, or days and weeks following the event. The focus is on preventing further victimization, enhancing comfort, and promoting recovery. Two of the more common techniques for crisis intervention are psychological first aid (PFA) and Robert's seven stage model (Roberts & Ottens, 2005):

Psychological First Aid. The WHO has promoted the use of PFA by professionals and community advocates after disasters or trauma (WHO, 2011). Psychological first aid does not replace the need for mental health professionals, but supports crisis responses and helps identify those who may need more specialized intervention. The key principles are look, listen, and link:

- Look – Professionals need to be aware of their own safety and threats to self; physical safety for the patient and/or the family; any immediate threats to physical health (breathing, circulation, neurological function); presence of any serious psychological distress, such as attempts at self-harm, tonic immobility, uncontrollable distress, threats to harm others or dissociation; and risks for lethality.
- Listen – Includes provision of privacy and comfort measures, carefully listening and attending to the patient's concerns, helping him or her identify any immediate needs or concerns, and providing positive support. Avoid phrases that imply disbelief or blame; reduce retraumatization by limiting the the number of times the patient is asked about the event. Establishment of a collaborative relationship is helpful as is reframing negative cognitions, such as self-blame or the belief that the person will never be safe again (Roberts & Ottens, 2005).
- Link – Includes identifying available resources to support the patient and connecting the person with these resources. Referrals may include patient advocates, counselors, legal resources, housing, pastoral services, victim services, or other resources in the community. Roberts and Ottens (2005) also suggest helping the patient to identify positive coping resources that he or she may have used in the past.

Restoration of a sense of control is important for victims of violence. If a person perceives having control over a situation, he or she has improved resilience to the adverse effects of the trauma (Davis & Reich, 2014). Lack of control is associated with blunted emotional responses and lack of awareness of what is happening; increased control is associated with increased awareness of emotions and attempts at resolution.

Safety and Suicide Prevention Planning

For some patients, returning home may be unsafe. However, victims of IPV have a high risk of lethality during the period around which they leave their partner (Weisz, Tolman, & Saunders, 2000). Advocates and local shelters are available to collaborate with the forensic nurse to assist patients in developing a safety plan.

Depression is common among victims of violence; suicide screening should be conducted on all victims of violence (Malouf, Jackson, & Borg, 2013). Sometimes, the event that precipitated the healthcare visit was a suicide attempt; the patient may still have medications in his or her system or injuries that need attention. A number of suicide screening tools are available. One scoring tool is the Nurses' Global Assessment of Suicide Risk (NGASR), which assigns a weight from 1 to 3 for each of a number of characteristics positively correlated with suicide risk (Mitchell, Kane, Havill, & Cassesse, 2013). Key factors include hopelessness, depression, presence of a suicide plan, stated intent, recent loss of a relationship (death, divorce, separation), prior suicide attempts, recent stress, persecutory thoughts, psychosis, withdrawal from others, alcohol or substance abuse, or terminal illness. Risks or concerns for suicide should be brought forward to the healthcare team.

Patient or family behaviors – such as increased speed or volume of speech or increased restlessness and motor movement – are signs of escalating risks for violent behavior (Isaacs, 2013). The forensic nurse should take precautions for the patient's safety and be familiar with strategies to de-escalate violence. If a patient or family member escalates and cannot be redirected, security or law enforcement may need to be contacted. The following de-escalation techniques may be of use:

- Ensure access to the exit for both the nurse and the patient (i.e., the nurse should not block the patient's exit)
- Maintain a distance of at least 4 body widths away from person (but not excessively more)
- Know the location of emergency bells or how to access additional resources
- Use a calm voice
- Offer comfort measures
- Set limits for inappropriate behavior or speech, and inform of the consequences
- Avoid arguing with or challenging the person
- Consider the use of anxiolytics (may prevent chemical or physical restraint later) (Isaacs, 2013).

Another potential source of safety risk is caring for patients who are in law enforcement custody. These patients may arrive in handcuffs from correctional facilities or police stations with injuries as either a victim or an assailant. Their health information is confidential and, ideally, they should be interviewed without guards present. Care of the patient in custody (e.g., handcuff removal, location of the officer during the examination) will depend upon policies of the correctional/law enforcement authority, as well as the healthcare facility.

Care and Treatment

Infection Prophylaxis. Guidelines for prevention or treatment of infection differ by country and by type of medication available. Recommendations from federal agencies (e.g., CDC-US or Public Health Agency of Canada) and local guidelines should be followed. General guidelines include:

- Tetanus – If the patient has a dirty wound or reason exists to believe that the wound may be contaminated, tetanus immunization should be considered if more than 5 years have elapsed since the patient's last immunization.
- Sexually transmitted infections (STI) – Many teams conduct baseline testing prior to treatment for gonorrhea, chlamydia, and syphilis after sexual assault; other teams prophylax without testing. Standard recommended protocols for STI typically treat gonorrhea and chlamydia. The forensic nurse should consult local and national protocols.

Pregnancy Prophylaxis. Emergency contraception (e.g., levonorgestrel) is typically provided within 5 days of unprotected vaginal penetration. It is safe for use even if the woman is taking another form of birth control. In some countries, it is available over-the-counter. Forensic nurses may have to advocate for patients to have access to emergency contraception.

Treatment of Other Injuries or Health Concerns. The patient may also require diagnostic imaging or interventions for injuries (e.g., head injury, wounds requiring sutures, fracture casting), or referrals to other specialities.

Evaluation

Evaluation is linked to identifying whether the desired outcomes for the patient were met. This phase consists of reevaluation. If needs are met, discharge planning commences. A number of factors can impinge discharge, such as patients who are not physically or mentally stable, or if safety issues exist. Social services and advocates are vital to the latter barriers.

Discharge Planning. Plans for discharge should be made in collaboration with the patient's wishes. Instructions should be both verbal and in writing (DOJ, 2013). The patient may not recall the instructions later. Having standardized discharge instructions that are individualized helps ensure that all aspects of the followup treatment are covered. The "Teach Back" method validates that the patient understands, and provides an opportunity for him or her to ask questions (Xu, 2012).

Quality Improvement

Quality Improvement. This process is the use of a deliberate and defined mechanism that focuses on activities to improve population health. The term refers to an ongoing effort to achieve measurable improvements that improve health care (Riley, Moran, Corso, Beitsch, & Bialek, 2010).

Peer/Team Review. Peer reviews are important, both as a learning tool and as a quality improvement (QI) measure, and are required according to the *National Sexual Assault Protocol* (DOJ, 2013). Peer review can be an effective tool in areas in which a limited number of cases occur (e.g., sexual assaults in rural areas) as a way to validate findings and educate providers. Another form of review is Team Review. This can be helpful both within nursing and with multidisciplinary teams. In addition, patient satisfaction is important to capture. Using a QI approach with patients offers them an opportunity to be heard. Lewis-O'Connor (in review) asked 359 patients who had experienced domestic and sexual assault what went well for them, what could have been better, and what two changes they would like to see. The findings identified a number of policy and procedures that would improve the service that patients receive.

CONCEPTS AND ISSUES

Mechanisms of Injury

If one understands the mechanism of the injury, one can anticipate the type, location, and severity of injuries. When an object contacts the body (or vice versa), a transfer of energy occurs and injury results. Greater speed on impact inflicts greater injury due to creating impact injury as well as acceleration and deceleration of internal organs. In addition, patient-specific variables affect risks for injury, such as age, sex, chronic health conditions, elasticity and health of tissues, location of injury, and medications. The type of injury also depends upon whether blunt or penetrating injury mechanisms were used.

Blunt Force Injury

Contact with a blunt object (e.g., fist, bat) or surface (e.g., wall) typically results in redness, bruising, abrasions, and/or lacerations. In addition, fractures, sprains, and strains may occur.

Redness Erythema. Redness is considered a nonspecific finding; it may be due to many factors. Reddened areas will blanch (whiten) if pressure is applied. The area of redness could also disappear quickly, so photographic documentation is recommended at the time of the acute event and subsequently in followup examination (serial photography). Redness may be difficult to note in darker skinned patients.

Bruises. Bruises result from the rupture of subcutaneous blood vessels in response to the application of blunt force without breaking the skin (See Figure 2.6). They are also called "contusions." The term "ecchymosis" should not be used for bruises as a different mechanism is involved (Nash & Sheridan, 2009; Primeau & Sheridan, 2013; Saukko & Knight, 2009). Ecchymoses are typically

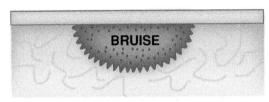

FIGURE 2.6 Bruise mechanism.

"nonpainful and nonindurated, lack distinct outer margins, and spread in the direction of gravity" (Primeau & Sheridan, 2013; p. 318). Ecchymoses may be noted in areas below or around bruises as the interstitial blood follows gravity directions through the fascia and spreads to areas beyond the original bruise. An example is a bruise to the cheek with ecchymotic spread to the lower jaw, or periorbital ecchymoses with a basal skull fracture. Key characteristics of bruising include:

- Variability of appearance – Appearance is affected by many factors, such as the amount of force, the type of tissue, the presence of underlying bone, and individual patient characteristics, such as health status, medications, and age.
- Pain – Bruises are usually painful, swollen in the acute phase, and may be indurated. They do not blanch with pressure as the blood cells remain in the area.
- Variability of color – Although color progresses as bruises age, color should not be used to age the bruise. The progression varies across patients and insufficient evidence exists to date bruises. Bruises are also sometimes difficult to detect on people with darker skin (Baker, Fargo, Shambley-Ebron, & Sommers, 2010) and new techniques are being explored to improve visualization, such as colorimetry to measure colors in an area of the skin (Scafide, Sheridan, Campbell, DeLeon, & Hayat, 2013).
- Varies with underlying tissues – Bruising is more likely to appear sooner in loose tissues (e.g., periorbital region, scrotum) than in bony areas (Lichenstein & Suggs, 2007; Saukko & Knight, 2009).

Timing. Deep bruises may take a few days to appear (Lichenstein & Suggs, 2007). Assessment should include palpation of all body surfaces as tenderness may be an early sign of deep bruising. Some bruises may be visualized with alternate light sources and enhanced photographic techniques. A followup examination to assess for the progression or healing of injuries is also useful.

Petechiae. Also called "Tardieu's spots," these are pinpoint areas of bleeding that appear as red dots, typically 1/10 mm to 2 mm in size (Saukko & Knight, 2009). Thin-walled venules rupture in areas above the level of compression, for instance, in the head and neck with strangulation attempts (See Figure 2.7) or in body parts above compression from a vehicle rollover. Key points include:

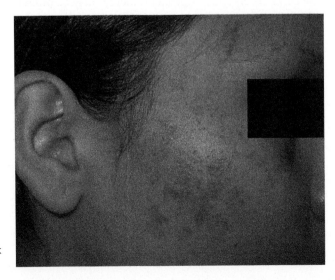

FIGURE 2.7 Petechiae on cheek poststrangulation attempt.

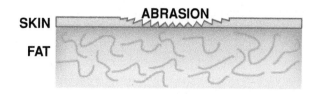

FIGURE 2.8   Abrasion mechanism.

- Blood vessels with limited structural support are most vulnerable to petechiae, such as in the skin of the upper eyelids, face, forehead, behind the ears, around the mouth, and in the sclera and conjuctivae of the eye.
- Some patients present with petechiae after prolonged episodes of vomiting or severe coughing: if so, they should be asked about these events.
- Areas of bleeding larger than 2 mm are called "purpura" and of 5 mm or more are known as "ecchymoses."
- Petechiae, purpura, and ecchymoses may be caused by other mechanisms, such as aging/fragile vessels, septic infections (e.g., meningococcal disease), blood dyscrasias (e.g., disseminated intravascular coagulation), and gravitational movement from a nearby bruise or injury (e.g., periorbital ecchymoses with basal skull fracture).
- Like bruises, petechiae, purpura, and ecchymoses will not blanch when pressure is applied.

Abrasions. Abrasions are superficial and result from the removal of some or all of the first layer of skin (i.e., the epidermis) (See Figure 2.8). This may be from either friction mechanisms (e.g., rug "burn," fall on pavement) or from compression/pressure (e.g., ligatures). Generally, abrasions do not bleed unless they extend deeper into the dermis, where the blood vessels are located.

Avulsions. The skin over an area is torn away by shearing or blunt forces in an avulsion, such as a fingernail torn off or a scalp torn by a windshield (Primeau & Sheridan, 2013). Generally, avulsions are deeper than they are long. They are particularly common over bony prominences but can occur anywhere.

Lacerations. Lacerations are tears in the skin that result after application of blunt force when the stretching of fibers is exceeded (See Figure 2.9).

- The term "lacerations" is often incorrectly used to refer to penetrating injuries or any open wound. Lacerations result only from blunt mechanisms.
- Lacerations are generally longer than they are deep.

The edges are typically ragged and uneven; may be bruised, abraded, and/or inverted; and may have bridging of connective tissue, hair, blood vessels, or nerves across the wound (See Figure 2.10).

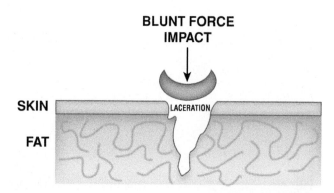

FIGURE 2.9   Lacerations.

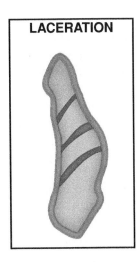

FIGURE 2.10   Cross-bridging.

Fractures (Deformities). Fractures may be caused by blunt trauma and result in acute deformities that can be observed or palpated:

- A step-off deformity may be palpable, such as with fractured ribs.
- Redness, swelling, and tenderness are associated with these acute deformities.
- Fractures may be simple (oblique), compound (open to the outside), comminuted (crushed), or spiral.

Penetrating Injury

Penetrating injuries include incised wounds, stab wounds, and gunshot wounds. In general, incised and stab wounds have the following characteristics:

- Clean cut margins
- No bruising or abrasions to the wound edges
- Deeper structures are evenly divided with no cross-bridging of tissue
- Usually free from foreign material

   These three types of wounds are addressed in greater detail below.

Incised Wounds. These wounds are wider than deep and are created by a sharp blade crossing the skin as shown on the upper portion of Figure 2.11. The penetrating or sharp object that causes them slices across the skin. The length of the wound is relevant, but the width is variable

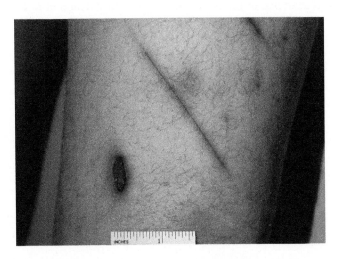

FIGURE 2.11   Penetrating injury – incised and stab.

depending on the location of the injury in relation to Langer's lines, lines across the skin similar to dermatomes in which there is limited skin flexibility (MedArt, 2008). If the incision is in the same direction as the line, the wound may not spread apart. This direction can make a stab or incised wound more difficult to notice; therefore, gentle traction of the skin is recommended when assessing for potential penetrating injury. If the incision is perpendicular to one of these lines, the wound will gape apart.

Stab Wounds. These are deeper than they are wide and are caused by a sharp object as shown on the lower left of Figure 2.11. A sharp, single-edged blade will sometimes cause a "V" shape to the wound and a rounded edge to the opposite side (a double-edged blade would have a "V" shape at both ends). Depth of penetration is less clear on soft tissue; the wound could be deeper than the weapon due to inward compression of the tissue. Bruises or abrasions from the handle of the knife may also sometimes be seen around the wound. The description of the wound (and/ or photographs) will aid in the investigation.

Gunshot Wounds. The characteristics of a gunshot injury will vary for a number of reasons, including the type of firearm or ammunition used and the tissue contacted. Gunshot wounds from the same distance with different ammunition or weapons can look vastly different. Exit and entrance wounds are typically misdiagnosed even by trauma physicians (Smock, 2007). Instead, the injury should be described and documented for forensic pathologists or firearm experts to interpret. Some characteristics help determine the distance between the firearm and the injury.

- A "contact" gunshot wound is created when the muzzle of the firearm is in contact with the skin (See Figure 2.12). The gases from the blast cause soot to be imbedded in the skin and inflict a burn. The wound may have a stellate (star-shaped) appearance. An exit wound may also have a stellate appearance, but would not have burns or soot. An abrasion may appear at the top of the wound from the edge of the firearm (See Figure 2.8). If an angle existed between the muzzle and skin, the wound would be more oval than round.
- A "near contact" wound exhibits tattooing of gunpowder imbedded in the skin around the injury.
- "Intermediate" contact wounds display a wider dispersion of tattooing, with the edges of the wound more jagged than with close contact wounds.
- "Distant" contact wounds have little or no tattooing and no burns at the injury site. The wound may have an abrasion rim (abrasion collar) formed with indentation of the skin as the bullet enters.

Burns

Burns may be from thermal, chemical, or electrical mechanisms. The severity of the burn is classified as shown in Table 2.8. Burns may be accidental or nonaccidental.

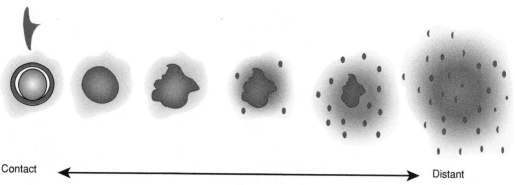

Contact ⟵――――――――――――――――――――――――⟶ Distant

FIGURE 2.12   Gunshot wounds.

TABLE 2.8 Burn Classifications

Depth	Description
Superficial thickness	• Formerly called "first degree" • Only the surface layer is involved, such as sunburn with redness and blistering
Partial thickness	• Deeper layers of the skin are involved; nerves are left damaged and exposed and are extremely painful
Full thickness	• Skin, underlying tissue/nerves, muscle, and even bone are involved; no pain exists in these areas as pain endings have been destroyed

Thermal Burns. Some characteristics of nonaccidental burns are identified below:

- Dry burns result from the application of hot objects to the skin (e.g., irons, hair curlers, cigarette lighters, or stove grills) (Lichenstein & Suggs, 2007). Nonaccidental burns may be patterned like an object (e.g., cigarette tip, stove element) and tend to be uniform in thickness across the burn. They may also appear as symmetrical, involving both sides of the body.
- Wet liquids create splash and irregular patterns with accidental burns while intentional burns are more likely to have a clear pattern (Duval, 2011). An example is immersion burns that have a "tide mark" or "stocking"-like appearance (See Figure 2.13). This type of pattern can be seen when a child is held in hot water. Accidental burns in hot water would be expected to have splash marks and be uneven.

"Donut" burns may be seen on buttocks when a person (typically a child) is held in a tub filled with hot water. The center of the buttocks in the compressed area will be spared, while the surrounding tissue will be burned from the hot water (DOJ, 2014).

The direction of the burn may be visible and perhaps inconsistent with the history provided. Wet burns leave a "V" shape, pointing in the direction of the spill (See Figure 2.14). This information may help support the determination of accidental versus nonaccidental burns, such as a child pulling a cup with hot liquid down from a counter; the "V" shape would be in a downward direction.

Electrical Burns. Electrical burns are more likely to occur with power sources greater than 100 V. Some key points related to electrical burns include:

- High voltage burns occur with voltages greater than 500 W and result in high morbidity and mortality.

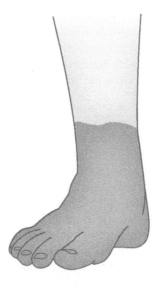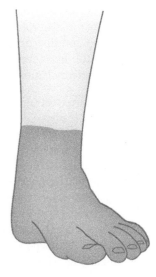

FIGURE 2.13 Stocking (immersion) burns.

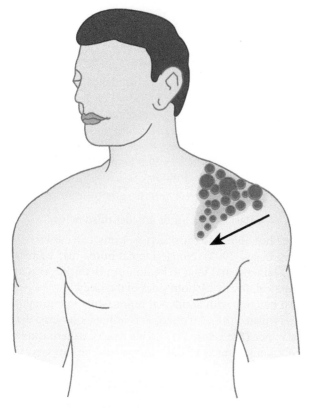

FIGURE 2.14 Burn direction.

- Alternating currents of 40 Hz to 110 Hz can cause tetany, spasm, and an inability to release the object, prolonging the length of contact.
- Direct current electricity (e.g., railroad lines) will throw the victim.
- The current passes through the body and electrothermal damage will be seen at the point of entrance and exit, as well as in the organs through which the current passes. Contact burns, electrical arcs, ignition of clothing, direct burns, or flash burns may occur.
- Wet skin is less resistant to electrical current; therefore, the risk of electrocution is greater. Most deaths from electrical currents are due to cardiac dysrhythmias, failure of the respiratory muscles (paralysis or brainstem damage), or complications from resulting burns (infection, shock). Muscle necrosis occurs and rhabdomyolysis may be seen (Duval, 2011).
- Lightning can also electrocute, striking the highest object or bouncing off a structure. The angle of impact and direction of the current determine the consequences – if the lightening travels through the heart, the consequences are most often fatal. Electrocution burns are typically feather-patterned burns that travel along the lines in which the lightening travelled over the skin.

Chemical Burns. Chemicals such as sulfuric acid, capsaicin oleum (pepper spray), or chloro-benzylidene (tear gas) can cause chemical burns. In addition, victims may experience eye irritation (tears, pain, eye muscle spasm, swelling, visual impairment), respiratory difficulty, and skin impairment. Pulmonary edema may occur in high concentrations. If an explosive device was used to deliver the agent, blunt or penetrating trauma or barotrauma may be present.

Both thermal and chemical burns may result in inhalation burns resulting in airway damage, swelling, thick saliva formation, and obstruction. Signs and symptoms may include soot or singeing of airways, stridor, hoarseness, and dyspnea (Dries & Endorf, 2013).

Toxic gases may be associated with burns. Cyanide poisoning can result from burning of synthetic materials, causing agitation, dizziness, and tachypnea at low levels; at higher levels, cyanide causes metabolic acidosis, seizures, and death (Dries & Endorf, 2013). Carbon monoxide poisoning

TABLE 2.9 Blast Injuries

Mechanism	Injuries
Pulmonary barotrauma (often fatal)	• Pulmonary contusion • Air embolism to brain or spinal cord • DIC, thrombosis • Poor pulmonary performance (hours to days) • ARDS from lung or other injuries
Inhalation	• Carbon monoxide poisoning (enclosed space)
Acoustic barotrauma	• Tympanic membrane rupture (common) • Hemotympanum • Ossicle fracture or dislocation
Thoracic barotrauma	• Decreased heart rate, stroke volume, cardiac index • Drop in BP with loss of systemic vascular resistance
Abdominal barotrauma	• Rupture of bowels
Penetrating trauma	• Puncture or stab wounds with debris/shrapnel (secondary trauma)
Blunt trauma	• Bruises, abrasions, fractures from impact with debris or being thrown
Burns or chemicals	• Burns to skin • Radiation contamination

occurs with fire or exhaust in enclosed areas (Duval, 2011). Carbon monoxide binds more easily to the hemoglobin molecule than oxygen, reducing the amount of oxygen available and shifting the oxyhemoglobin curve to the left. Oximeters are unreliable with carbon monoxide poisoning since the heme sites will be saturated, but with carbon monoxide rather than oxygen. At lower to moderate levels, patients will have tachypnea, tachycardia, and seizures. At higher levels (e.g., above 60% blood levels), the patient may develop shock, apnea, coma, and death.

Blasts

Explosions cause a wave of compression through the air or water. The velocity is greatest near the center of the blast and decreases as the waves spread outward. A wave of low pressure follows, again causing pressure changes in the body (Saukko & Knight, 2009). Injuries differ by location of the blast and the organs or tissue affected:

- The greatest injuries occur to air-filled organs (e.g., tympanic membrane, lungs, bowel). Examples of blast injuries are shown in Table 2.9.
- Injuries may be primary, secondary, tertiary, or quaternary.
  - Primary injuries are caused by the direct effect of the explosive overpressure on the tissue; may create pulmonary barotrauma and is more likely to be fatal than secondary injuries.
  - Secondary injuries are caused by propelled objects that strike the body; injuries include bleeding, burns, blunt and penetrating injury from debris, and compression injuries from the collapse of structures or objects landing on the victim.
  - Tertiary injuries are caused by high-energy blasts; injuries occur when the body is propelled through the air and strikes other objects.
  - Quaternary injuries involve all other injuries caused by explosives.

Descriptions of injuries should include the consistent use of terms as well as descriptions of the characteristics of the injury, such as size, color, shape, presence of any pattern, bleeding, and any signs of healing such as granulation tissue. This standardization is important for both a shared understanding of the injury and mechanisms, but also for moving research forward toward an improved understanding of patterns of injury with various types of violence.

Evidence-Informed Practice

Evidence-informed nursing practice requires the integration and consideration of three components: the highest quality research, clinical expertise, and the patient's values and circumstances (Strauss & Haynes, 2009). Evidence-informed practice is also important in court proceedings.

Evidence Quality. Professional nursing practice must ensure that practices are based on robust, quality evidence. In some areas of practice, little or no research is available. In such instances, practice should be guided by expert opinion. The goal, however, is to base practice on systematic reviews: rigorous replicable reviews of all available studies on a particular topic, which employ analytic techniques such as meta-analyses (quantitative studies) or meta-syntheses (qualitative studies).

Rules of Evidence and Evidence-Based Practice. Evidence that is presented in court must be of high quality. This includes theories and techniques that have been scientifically tested. The forensic nurse should use the best evidence available to guide both practice and testimony. Knowledge of the quality of evidence is important for forensic nurses. Nurses should seek legal guidance from the institutions in which they are employed.

Ethical Concerns

Ethical Principles. Forensic nurses are governed by the code of ethics for nursing practice within their practice area. Principle of ethics aid in decision making about interventions and provide a context for care that is critical for working with vulnerable populations. Examples of ethical issues in the clinical setting include:

- Informed consent, informed refusal, age of consent
- Incapacitated patients
- End-of-life decisions
- Organ donation/transplant

Research Ethics. Evidence-based practice requires the generation of research and new knowledge. Concerns have been raised that involvement in research may create further trauma for vulnerable patients (Edwards, Sylaska, & Gidycz, 2014). Studies have demonstrated, however, that research participation is well tolerated and even a positive experience in populations such as victims of IPV and physical assault (Griffin, Resick, Waldrop, & Mechanic, 2003) and victims of sexual assault (Campbell, Adams, Wasco, Ahrens, & Sefl, 2010; Griffin, Resick, Waldrop, & Mechanic, 2003). The forensic nurse should ensure that research that is conducted on patients adheres to ethics approvals and does not cause the patient distress.

Catastrophic, Biochemical, and Terrorist Responses

Disasters and terrorism can quickly overwhelm the resources of the clinical setting, the community, and the individuals in the community. The clinical setting may be faced with a loss of electricity, limited communications, limited supplies, structural damage, and inadequate staff (Williams & Williams, 2013), all of which pose challenges for assessment and care, and evidence collection and preservation. Potential safety concerns exist in the midst of chaos involving agitated and distraught patients and families. The role of the forensic nurse in a disaster is to provide trauma and emergency nursing care, crisis intervention, mental health and critical incident stress management, public health nursing, and perhaps death investigation (IAFN, n.d.b).

The impact of violence in disasters is compounded by the loss of family and friends as support networks; concerns about safety; challenges in meeting basic needs; and financial concerns (Pittaway, Bartolomia, & Rees, 2007; West, 2006). These issues and loss of support can increase the risk for violence and reduce the victim's resilience to the trauma. The IAFN has developed a checklist for sexual assault services during disasters (IAFN, n.d.a). West (2006) recommends some key actions that forensic nurses may implement to address gaps in victim services after disasters:

- Work with community partners to advocate for uniform reporting systems during disasters
- Create an evidence preservation toolkit to use during a disaster, including documentation systems
- Establish support teams that are culturally competent, will be available during disasters, and which are integrated with victim services/advocate units
- Advocate for funding to support trauma-informed models to meet the short- and long-term needs of individuals, families, and communities
- Work to educate media services on trauma-informed approaches, such as which messages will empower versus retraumatize and the impact of repetitive violent images

Violence Prevention in the Clinical Setting. Prevention of violence is critical for forensic nurses, particularly given the vast number of health consequences associated with violence. The perpetuation of violence across the lifespan provides further emphasis for the need for prevention (Wilkins, Tsao, Hertz, Davis, & Klevens, 2014).

Examples of primary, secondary, and tertiary prevention in the clinical setting are:

- Primary – Dating violence programs focused on healthy relationships and sexual assault awareness education or awareness
- Secondary – Programs to help identify potential human trafficking victims and provide services
- Tertiary – Predischarge planning, such as safety planning, linking the patient to external support agencies and networks, and assisting the patient in exploring effective coping strategies to use after discharge

FUTURE ISSUES

Career Opportunities

Forensic nursing knowledge can be invaluable in the clinical setting. Forensic nurse examiners are being employed in many clinical settings to care for victims of violence and collect evidence, particularly where an insufficient number of physicians exists (Lynch, 2011b).

Forensic nurse examiners have been placed in advisory positions in clinical settings, helping develop protocols for violence, safety, and disaster planning. They can serve on-call to assist with specific situations, such as responding to a call the operating room to help retrieve a bullet or other evidence from the surgical team, or consulting with medical unit staff regarding an older adult patient who may have experienced abuse.

Forensic roles have expanded in the last 20 years and more opportunities are emerging for forensic nurses.

Involvement with Government and Policy Makers

Moving forward, nurses are encouraged to interact with governmental agencies and policy makers to raise awareness of the effectiveness of forensic nurses and their impact on the health of the community. To do this, nurses need to be prepared to present policy briefing papers and conduct cost-benefit analyses to support the creation of forensic nursing services in the community. Forensic nurses can use the growing body of literature to show links between current violence and future health issues and repeat hospital visits that occur without compassionate, comprehensive services. Millions of dollars are spent yearly on the long-term effects of IPV, but every dollar spent on prevention yields 6 dollars of savings (Wells, Emery, & Boodt, 2012). Forensic nurses need to arm themselves with this information and build a case for the importance of forensic nursing in preventing violence and its deleterious effects.

Worldwide, significant variability exists in protective agencies and legislation for vulnerable individuals. Forensic nurses have begun to work internationally to assist nursing colleagues in providing forensic nursing care to vulnerable populations. Opportunities are available to expand this work and to advocate for international standards for the protection of vulnerable populations and the provision of trauma-informed, patient-centered forensic care.

Education

Expansion of forensic nursing in clinical settings relies upon access to high-quality education programs. The forensic nursing roles in some specialty areas developed before the educational programs (Kent-Wilkinson, 2010). The number of forensic courses, programs, and degrees has increased over time. However, some educational institutions have been challenged to maintain their forensic programs due to government budget cuts. Again, forensic nurses must become active in lobbying for violence prevention and their role in it, and actively participate in establishing policy and professional nursing standards for caring for victims of trauma and violence.

A need exists to educate nonspecialized healthcare personnel and the community in violence prevention and intervention, especially while a gap persists in available forensic nursing services. Forensic nurses can lead this initiative. For instance, most emergency nurses are uncomfortable with caring for victims of sexual assault, even if a sexual assault nurse is enroute. Rural nurses have requested short programs so they can work within their scope of practice in partnership with physicians to improve services and response times (Jakubec, Carter-Snell, Ofrim, & Skanderup, 2013), leading to the development of an Enhanced Emergency Sexual Assault Services (EESAS) online program and resources. Another innovative approach is a program for American Indian and Alaskan women in which local women are trained to provide cultural and spiritual support, first aid, culturally competent support, and forensic examinations (SafeStar, 2014).

Forensic nurses have a key role in the clinical setting, taking a lead in working with patients who have been exposed to violence and trauma. Forensic nurses bring an index of suspicion in working with patients who may be victims of violence, yet present with seemingly unrelated complaints. Forensic nurses are also equipped with the knowledge of physical and psychological findings seen with violence, and an understanding of the legal system. Further research is required in many areas to support evidence-based practice and decision making. Forensic nurses can provide leadership in the clinical setting by supporting other healthcare staff, law enforcement personnel, counselors, and community agencies in their care and understanding of patients who are exposed to violence.

Future Research

Since the 1990s, the body of research in forensic nursing practice has grown. Yet, significant gaps or areas for growth related to clinical forensic nursing remain. Some suggestions for research foci are:

- Replication of existing studies – It is difficult to conduct randomized controlled trials in clinical settings. Therefore, studies are often characterized by small sample sizes and convenience samples, which limit the generalizability of the findings. Replication of research in multiple settings strengthens the confidence in the findings and allows for systematic reviews of the research and a higher level of filtered information.
- Injury patterns – As noted earlier, much variability exists in injury nomenclature and documentation and only limited data exists on patterns of injury with various types of violence.
- Effective interventions – Outcome studies are limited, related to the effectiveness of trauma-informed, PCC, and specific interventions. For instance, negative reactions to disclosure can worsen risks for health outcomes, but do positive responses decrease risks? What types of positive responses or crisis interventions are most effective and in what context? How can forensic nurses work best with patients to create positive outcomes for health and well-being?

- Evidence protocols – Forensic laboratories research best methods to analyze evidence collected, but limited data exist regarding the best methods of collection and preservation in the clinical setting. Variations abound for storage of evidence in clinical units, such as drying kits, freezing or refrigerating, types of swabs used, techniques for the collection of swabs, application of dyes, and techniques such as colorimetry or using alternate light source to detect bruising and fluids.
- Violence prevention – A need exists to continue to explore the most effective ways to prevent various forms of violence. Bystander intervention, patient resistance, and offender interventions are three examples of approaches for intimate partner and sexual violence. The evidence is varied and although some approaches are more predominant than others, a clear picture has not yet emerged of the most effective model or impact of context. Effectiveness and implementation of universal screening across ages and genders is also recommended. Recognition of victims is required to stop the cycle and prevent further violence (WHO, 2014a).

CASE STUDY

Ella is a 19-year-old female patient whose roommate brings her to the emergency department. Ella reports that she and her boyfriend had "quite a few drinks" and then argued approximately 8 hours ago. He struck her in the face with his fist and she fell to the ground. He then got on top of her and restrained her arms above her head and penetrated her vaginally with his penis multiple times. She does not recall many other events; she reports that she "kind of went blank." She does recall that, afterward, he "passed out" and she got her clothes and went home to her roommate. She states that she is "sore," but does not believe that she is injured nor likely needs an examination. She does not want police to be involved because she states it is her fault for making him angry and for drinking so much. Ella is requesting pregnancy protection. She is still wearing the clothes she put on at her boyfriend's place.

REVIEW QUESTIONS

1. This assault must be reported to the police.
   a. True
   b. False

2. If Ella does not think she has injuries, she does not need an examination.
   a. True
   b. False

3. Which of the following samples would you recommend be obtained (list all)?
   a. Anal
   b. External genitalia
   c. Nipple/breast swab
   d. Oral
   e. Rectal
   f. Vaginal/cervical

4. Which is an accurate statement about treatment?
   a. Emergency contraception is contraindicated.
   b. She does not need STI treatment as this incident involved her boyfriend.
   c. She should be offered routine treatment for HIV.
   d. She should be offered STI treatments for gonorrhea and chlamydia.

5. When taking the history, the nurse informs a colleague, "I've got Ella's story." Ella observes the nurse document the phrase "alleged sexual assault." What risk does the patient face during this emergency department visit?
   a. Dissociation
   b. Revictimization
   c. Secondary victimization
   d. Vicarious violence

6. Which statement is correct to consider while assessing her injuries?
   a. A symmetrical burn pattern is consistent with nonaccidental injury.
   b. An ecchymosis and a bruise are the same.
   c. Bruises show patterns more clearly than abrasions.
   d. The terms "laceration" and "incised wound" are interchangeable.

7. The nurse is asked to provide opinion testimony related to injuries found on Ella and their significance. He chooses to provide his opinion based on the 1,100 cases of physical and sexual assault in which he has provided care rather than the available research. His argument is that the research is only quasi-experimental and does not reflect randomized controlled trials. This is a valid rationale for using his opinion and he should proceed.
   a. True
   b. False

REFERENCES

Abbey, A., Saenz, C., & Buck, P. O. (2005). The cumulative effects of acute alcohol consumption, individual differences, and situational perceptions on sexual decision making. *Journal of Studies on Alcohol, 66*(1), 82–90.

Adams, J. A., Harper, K., Knudson, S., & Revilla, J. (1994). Examination findings in legally confirmed child sexual abuse: It's normal to be normal. *Pediatrics, 94*(3), 310–317.

Allen, N. E., Larsen, S. E., Javdani, S., & Lehrner, A. (2012). Council-based approaches to reforming the health care response to domestic violence: Promising findings and cautionary tales. *American Journal of Community Psychology, 50*, 50–63.

Ambuel, B., Trent, B. K., Lenehan, P., Cronholm, P., Downing, D., Jelley, M.,...Block, R. (2011). *Competencies needed by health professionals for addressing exposure to violence and abuse in patient care.* Eden Prairie, MN: Academy on Violence and Abuse.

American Academy of Pediatrics (AAP). (n.d.). *The resilience project.* Retrieved July 10, 2015, from https://www.aap.org/en-us/advocacy-and-policy/aap-health-initiatives/Medical-Home-for-Children-and-Adolescents-Exposed-to-Violence/Pages/About-the-Project.aspx.

American Nurses Association (ANA). (2015). *Code of ethics for nurses with interpretive statements.* Silver Spring, MD: Nursesbooks.org. Retrieved from http://www.nursingworld.org/MainMenuCategories/EthicsStandards/CodeofEthicsforNurses/Code-of-Ethics-For-Nurses.html

American Psychiatric Association. (2013). *Posttraumatic stress disorder.* Retrieved from http://www.dsm5.org/Documents/PTSD%20Fact%20Sheet.pdf

Anastario, M., Shehab, N., & Lawry, L. (2009). Increased gender-based violence among women internally displaced in Mississippi 2 years post-Hurricane Katrina. *Disaster Medicine and Public Health Preparedness, 3*(1), 18–26. doi: 10.1097/DMP.0b013e3181979c32

Anderson, S. L., McClain, N., & Riviello, R. J. (2006). Genital findings of women after consensual and nonconsensual intercourse. *Journal of Forensic Nursing, 2*(2), 59–65.

Anderson, S. L., Parker, B. J., & Bourguignon, C. M. (2009). Predictors of genital injury after non-consensual intercourse. *Advanced Emergency Nursing Journal, 31*(3), 236–247.

Archambault, J. (2005), May 19. Time limits for conducting a forensic examination: Can biological evidence be recovered 24, 36, 48, 72, 84, or 96 hours following a sexual assault? *SATI e-news* May 19. Retrieved from http://www.mysati.com/enews/May2005/practices_0505.htm

Baker, R. B., Fargo, J. D., Shambley-Ebron, D., & Sommers, M. S. (2010). A source of healthcare disparity: Race, skin color, and injuries after rape among adolescents and young adults. *Journal of Forensic Nursing, 6*(3), 144–150.

Bellis, M. A., Hughes, K., Leckenby, N., Hardcastle, K. A., Perkins, C., & Lowey, H. (2014a). Measuring mortality and the burden of adult disease associated with adverse childhood experiences in England: A national survey. *Journal of Public Health, 1*–10. doi:10.1093/pubmed/fdu065

Bellis, M. A., Hughes, K., Leckenby, N., Jones, L., Baban, A., Kachaeva, M.,...Terzic, N. (2014b). Adverse childhood experiences and associations with health-harming behaviours in young adults: Surveys in eight eastern European countries. *Bulletin of the World Health Organization, 92*(9), 641–655.

Bennett Cattaneo, L., & Goodman, L. A. (2003). Victim-reported risk factors for continued abusive behavior: Assessing the dangerousness of arrested batterers. *Journal of Community Psychology, 31,* 349.

Bicknell-Hentges, L., & Lynch, J. J. (2009). *Everything counselors and supervisors need to know about treating trauma.* Paper based on a presentation at the American Counseling Association Annual Conference and Exposition, Charlotte, NC.

Black, M. C., Basile, K. C., Brieding, M. J., Smith, S. G., Walters, M. L., Merrick, M. T., Chen, J., & Stevens, M. R. (2011). *The national intimate partner and sexual violence survey (NISVS): 2010 summary report.* Atlanta, GA: National Center for Injury Prevention and Control, Centers for Disease Control and Prevention.

Bonomi, A. E., Anderson, M. L., Rivara, F. P., & Thompson, R. S. (2009). Women who suffer abuse use mental health care services more than women who have never been abused. *AHRQ Research Activities, 44*(3), 16.

Bovin, M. J., Jager Hyman, S., Gold, S. D., Marx, B. P., & Sloan, D. M. (2008). Tonic immobility mediates the influence of peritraumatic fear and perceived inescapability on posttraumatic stress symptom severity among sexual assault survivors. *Journal of Traumatic Stress, 21*(4), 402–409.

Bracha, H. S. (2004). Freeze, flight, fight, fright, faint: Adaptationist perspectives on the acute stress response spectrum. *CNS Spectrum, 9*(9), 679–685.

Bryant, R. A. (2011). Acute stress disorder as a predictor of posttraumatic stress disorder: A systematic review. *Journal of Clinical Psychiatry, 72*(2), 233–239.

Bryant, R. A. (2013). An update of acute stress disorder. *PTSD Research Quarterly, 24*(1), 1–6.

Bryant, R. A., Friedman, M. J., Spiegel, D., Ursano, R., & Strain, J. (2010). A review of acute stress disorder in DSM-5. *Depression and Anxiety, 28*(9), 802–817.

Burgess, A. W. (1983). Rape trauma syndrome. *Behavioral Sciences and the Law, 1*(3), 97–113.

Burgess, A. W., & Holmstrom, L. L. (1974). Rape trauma syndrome. *American Journal of Psychiatry, 131*(9), 981–986.

Burgess, A. W., Roberts, A. R., & Regehr, C. (2010). Victim services, legislation and treatment. In A.W. Burgess, C. Regehr, & A. R. Roberts (Eds.), *Victimology: Theories and application* (pp. 67–100). Sudbury, MA: Jones and Bartlett Publishers.

Burri, A., & Maercker, A. (2014). Differences in prevalence rates of PTSD in various European countries explained by war exposure, other trauma and cultural value orientation. *BMC Research Notes, 7*(407), 1–11. Retrieved from http://www.biomedcentral.com/content/pdf/1756-0500-7-407.pdf

Campbell, J, C. (1981). Misogyny and homicide of women. *Advances in Nursing Science, 3,* 67–85.

Campbell, R. (2006). Rape survivors' experiences with the legal and medical systems: Do rape victim advocates make a difference? *Violence Against Women, 12,* 30–45.

Campbell, R. (2012). *The neurobiology of sexual assault* [Webinar]. U.S. Department of Justice. Retrieved from http://nij.gov/multimedia/presenter/presenter-campbell/Pages/welcome.aspx

Campbell, R., Adams, A. E., Wasco, S. M., Ahrens, C. E., & Sefl, T. (2010). "What has it been like for you to talk with me today?" The impact of participating in interview research on rape survivors. *Violence Against Women, 16*(1), 60–83.

Canadian Bar Association. (2012). *Children and consent to medical care.* British Columbia, Canada: Canadian Bar Association. Retrieved from http://www.cba.org/bc/public_media/health/422.aspx

Canadian Centre for Elder Law. (2011). *A practical guide to elder abuse and neglect law in Canada.* Vancouver, Canada: British Columbia Law Institute. Retrieved from http://www.bcli.org/sites/default/files/Practical_Guide_English_Rev_JULY_2011.pdf

Cannon, W. B. (1929). *Bodily changes in pain, hunger, fear and rage.* New York, NY: Appleton.

Carnochan, J., Butchart, A., Feucht, T., Mikton, C., & Shepherd, J. (2010). *Violence prevention: An invitation to intersectoral action.* Geneva, Switzerland: World Health Organization.

Carpenito, L. J. (2013). *Nursing diagnosis: Application to clinical practice* (14th ed.). Philadelphia, PA: Lippincott Williams & Wilkins/Wolters Kluwer.

Carter-Snell, C. J. (2007). *Understanding women's risks for injury from sexual assault.* (Unpublished doctoral dissertation). Edmonton, Canada: University of Alberta.

Carter-Snell, C. J. (2011). Injury documentation: Using the BALD STEP mnemonic and the RCMP sexual assault kit. *Outlook, 34*(1), 15–20.

Carter-Snell, C., & Soltys, K. (2005). Forensic ultraviolet lights in clinical practice: Evidence for the evidence. *Canadian Journal of Police and Security Services, 3*(2), 90–96.

Catalano, S. (2011). *Criminal victimization, 2005.* Washington, DC: U.S. Department of Justice. Retrieved from www.bjs.gov/content/pub/pdf/cv05.pdf

Centers for Disease Control and Prevention (CDC). (2012). *Adverse childhood experiences: Looking at how ACEs affect our lives and society.* Atlanta, GA: CDC. Retrieved from http://vetoviolence.cdc.gov/apps/phl/images/ACE_Accessible.pdf

Centers for Disease Control and Prevention (CDC). (2014). *Intimate partner violence: Consequences.* Atlanta, GA: CDC. Retrieved from http://www.cdc.gov/violenceprevention/intimatepartnerviolence/consequences.html

Charmandari, E., Tsigos, C., & Chrousos, G. (2005). Endocrinology of the stress response. *Annual Review of Physiology, 67*, 259–284.

Cherpitel, C. J., Ye, Y., Bond, J., Borges, G., & Monteiro, M. (2015). Relative risk of injury from acute alcohol consumption: Modeling the dose-response relationship in emergency department data across 18 countries. *Addiction, 110*(2), 279–288.

Christian, C. W. (2011). Timing of the medical examination. *Journal of Child Sexual Abuse, 20*(5), 505–520.

Christiansen, D. M., & Hansen, M. (2015). Accounting for sex differences in PTSD: A multi-variable mediation model. *European Journal of Psychotraumatology, 19*(6), 1–10. Retrieved from http://dx.doi.org/10.3402/ejpt.v6.26068

Classen, C. C., Palesh, O. G., & Aggarwal, R. (2005). Sexual revictimisation: A review of the empirical literature. *Trauma, Violence and Abuse, 6*(2), 103–129.

Cohen, M. (2013). A process of validation of a three-dimensional model of the identification of abuse in older adults. *Archives of Gerontology and Geriatrics, 57*(3), 243–249.

Cohen, R. A., Paul, R. H., Stroud, L., Gunstad, J., Hitsman, B. L., McCaffery, J., . . . Gordon, E. (2006). Early life stress and adult emotional experience: An international perspective. *International Journal of Psychiatry in Medicine, 36*(1), 35–52.

Connor-Smith, J. K., Henning, K., Moore, S., & Holdford, R. (2011). Risk assessments by female victims of intimate partner violence: Predictors of risk perceptions and comparison to actuarial measure. *Journal of Interpersonal Violence, 26*, 2517.

Cooper, C., Selwood, A., & Livingston, G. (2008). The prevalence of elder abuse and neglect: A systematic review. *Age and Ageing, 37*(2), 151–160. doi: 10.1093/ageing/afm194

Coxell, A. W., & King, M. B. (2010). Adult male rape and sexual assault: Prevalence, re-victimisation and the tonic immobility response. *Sexual and Relationship Therapy, 25*(4), 372–379.

Coxell, A. W., King, M. B., Mesey, G. C., & Gordon, D. (1999). Lifetime prevalence, characteristics, and associated problems of non-consensual sex in men: A cross-sectional survey. *British Medical Journal, 318*, 846–850.

Craig, W., & McCuaig, H. (2012). *Bullying and fighting.* Ottawa, Canada: Public Health Agency of Canada. Retrieved from http://www.phac-aspc.gc.ca/hp-ps/dca-dea/publications/hbsc-mental-mentale/bullying-intimidation-eng.php

Curtis, T., Miller, B. C., & Berry, E. H. (2000). Changes in reports and incidence of child abuse following natural disasters. *Child Abuse and Neglect, 24*(9), 1151–1162.

Darnell, C. (2011). *Forensic science and healthcare: Caring for patients, preserving the evidence.* Boca Raton, FL: CRC Press.

Davis, M. C., & Reich, J. W. (2014). *The resilience handbook: Approaches to stress and trauma.* New York, NY: Taylor & Francis.

Department of Justice. (2015). *Aboriginal victimization in Canada: A summary of the literature.* Ottawa, Canada: Government of Canada. Retrieved from http://www.justice.gc.ca/eng/rp-pr/cj-jp/victim/rd3-rr3/p3.html

Dhai, A., & Payne-James, J. (2013). Problems of capacity, consent and confidentiality. *Best Practices and Research: Clinical Obstetrics and Gynaecology, 27*(1), 59–75.

Dries, D. J., & Endorf, F. W. (2013). Inhalation injury: Epidemiology, pathology, treatment strategies. *Scandinavian Journal of Trauma, Resuscitation and Emergency Medicine, 21*, 31–46.

Du Mont, J., Macdonald, S., Rotbard, N., Bainbridge, D., Asilani, E., Smith, N., & Cohen, M. M. (2010). Drug-facilitated sexual assault in Ontario, Canada: Toxicological and DNA findings. *Journal of Forensic and Legal Medicine, 17*(6), 333–338.

Du Mont, J., Macdonald, S., White, M., Turner, L., White, D., Kaplan, S., & Smith, T. (2014). Client satisfaction with nursing-led sexual assault and domestic violence services in Ontario. *Journal of Forensic Nursing, 10*(3), 122–134.

Duffy, J. Y., Hughes, M., Asnes, A. G., & Leventhal, J. M. (2014). Child maltreatment and risk patterns among participants in a child abuse prevention program. *Child Abuse and Neglect, 44*, 184–193. doi: 10.1016/j.chiabu.2014.11.005

Duke, N. N., Pettingell, S. L., McMorris, B. J., & Borowsky, I. W. (2010). Adolescent violence perpetration: Associations with multiple types of adverse childhood experiences. *Pediatrics, 125*(4), e778–e786.

Dunlap, H., Brazeau, P., Stermac, L., & Addison, M. (2004). Acute forensic medical procedures used following a sexual assault among treatment-seeking women. *Women and Health, 40*(2), 53–65.

Duval, J. B. (2011). Electrical, thermal and inhalation injuries. In V. A. Lynch, & J. B. Duval (Eds.), *Forensic nursing science* (2nd ed.). (pp. 331–339). St. Louis, MO: Elsevier/Mosby.

Edwards, K. M., Sylaska, K. M., & Gidycz, C. A. (2014). Women's reactions to participating in dating violence research: A mixed methodological study. *Psychology of Violence, 4*(2), 224–239.

El Sohly, M. A., & Salamone, S. J. (1999). Prevalence of drugs used in cases of alleged sexual assault. *Journal of Analytical Toxicology, 23*(3), 141–146.

Espelage, D. L., Low, S., Rao, M. A., Hong, J. S., & Little, T. D. (2014). Family violence, bullying, fighting and substance use among adolescents: A longitudinal mediational model. *Journal of Research on Adolescence, 24*(2), 337–349.

Eulitt, P. J., Tomberg, R. J., Cunningham, T. D., Counselman, F. L., & Palmer, R. M. (2014). Screening elders in the emergency department at risk for mistreatment: A pilot study. *Journal of Elder Abuse, 26*, 424–435.

Falb, K. L., McCauley, H. L., Decker, M. R., Gupta, J., Raj, A., & Silverman, J. G. (2011). School bullying perpetration and other childhood risk factors as predictors of adult intimate partner violence perpetration. *Archives in Pediatric Adolescent Medicine, 165*(10), 890–894.

Faugno, D., Waszak, D., Strack, G. B., Brooks, M. A., & Gwinn, C. G. (2013). Strangulation forensic examination: Best practice for care providers. *Advanced Emergency Nursing Journal, 35*(4), 314–317.

Federal Bureau of Investigation. (2011). *Crime in the United States, 2011: Murder victims 2007–2011*. Retrieved on March 3, 2015, from http://www.fbi.gov/about-us/cjis/ucr/crime-in-the-u.s/2011/crime-in-the-u.s.-2011/tables/expanded-homicide-data-table-8

Felitti, V., Anda, R., Nordenberg, D., Williamson, D. F., Spitz, A. M., Edwards, V., Koss, M. P., & Marks, J. S. (1998). The relationship of adult health status to childhood abuse and household dysfunction. *American Journal of Preventive Medicine, 14*, 245–258.

Finsterwald, C., & Alberini, C. M. (2014). Stress and glucocorticoid-receptor dependent mechanisms in long term memory: From adaptive responses to psychopathologies. *Neurobiology of Learning and Memory, 112*, 17–29.

Fishman, P. A., Bonomi, A. E., Anderson, M. L., Reid, R. J., & Rivara, F. P. (2010). Changes in health care costs over time following the cessation of intimate partner violence. *Journal of General Internal Medicine, 25*(9), 920–925.

Flaherty, E. G., Perez-Rossello, J. M., Levine, M. A., Hennrikus, D. W. L., American Academy of Pediatrics Committee on Child Abuse and Neglect, Section on Radiology, Section on Endocrinology, and Section on Orthopaedics & Society for Pediatric Radiology. (2014). Evaluating children with fractures for child physical abuse. *Pediatrics, 133*(2), e477–e489.

Foshee, V. A., Reyes, H. L., Ennett, S. T., Suchindran, C., Mathias, J. P., Karriker-Jaffe, K., Bauman, K. E., & Benefield, T. S. (2011). Risk and protective factors distinguishing profiles of adolescent peer and dating violence perpetration. *Journal of Adolescent Health: Official Publication of the Society for Adolescent Medicine, 48*, 344–350.

Fulmer, T., Guadagno, L., Dyer, C. B., & Connolly, M. T. (2004). Progress in elder abuse screening and assessment instruments. *Journal of the American Geriatrics Society, 52*, 297–304.

Gall, J., Goldney, R., & Payne-James, J. J. (2011). Self-inflicted injuries and associated psychological profiles. In J. Gall & J. Payne-James (Eds.), *Current practice in forensic medicine* (p. 262). Oxford, England: John Wiley & Sons.

Gerth, J., Rossegger, A., Urbaniok, F., & Endrass, J. (2014). The Ontario Domestic Assault Risk Assessment (ODARA) - Validated and authorized German translation of an intimate partner violence screening tool. *Fortschritte der Neurologie-Psychiatrie, 82*(11), 616–626.

Gittins, C. B., Paterson, H. M., & Sharpe, L. (2015). How does immediate recall of a stressful event predict psychological response to it? *Journal of Behavior Therapy and Experimental Psychiatry, 46*, 19–26.

Glass, N. A., Laughon, K., Campbell, J., Wolf, A. D., Block, C. R., Hanson, G., Sharps, P. W., & Taliaferro, E. (2008). Non-fatal strangulation is an important risk factor for homicide of women. *Journal of Emergency Medicine, 35*(3), 329–335.

Gorham, L., & Brown, S. L. (2008). SANE peer review: What is it? Do we need it? *Forensic Examiner, 17*(1), 20.

Government of Canada. (2012). *Bullying prevention programs*. Ottawa, Canada: Government of Canada. Retrieved from http://healthycanadians.gc.ca/healthy-living-vie-saine/bullying-intimidation/prevention-eng.php

Griffin, M. G., Resick, P. A., Waldrop, A. E., & Mechanic, M. B. (2003). Participation in trauma research: Is there evidence of harm? *Journal of Traumatic Stress, 16*(3), 221–227.

Hack, J. B., & Hoffman, R. S. (2011). General management of poisoned patients. In D. M. Cline, O. J. Ma, R. K. Cydulka, G. D. Meckler, D. A. Handel, & S. H. Thomas (Eds.), *Tintinalli's emergency medicine: A comprehensive study guide* (7th ed.). New York, NY: McGraw-Hill.

Hall, E., & Ballantyne, J. (2003). Novel Y-STR typing strategies reveal the genetic profile of the semen donor in extended interval post-coital cervicovaginal samples. *Forensic Science International, 136*(1–3), 58–73.

Hamby, S., Finkelhor, D., & Turner, H. (2012). Teen dating violence: Co-occurrence with other victimizations in the National Survey of Children's Exposure to Violence (NatSCEV). *Psychology of Violence, 2*(2), 111–124.

Hanson, R. K., Helmus, L., & Bourgon, G. (2007). *The validity of risk assessments for intimate partner violence: A meta-analysis*. Ontario, Canada: Public Safety Canada. Retrieved from https://www.publicsafety.gc.ca/cnt/rsrcs/pblctns/ntmt-prtnr-vlnce/ntmt-prtnr-vlnce-eng.pdf

Haskell, L. (2003). *First stage trauma treatment: A guide for mental health professionals working with women*. Toronto, Canada: Centre for Addiction and Mental Health.

Humphreys, K. L., Sauder, C. L., Martin, E. K., & Marx, B. P. (2010). Tonic immobility in childhood sexual abuse survivors and its relationship to posttraumatic symptomatology. *Journal of Interpersonal Violence, 25*(2), 358–373.

Hussain, N., Sprague, S., Madden, K., Hussain, F. N., Pindiprolu, B., & Bhandari, M. (2013). A comparison of the types of screening tool administration methods used for the detection of intimate partner violence: A systematic review and meta-analysis. *Trauma, Violence and Abuse, 16*(1), 60–69.

Institute for Patient- and Family-Centered Care. (2010). *Frequently asked questions*. Retrieved from http://www.ipfcc.org/faq.html

International Association of Forensic Nurses (IAFN). (n.d.a). *Forensic nursing in disasters.* Retrieved from http://www.forensicnurses.org/?page=FNinDisasters

International Association of Forensic Nurses (IAFN). (n.d.b). *Frequently asked questions.* Elkridge, MD: IAFN. Retrieved from http://www.forensicnurses.org/?page=FNFAQs

International Council of Nurses (ICN). (2012). *ICN code of ethics for nurses.* Geneva, Switzerland: ICN. Retrieved from http://www.icn.ch/images/stories/documents/about/icncode_english.pdf

Isaacs, E. (2013). The violent patient. In J. G. Adams (Ed.), *Emergency medicine* (2nd ed.) (pp. 1630–1638). Philadelphia, PA: Elsevier.

Jakubec, S., Carter-Snell, C., Ofrim, J., & Skanderup, J. (2013). Identifying rural sexual assault service strengths, concerns, and educational needs in rural and remote communities in Alberta, Canada. *Enfermeria Global, 12*(31), 427–442.

Johnson, H. (2006). *Measuring violence against women.* Ottawa, Canada: Statistics Canada. Retrieved from http://www.statcan.gc.ca/pub/85-002-x/2013001/article/11766-eng.pdf

Joki-Erkkila, M., Tuomisto, S., Seppanen, M., Huhtala, H., Ahola, A., Raino, J., & Karhunen, P. J. (2014). Clinical forensic sample collection techniques following consensual intercourse in volunteers-cervical canal brush compared to conventional swab. *Journal of Forensic and Legal Medicine, 27,* 50–54.

Joubert, L., & Posenelli, S. (2009). Responding to a "window of opportunity": The detection and management of aged abuse in an acute and subacute health care setting. *Social Work in Health Care, 48*(7), 702–714. Retrieved from http://search.ebscohost.com/login.aspx?direct=true&AuthType=ip,url,cookie,uid&db=rzh&AN=2010495493&site=ehost-live

Kapur, N. A., & Windish, D. M. (2011). Optimal methods to screen men and women for intimate partner violence: Results from an internal medicine residency continuity clinic. *Journal of Interpersonal Violence, 26*(12), 2335–2352. doi: 10.1177/0886260510383034

Kelly, D. L., Larkin, H. J., Cosby, C. D., & Paolinetti, L. A. (2013). Derivation of the Genital Injury Severity Scale (GISS): A concise instrument for description and measurement of external female genital injury after sexual intercourse. *Journal of Forensic and Legal Medicine, 20*(6), 724–731.

Kent-Wilkinson, A. (2010). Forensic nursing educational development: An integrated review of the literature. *Journal of Psychiatric and Mental Health Nursing, 18*(3), 236–246.

Kilpatrick, D. G., Resnick, H. S., Milanak, M. E., Miller, M. W., Keyes, K. M., & Friedman, M. J. (2013). National estimates of exposure to traumatic events and PTSD prevalence using DSM-IV and DSM-5 criteria. *Journal of Traumatic Stress, 26,* 537–547.

Kilpatrick, D. G., Ruggiero, K. J., Acierno, R., Saunders, B. E., Resnick, H. S., & Best, C. (2003). Violence and risk of PTSD, major depression, substance abuse/dependence and comorbidity: Results from the National Survey of Adolescents. *Journal of Consulting and Clinical Psychology, 71*(4), 692–700.

Kolbe, A. R., Hutson, R. A., Shannon, H., Trzcincksi, E., Miles, B., Levitz, N., Puccio, M., James, L., . . . Muggah, R. (2010). Mortality, crime and access to basic needs before and after the Haiti earthquake: A random survey of Port-au-Prince households. *Medicine, 26*(4), 281–297.

Krebs, C. P., Lindquist, C. H., Warner, T. D., Fisher, B. S., & Martin, S. L. (2007). *The campus sexual assault study.* Washington, DC: U.S. Department of Justice.

La Bash, H., & Papa, A. (2014). Shame and PTSD symptoms. *Psychological Trauma; Theory, Research, Practice and Policy, 6*(2), 159–166.

Lam, S. W., Engebretsen, K. M., & Bauer, S. R. (2011). Toxicology today: What you need to know now. *Journal of Pharmacy Practice, 24*(2), 174–188.

Larkin, H. J., Cosby, C. C., Kelly, D., & Paolinetti, L. A. (2012). A pilot study to test the differential validity of a genital injury severity scale in development for use in forensic sexual assault examinations. *Journal of Forensic Nursing, 8*(1), 30–38.

Ledray, L. E. (2001). *Evidence collection and care of the sexual assault survivor: The SANE-SART response.* Enola, PA: National Sexual Violence Resource Center. Retrieved from http://www.nsvrc.org/publications/guides/evidence-collection-and-care-sexual-assault-survivor-sane-sart-response

Ledray, L. E. (2008). Consent to photograph: How far should disclosure go? *Journal of Forensic Nursing, 4*(4), 188–189.

Lehrer, J. A., Lehrer, E. L., & Zhao, Z. (2010). Physical dating violence victimization in college women in Chile. *Journal of Women's Health, 19*(5), 893–902.

Lewis-O'Connor, A. (2007). *When push comes to shove: Screening mothers for intimate partner violence during their child's pediatric visit* (Unpublished doctoral dissertation). Boston College, Boston, MA. Retrieved from http://gradworks.umi.com/32/83/3283887.html

Lichenstein, R., & Suggs, A. H. (2007). Child abuse/assault. In J. S. Olshaker, M. C. Jackson, & W. S. Smock (Eds.), *Forensic emergency medicine* (2nd ed.) (pp 157–173). Philadelphia, PA: Lippincott, Williams & Wilkins.

Linden, J. A., Lewis-O'Connor, A., & Jackson, M. C. (2007). Forensic examination of adult victims and perpetrators. In J. S. Olshaker, M. C. Jackson, & W. S. Smock (Eds.), *Forensic emergency medicine* (2nd ed.) (pp. 85–125). Philadelphia, PA: Lippincott, Williams & Wilkins.

Lloyd, J. (2014). Violent and tragic events: The nature of domestic violence related homicide cases in central Australia. *Australian Aboriginal Studies, 2014*(1), 99–110.

Lonsway, K. A., & Archambault, J. (2013). *Effective victim advocacy in the criminal justice system.* Addy, WA: End Violence Against Women International. Retrieved from http://www.evawintl.org/Library/DocumentLibraryHandler.ashx?id=32

Lynch, V. A. (2011a). Evolution of forensic nursing science. In V. A. Lynch, & J. B. Duval (Eds.), *Forensic nursing science* (2nd ed.; pp. 1–9). St. Louis, MO: Elsevier/Mosby.

Lynch, V. A. (2011b). Global expansion and future perspectives. In V. A. Lynch, & J. B. Duval (Eds.), *Forensic nursing science* (2nd ed.; pp. 617–629). St. Louis, MO: Elsevier/Mosby.

Lynch, V. A. (2014). Enrichment of theory through critique, restructuring, and application. *Journal of Forensic Nursing, 10*(3), 120–121.

Lynch, V. A., & Duval, J. B. (2006). *Forensic nursing.* St. Louis, MO: Elsevier/Mosby.

Macdonald, S. & Norris, P. (2007). *Guidelines for the collection of forensic evidence from the person who is unable to provide consent.* Toronto, Canada: Ontario Network of Sexual Assault & Domestic Violence Treatment Centres (SA/DVTC). Retrieved from http://www.satcontario.com/files/Guidelines_for_Collection___unable_to_consent.pdf

Maguire, S. A., Upadhyaya, M., Evans, A., Mann, M. K., Haroon, M. M., Tempest, V., Lumb, R. C., & Kemp, A. M. (2013). A systematic review of abusive visceral injuries in childhood: Their range and recognition. *Child Abuse and Neglect, 37*(7), 430–435.

Maguire, S. A., Watts, P. O., Shaw. A. D., Holden, S., Taylor, R. H., Watkins, W. J., Mann, W. K., Tempest, V., & Kemp, A. M. (2013). Retinal hemorrhages and related findings in abusive and non-abusive head trauma: A systematic review. *Eye, 27*(1), 28–36.

Maier, S. L. (2008). "I have heard horrible stories." Rape victim advocates' perceptions of the revictimization of rape victims by the police and medical system. *Violence Against Women, 14*(7), 786–808.

Malouf, N. E., Jackson, B. F., & Borg, K. (2013). Self-harm and danger to others. In J. G. Adams (Ed.), *Emergency medicine* (2nd ed.; pp. 1639–1643). Philadelphia, PA: Elsevier.

Martsolf, D. S., & Draucker, C. B. (2008). The legacy of childhood sexual abuse and family adversity. *Journal of Nursing Scholarship, 40*(4), 333–340. Retrieved from http://search.ebscohost.com/login.aspx?direct=true&AuthType=ip,url,cookie,uid&db=rzh&AN=2010143911&site=ehost-live

Mayntz-Press, K. A., Sims, I. M., Hall, A., & Ballantyne, J. (2008). Y-STR profiling in extended interval (> or = 3 days) postcoital cervicovaginal samples. *Journal of Forensic Science, 53*(2), 342–348.

McClennan, S., Worster, A., & MacMillan, H. (2008). Caring for victims of intimate partner violence: A survey of Canadian emergency departments. *Canadian Journal of Emergency Medicine, 10*(4), 325–328.

McCusker, J., Bellevance, F., Cardin, S., Trepanier, S., Verdon, J., & Ardman, O. (1999). Detection of older people at risk of adverse health outcomes after an emergency visit: The ISAR screening tool. *Journal of the American Geriatrics Society, 47*(10), 1229–1237.

McLaughlin, K. A., Koenen, K. C., Hill, E. D., Petukhova, M., Sampson, N. A., Zaslavsky, A. M., & Kessler, R. C. (2013). Trauma exposure and posttraumatic stress disorder in a national sample of adolescents. *Child and Adolescent Psychiatry, 52*(8), 815–830.

McWhinney-Delaney, L. (2006). *The development and psychometric testing of the Risk for Abuse Assessment Scale and the Abuse Assessment Tool for use in Jamaican women* (Unpublished doctoral dissertation). Atlanta, GA: Emory University.

MedArt. (2008). *Langer's lines.* Retrieved from http://www.med-ars.it/galleries/langer.htm

Meinbresse, M., Brinkley-Rubinstein, L., Grassette, A., Benson, J., Hall, C., Hamilton, R., Malott, M., & Henkins, D. (2014). Exploring the experiences of violence among individuals who are homeless using a consumer-led approach. *Violence and Victims, 29*(1), 122–136.

Messing, J. T., Amanor-Boadu, Y., Cavanaugh, C. E., Glass, N. E., & Campbell, J. C. (2013). Culturally competent intimate partner violence risk assessment: Adapting the Danger Assessment for immigrant women. *Social Work Research, 37*(3), 263–275.

Messman-Moore, T. L., Ward, R. M., & Brown, A. L. (2009). Substance use and PTSD symptoms impact the likelihood of rape and revictimization in college women. *Journal of Interpersonal Violence, 24*(3), 499–521.

Millar, G., Stermac, L., & Addison, M. (2002). Immediate and delayed treatment seeking among adult sexual assault. *Women and Health, 35*(1), 53–64.

Mitchell, A. M., Kane, I., Havill, A., & Cassesse, C. (2013). Self-directed violence and the forensic nurse. In R. Constantino, P. A. Crane & S. E. Young (Eds.), *Forensic nursing: Evidence-based principles and practice* (pp. 176–194). Philadelphia, PA: F.A. Davis.

Mok, J. Y. (2008). Non-accidental injury in children: An update. *Injury, 39*(9), 978–985.

Moor, A., Ben-Meir, A., Golan-Shapira, D., & Farchi, M. (2013). Rape: A trauma of paralyzing dehumanization. *Journal of Aggression, Maltreatment and Trauma, 22*(10), 1051–1069.

Morgan, J. A. (2008). Comparison of cervical os versus vaginal evidentiary findings during sexual assault exam. *Journal of Emergency Nursing, 34*(2), 102–105.

Moscardino, U., Scrimin, S., Capello, F., & Altoe, G. (2014). Brief report: Self-blame and PTSD symptoms in adolescents exposed to terrorism: Is school connectedness a mediator? *Journal of Adolescence, 37*(1), 47–52.

Nash, K. R., & Sheridan, D. J. (2009). Can one accurately date a bruise? State of the science. *Journal of Forensic Nursing, 5*(1), 31–37.

National Sexual Violence Resource Center. (2015). *SART history.* Retrieved from http://www.nsvrc.org/projects/sart-history

NCAI Policy Research Center. (2013). *Policy insights brief: Statistics on violence against Native Women.* Retrieved from http://www.ncai.org/attachments/PolicyPaper_tWAjznFslemhAffZgNGzHUqIWMRPkCDjpFtxeKEUVKjubxfp-GYK_Policy%20Insights%20Brief_VAWA_020613.pdf

Neale, A. V., Hwalek, M. A., Scott, R. O., Sengstock, M. C., & Stahl, C. (1991). Validation of the Hwalek-Sengstock elder abuse screening test. *Journal of Applied Gerontology, 10*(4), 406–418.

Nelson, H. D., Bougatsos, C., & Blazina, I. (2012). Screening women for intimate partner violence: A systematic review to update the U.S. preventive services task force recommendation. *Annals of Internal Medicine, 156*(11), 796–808. Retrieved from http://search.ebscohost.com/login.aspx?direct=true&AuthType=ip,url,cookie,uid&db=a9h&AN=76450242&site=ehost-live

Norris, F. H., & Slone, L. B. (2013). Understanding research on the epidemiology of trauma and PTSD. *PTSD Research Quarterly, 24*(2–3), 1–5.

Office for Victims of Crime. (2011). *Learn about SARTs: How did SARTs evolve?* Retrieved from http://ovc.ncjrs.gov/sartkit/about/about-evolve-print.html#hs

Olson, K. L., Marc, D. T., Grude, L. A., McManus, C. J., & Kellerman, G. H. (2011). The hypothalamic-pituitary-adrenal axis: The actions of the central nervous system and potential biomarkers. *Anti-aging therapeutics, XIII* (pp. 91–100). Chicago, IL: American Academy of Anti-Aging Medicine.

Ozbay, F., Johnson, D. C., Dimoulas, E., Morgan, C. A., Charney, D., & Southwick, S. (2007). Social support and resilience to stress: From resiliency to clinical practice. *Psychiatry, 4*(5), 35–40.

Ozer, E. J., Best, S. R., Lipsey, T. L., & Weiss, D. S. (2003). Predictors of posttraumatic stress disorder and symptoms in adults: A meta-analysis. *Psychological Bulletin, 129*(1), 52–73.

Pasqualone, G. (2011). Forensic photography. In V. A. Lynch & J. B. Duval (Eds.), *Forensic nursing science* (2nd ed.) (pp. 61–79). St. Louis, MO: Elsevier/Mosby.

Pitman, R. K., Shin, L. M., & Rauch, S. L. (2001). Investigating the pathogenesis of posttraumatic stress disorder with neuroimaging. *Journal of Clinical Psychiatry, 62*(Suppl 17), 47–54.

Pittaway, E., Bartolomei, L., & Rees, S. (2007). Gendered dimensions of the 2005 tsunami and a potential social work response in post-disaster situations. *International Social Work, 50,* 307–319.

Primeau, A., & Sheridan, D. J. (2013). Evidence: Forensic nursing in the emergency and acute care departments. In R. Constantino, P. A. Crane, & S. E. Young (Eds.), *Forensic nursing: Evidence-based principles and practice* (pp. 308–325). Philadelphia, PA: F.A. Davis.

Raposo, S. M., Mackenzie, C. S., Henriksen, C. A., & Afifi, T. O. (2014). Time does not heal all wounds: Older adults who experienced childhood adversities have higher odds of mood, anxiety and personality disorders. *American Journal of Geriatric Psychiatry, 22*(11), 1241–1250.

Reis, M. (2000). The IOA screen: An abuse-alert measure that dispels myths. *Generations, 24*(2), 13–16.

Reis, M., & Nahmiash, D. (1995). When seniors are abused: An intervention model. *Gerontologist, 35*(5), 666–671.

Renke, W. (2005). The constitutionality of mandatory reporting of gunshot wounds legislation. *Health Law Review, 14*(1), 3–8.

Riley, W., Moran, J., Corso, L., Beitsch, L., & Bialek, R., (2010). Defining quality improvement in public health. *Journal of Public Health Management and Practice, 16*(1), 5–7.

Roach, J. P., Acker, S. N., Bensard, D. D., Sirotnak, A. P., Karrer, F. M., & Partrick, D. A. (2014). Head injury patterns in children can help differentiate accidental from non-accidental trauma. *Pediatric Surgery International, 30*(11), 1103–1106.

Roberts, A. R., & Ottens, A. J. (2005). The seven-stage crisis intervention model: A road map to goal attainment, problemsolving, and crisis resolution. *Brief Treatment and Crisis Intervention, 5*(4), 329–339.

Rodriguez, M. A., Wallace, S. P., Woolf, N. H., & Mangione, C. M. (2006). Mandatory reporting of elder abuse: Between a rock and a hard place. *Annals of Family Medicine, 4*(5), 403–409.

Royal Canadian Mounted Police (RCMP) Laboratory. (2014). *Health care practitioner's guide: For use with the RCMP sexual assault evidence kit* (SAEK-Biology). Ottawa, Canada: RCMP.

Rutty, J. E. (2006). Does England need a new genesis of forensic nursing? *Forensic Science, Medicine and Pathology, 2*(3), 149–155.

Sachs, C. J., Benson, A., Schriger, D. L., & Wheeler, M. (2011). Reliability of female genital injury detection after sexual assault. *Journal of Forensic Nursing, 7*(4), 190–194.

SafeStar. (2014). *SafeStar: Sexual assault forensic examinations, support, training, access and resources.* Retrieved from http://www.safestar.net/faq.html

Saukko, P., & Knight, B. (2009). *Knight's forensic pathology* (3rd ed.). London, England: Hodder Arnold.

Scafide, K. R., Sheridan, D. J., Campbell, J., Deleon, V. B., & Hayat, M. J. (2013). Evaluating change in bruise colorimetry and the effect of subject characteristics over time. *Forensic Science, Medicine, and Pathology, 9*(3), 367–376. doi: 10.1007/s12024-013-9452-4

Schwabe, L., & Wolf, O. T. (2014). Timing matters: Temporal dynamics of stress effects on memory retrieval. *Cognitive, Affective and Behavioral Neuroscience, 14*(3), 1041–1048.

Scott, J. C., Matt, G. E., Wrocklage, K. M., Crnich, C., Jordan, J., Southwick, S. M., Krystal, J. H., & Schweinsburg, B. C. (2014). A quantitative meta-analysis of neurocognitive functioning in posttraumatic stress disorder. *Psychological Bulletin.* Advance online publication. http://dx.doi.org/10.1037/a0038039

Selye, H. (1976). Forty years of stress research: Principal remaining problems and misconceptions. *Canadian Medical Association Journal, 115*(1), 53–56.

Sheridan, D. J. (2007). Treating survivors of intimate partner abuse: Forensic identification and documentation. In J. S. Olshaker, M. C. Jackson, & W. S. Smock (Eds.), *Forensic emergency medicine* (2nd ed.) (pp. 202–222). Philadelphia, PA: Lippincott, Williams & Wilkins.

Silverman, E. M., & Silverman, A. G. (1978). Persistence of spermatozoa in the lower genital tracts of women. *Journal of the American Medical Association, 240*(17), 1875–1877.

Silverman, J., Raj, A., Mucci, L., & Hathaway, J. (2001). Dating violence against adolescent girls, associated substance use, unhealthy weight control, sexual risk behavior, pregnancy, and suicidality. *Journal of the American Medical Association, 286,* 572–579.

Sinha, M. (2012). *Family violence in Canada: A statistical profile, 2010* (No. 85–002-X). Ottawa, Canada: Statistics Canada.

Sinha, M. (2013). *Measuring violence against women: A statistical profile* (No. 85-002-X). Ottawa, Canada: Statistics Canada. Retrieved from http://www.statcan.gc.ca/pub/85-002-x/2013001/article/11766-eng.pdf.

Slatore, C. G., Hansen, L., Ganzini, L., Press, N., Osborne, M. L., Chesnutt, M. S., & Mularski, R. A. (2012). Communication by nurses in the intensive care unit: Qualitative analysis of domains of patient-centered care. *American Journal of Critical Care, 21*(6), 410–481.

Sledjeski, E. M., Speisman, B., & Dierker, L. C. (2008). Does number of lifetime traumas explain the relationship between PTSD and chronic medical conditions? Answers from the National Comorbidity Survey-Replication (NCS-R). *Journal of Behavioral Medicine, 31*(4), 341–349.

Smock, W. S. (2007). Penetrating trauma. In J. S. Olshaker, M. C. Jackson, & W. S. Smock (Eds.), *Forensic emergency medicine* (2nd ed.) (pp. 53–71). Philadelphia, PA: Lippincott, Williams & Wilkins.

Smock, W., & Besant-Matthews, P. (2007). Forensic photography in the emergency department. In J. S. Olshaker, M. C. Jackson, & W. S. Smock (Eds.), *Forensic emergency medicine* (2nd ed.) (pp. 268–291). Philadelphia, PA: Lippincott, Williams & Wilkins.

Snell, D., McCracken, L., & Lind, C. (2012). Should nurses assess for domestic violence. *Alberta Association of Registered Nurses, 68*(2), 14–15.

Soler, L., Kirchner, T., Paretilla, C., & Forns, M. (2013). Impact of poly-victimization on mental health: The mediator and/or moderator role of self-esteem. *Journal of Interpersonal Violence, 28*(13), 2695–2712.

Sommers, M. S., Brunner, L. S., Brown, K. M., Buschur, C., Fargo, J. D., Fisher, B. S., Hinkle, C., & Zink, T. M. (2012). Injuries from intimate partner and sexual violence: Significance and classification systems. *Journal of Forensic and Legal Medicine, 19*(5), 250–263.

Sonik, A., Stein-Wexler, R., Rogers, K. K., Coulter, K. P., & Wootton-Gorges, S. L. (2010). Follow-up skeletal surveys for suspected non-accidental trauma: Can a more limited survey be performed without compromising diagnostic information? *Child Abuse and Neglect, 34*(10), 804–806.

Srabstein, J. C., & Leventhal, B. L. (2010). Prevention of bullying-related morbidity and mortality: A call for public health policies. *Bulletin of the World Health Organization, 88,* 403–403. Retrieved from http://www.who.int/bulletin/volumes/88/6/10-077123/en/

Stark, S. (2012). Elder abuse: Screening, intervention and prevention. *Nursing, 42*(10), 24–25. Retrieved from http://dx.doi.org/10.1097/01.NURSE.0000419426.05524.45

Stoltenborgh, M., Bakermans-Kranenburg, M. J., & van Ijzendoom, M. H. (2012). The universality of childhood emotional abuse: A meta-analysis of worldwide prevalence. *Journal of Aggression, Maltreatment and Trauma, 21*(8), 870–890.

Stoltenborgh, M., Bakermans-Kranenburg, M. J., van Ijzendoom, M. H., & Alink, L. R. (2013). Cultural-geographical differences in the occurrence of child physical abuse? A meta-analysis of global prevalence. *International Journal of Psychology, 48*(2), 81–94.

Stoltenborgh, M., van Ijzendoom, M. H., Euser, E. M., & Bakermans-Kranenburg, M. J. (2011). A global perspective on child sexual abuse: Meta-analysis of prevalence around the world. *Child Maltreatment, 16*(2), 79–101.

Straus, M. A. (2004). Prevalence of violence against dating partners by male and female university students worldwide. *Violence Against Women, 10*(7), 790–811.

Strauss, S., & Haynes, R. B. (2009). Managing evidence-based knowledge: The need for reliable, relevant and readable resources. *Canadian Medical Association Journal, 180*(9), 942–945.

Substance and Mental Health Services Administration (SAMHSA). (2011). *Trauma-informed approach and trauma-specific interventions.* Retrieved from http://www.samhsa.gov/traumajustice/traumadefinition/index.aspx

Sweet, D., Lorente, M., Lorente, J. A., Valenzuela, A., & Villanueva, E. (1997). An improved method to recover saliva from human skin: The double swab technique. *Journal of Forensic Science, 42*(2), 320–322.

Thackeray, J. D., Hornor, G., Benzinger, E. A., & Scribano, P. V. (2011). Forensic evidence collection and DNA identification in acute child sexual assault. *Pediatrics, 128*(2), 227–232.

Tiller, J., & Baker, L. (2014). *The neurobiology of sexual assault.* Learning Network Brief (14). London, Ontario: Learning Network, Centre for Research and Education on Violence Against Women and Children. Retrieved March 3,

2015, from http://www.vawlearningnetwork.ca/sites/learningtoendabuse.ca.vawlearningnetwork/files/L_B_14. pdf

TIP Project Team. (2013). *Trauma-informed practice guide.* British Columbia, Canada: Provincial Mental Health and Substance Abuse Planning Council. Retrieved from http://bccewh.bc.ca/wp-content/uploads/2012/05/2013_TIP-Guide.pdf

Touza, C., Prado, C., & Segura, M. P. (2012). Detection scales for the risk of domestic abuse and self-negligent behavior in elderly persons. *Journal of Elder Abuse & Neglect, 24*(4), 312–325. Retrieved from http://dx.doi.org/10.1080/08946566.2012.661682

Trickett, P. K., Noll, J. G., & Putnam, F. W. (2011). The impact of sexual abuse on female development: Lessons from a multigenerational, longitudinal research study. *Development and Psychopathology, 23*(2), 453–476.

Truman, J. L., & Langton, L. (2014). *Criminal victimization, 2013* (revised). Washington, DC: U.S. Department of Justice. Retrieved from http://www.bjs.gov/index.cfm?ty=pbdetail&iid=5111

U.S. Department of Defense. (2004). *Task force report on care for victims of sexual assault.* Retrieved from http://www.defense.gov/News/May2004/d20040513SATFReport.pdf

U.S. Department of Justice (DOJ). (2013). *A national protocol for sexual assault medical forensic examinations adults/adolescents* (2nd ed.). Washington, DC: DOJ. Retrieved from https://www.ncjrs.gov/pdffiles1/ovw/241903.pdf

U.S. Department of Justice (DOJ). (2014). *Recognizing when a child's injury or illness is caused by abuse.* Washington, DC: DOJ. Retrieved from http://ojjdp.gov/pubs/243908.pdf

U.S. Preventive Services Task Force. (2013). *Intimate partner violence and abuse of elderly and vulnerable adults: Screening.* Retrieved March 3, 2015, from http://www.uspreventiveservicestaskforce.org/uspstf12/ipvelder/ipvelderfinalrs.htm

Ullman, S. E., & Peter-Hagene, L. (2014). Social reactions to sexual assault disclosure, coping, perceived control and PTSD symptoms in sexual assault victims. *Journal of Community Psychology, 42*(4), 495–508.

United Nations (UN). (2011). *Guidelines for the forensic analysis of drugs facilitating sexual assault and other criminal acts.* Vienna, Austria: UN Office on Drugs and Crime Laboratory and Scientific Section.

Uvnas-Moberg, K., Arn, I., & Magnusson, D. (2005). The psychobiology of emotion: The role of the oxytocinergic system. *International Journal of Behavioral Medicine, 12*(2), 59–65.

Valentine, J. L. (2014). Why we do what we do: A theoretical evaluation of the integrated practice model for forensic nursing science. *Journal of Forensic Nursing, 10*(3), 113–119.

Van Stegeren, A. H. (2009). Imaging stress effects on memory: A review of neuroimaging studies. *Canadian Journal of Psychiatry, 54*(1), 16–27.

Vertamatti, M. A., deAbreu, L. C., Otsuka, F. C., Costa, P. R., Ferreira, J. D., Tavares, C., Santos, M. E., & Barbosa, C. P. (2012). Factors associated to time of arrival at the health service after sexual violence. *Health Medicine, 6*(1), 37–41.

Walker, L. E. (1984). *The battered woman syndrome.* New York, NY: Springer.

Walker, L. E. (2006). Battered woman syndrome. *Annals of the New York Academy of Sciences, 1087*(1), 142–157.

Walsh, C. A., & Yon, Y. (2012). Developing an empirical profile for elder abuse research in Canada. *Journal of Elder Abuse and Neglect, 24*(2), 104–119.

Wangmo, T., Teaster, P. B, Grace, J., Wong, W., Mendiondo, M. S., Blandford, C., Fisher, S., & Fardo, D. W. (2014). An ecological systems examination of elder abuse: A week in the life of adult protective services. *Journal of Elder Abuse and Neglect, 26*(5), 440–457.

Weisz, A., Tolman, R., & Saunders, D. G. (2000). Assessing the risk of severe domestic violence. *Journal of Interpersonal Violence, 15*(1), 75–90.

Wells, L., Emery, J. C., & Boodt, C. (2012). Preventing domestic violence in Alberta: A cost savings perspective. School of Public Policy, University of Calgary. *SPP Research Papers, 5*(17). Retrieved March 5, 2015, from http://papers.ssrn.com/sol3/papers.cfm?abstract_id = 2088960

West, H. (2006). *After the crisis initiative: Healing from trauma after disasters.* Retrieved from http://gainscenter.samhsa.gov/atc/text/papers/victims_paper.htm

White, C. (2013). Genital injuries in adults. *Best Practices and Research: Clinical Obstetrics and Gynaecology, 27*(1), 113–130.

Wibbenmeyer, L., Liao, J., Heard, J., Kealey, L., Kealey, G., & Oral, R. (2014). Factors related to child maltreatment in children presenting with burn injuries. *Journal of Burn Care and Research, 35*(5), 374–381.

Wilkins, N., Tsao, B., Hertz, M., Davis, R., & Klevens, J. (2014). *Connecting the dots: An overview of the links among multiple forms of violence.* Atlanta, GA: National Center for Injury Prevention and Control, Centers for Disease Control and Prevention.

Williams, J., & Williams, D. (2013). Disaster forensic nursing. In R. Constantino, P. A. Crane, & S. E. Young (Eds.), *Forensic nursing: Evidence-based principles and practice* (pp. 391–416). Philadelphia, PA: F.A. Davis.

Williams, S., Panacek, E., Green, W., Kanthaswamy, S., Hopkins, C., & Calloway, C. (2014). Recovery of salivary DNA from the skin after showering. *Forensic Science, Medicine and Pathology, 4*, 1–6. doi:10.1007/s12024-014-9635-7

Wolitzky-Taylor, K. B., Ruggiero, K. J., Danielson, C. K., Resnick, H. S., Hanson, R. F., Smith, D. W., Saunders, B. E., & Kilpatrick, D. G. (2008). Prevalence and correlates of dating violence in a national sample of adolescents. *Journal of the American Academy of Child and Adolescent Psychiatry, 47*(7), 755–762.

Wong, C. F., Clark, L. F., & Marlotte, L. (2014). The impact of specific and complex trauma on the mental health of homeless youth. *Journal of Interpersonal Violence.* Electronic publication.

World Health Organization (WHO). (2005). *WHO multi-country study on women's health and domestic violence against women: Summary report of initial results on prevalence, health outcomes and women's responses.* Geneva, Switzerland: WHO.

World Health Organization (WHO). (2009). *Violence prevention: The evidence. Preventing violence by reducing the availability and harmful use of alcohol.* Geneva, Switzerland: WHO.

World Health Organization (WHO). (2011). *Psychological first aid: Guide for field workers.* Retrieved from http://www.who.int/mental_health/publications/guide_field_workers/en/

World Health Organization (WHO). (2013). Guidelines for the management of conditions specifically related to stress. Geneva, Switzerland: WHO.

World Health Organization (WHO). (2014a). *Global status report on violence prevention.* Retrieved from www.who.int/violence_injury_prevention/violence/status_report/2014

World Health Organization (WHO). (2014b). *Violence against adults and children with disabilities.* Geneva, Switzerland: WHO.

Xu, P. (2012). Using teach-back for patient education and self-management. *American Nurse Today, 7*(3). E-publication. Retrieved from http://www.americannursetoday.com/using-teach-back-for-patient-education-and-self-management/

Zink, T., Fargo, J. D., Baker, R. B., Bushur, C., Fisher, B. S., & Sommers, M. S. (2010). Comparison of methods for identifying ano-genital injury after consensual intercourse. *Journal of Emergency Medicine, 39*(1), 113–118.

CHAPTER 3

Forensic Nursing and the Deceased

Pamela D. Tabor
Bobbi Jo O'Neal

OBJECTIVES

At the completion of this chapter, the learner will be able to:

- Synthesize the history and theory of death investigation.
- Comprehend the intersecting systems and services involved in death investigation.
- Apply current practice and prevention standards to death investigations.
- Characterize populations at risk.
- Analyze the concepts and issues associated with death investigation.
- Recognize future issues regarding death investigation.

KEY TERMS

Algor mortis: Latin – algor, "coldness"; mortis, "of death."

Asphyxia: Greek – α, "without" and sphyxis "heartbeat" as a result of a lack of oxygen or excess carbon dioxide.

Autopsy: Greek – meaning "seeing with one's own eyes"; the prefix "auto" refers to an organism that is self-sustaining and "opsy" refers to a medical examination.

Cause of death (COD): The official determination of the disease or injury and the sequence of events responsible for the occurrence that leads to an individual's death; the internal or external factors that set in motion the event(s) that caused the death.

Death: The cessation of all biological functions; determined when a person has irreversible cessation of all brain functions, including the brainstem. The determination of death needs to be made via accepted medical practice.

Livor mortis: Latin – livor, "bluish color"; mortis, "of death."

Manner of death (MOD): The description used to classify the conditions that caused a death and the circumstances by which they occur; explains how the cause of death arose through determining factors that set the cause of death into motion. Manner of death is classified by one of the following five categories: natural, accident, suicide, homicide, and undetermined.

Mechanism of death: Refers to the changes in physiology and biochemistry resulting in death, or the agent used to cause death.

Mortality rate: Usually expressed per 100,000 or 10,000 of a given population, except for infants, which are expressed per 1,000 live births.

Necropsy: Greek – "Looking at the dead"; this term in the strictest sense refers to autopsies performed on nonhuman animals.

Pallor mortis: Latin – pallor, "paleness"; mortis, "of death."

Postmortem rise: Used to help determine the time of death by analyzing the vitreous humor for a rise of potassium and fall in sodium concentration.

Putrefaction: Final stage of death; decomposition is caused by bacterial enzymes.

Rigor mortis: Latin – rigor, "stiffness"; mortis, "of death."

Statutory authority: A set of laws enforcing legislation on behalf of the state/province. In the United States, individual statutes dictate whether a coroner or medical examiner has jurisdiction over a death scene investigation (DSI), their roles and responsibilities, and who may determine cause and manner of death (MOD). In other countries, the jurisdiction is exercised within the geographic area and/or legal system that has authority (Bader & Gabriel, 2010; Bailey, 2014; Elrouby, 2013; Hanzlick, 2007; Hammer, Moynihan, & Pagliaro, 2013; National Institute of Justice, 2009; Venes & Taber, 2013).

HISTORY AND THEORY

In the eighteenth century, it was observed that bodily changes occurred after death. The sequential categories of mortis were identified: pallor, algor, rigor, and livor (Hanzlick, 1997). Historically, death investigation in the United States (US) (and other countries that were once under English law) began with the English system of "Crowner" (National Research Council of the National Academy of Sciences, 2009). This system, introduced to the American Colonies by English settlers, was first established as a legal investigative function to ensure the Crown received its decreed share of proceeds from the estates of the deceased. The name was changed to "Coroner" and the investigation into the causes of death (COD) and manner of death (MOD) evolved as the office's primary function (National Research Council of the National Academy of Sciences, 2009).

In colonial America, not all autopsies were performed to determine COD some were conducted out of curiosity. Examples include those to determine whether conjoined twins had one or two souls, or if death occurred as a result of witchcraft (Iserson, 2003).

The Model Post-Mortem Examination Act (1954) recommended that a forensic examination be completed for all deaths that were:

- violent;
- sudden or unexpected;
- suspicious;
- employment-related;
- where the body was to be cremated, dissected, buried at sea, or unavailable for later examination;
- of prisoners or psychiatric inmates; or
- a threat to public health (Iserson, 2003).

In the mid-nineteenth century, US citizens demanded more scientific approaches to death investigation. For instance, Maryland legislated that coroners could require a physician to assist in inquests (American Bar Association, Office for Victims of Crime, 2005; Bader & Gabriel, 2010; Hanzlick, 1997; National Research Council of the National Academy of Sciences, 2009). In 1877, Massachusetts became the first state to initiate the medical examiner system using medical doctors to replace coroners (Iserson, 2003).

In the 21st century across the US, a fragmented system of coroners and medical examiners exists with variance between states and jurisdictions. Other examples of jurisdiction include Canada, which is dictated by provincial or territorial governments; Wales and the United Kingdom are under the jurisdiction of the Ministry of Justice.

Despite the locale, the jurisdictional authority tends to dictate:

- who has jurisdiction over death scene investigations (DSIs);
- roles and responsibilities of coroners and medical examiners;
- who may determine COD and MOD; and
- who may complete a death certificate (National Institute of Justice, 2009).

Medical Examiner System

This system is usually administered under the direction of a "medical examiner" who:

- typically is an appointed official;
- usually is a physician; and
- has additional training in pathology or forensic pathology (O'Hear, 2013).

Coroner System

- Usually administered by an elected or appointed official, referred to as the "coroner."
- The requirements to hold office vary from state to state, and may or may not include medical training.

Mixed or Medical Examiner/Coroner (ME/C) Systems

Some states and countries operate under a mixed system of coroners, Justices of the Peace, and medical examiners. The make-up and administration of these systems vary from state to state, jurisdiction to jurisdiction, and country to country and may:

- use county, state, command, or regionalized area medical examiners and/or coroners, or have a decentralized state or territorial system; or
- have coroners who perform DSIs and determine the COD and MOD; and
- have MEs who perform autopsies (e.g., homicides, suspicious circumstances, undetermined deaths) and have authority for the final determination of the COD and the MOD (National Research Council of the National Academy of Sciences, 2009). Table 3.1 provides a chronological sequence of events related to medicolegal death investigations.

Theories

- Nurses have a solid knowledge base for application to forensics with mastery of core concepts such as:
  - anatomy and physiology;
  - physical assessment and examination;
  - obtaining indepth health, psychosocial, and family histories;
  - evaluation of trauma;
  - holistic care of patients and families; and
  - experience working and communicating with multiple disciplines (Occupational Safety and Health Administration, 2015).
- Forensic nurses work with multiple disciplines; therefore, multiple theories apply:
  - descriptive theory;
  - prescriptive theory;
  - practice theory;
  - role theory (health care and law); and
  - Integrated Practice Model for Forensic Nursing Science (Lynch & Duval, 2011).

Additional theories from nursing, forensic science, and criminal justice can be drawn upon as well.

TABLE 3.1 Timeline of Changes Associated with Death and DSI

18th Century	Stages of mortis recognized
Colonial America	Crowner $\Rightarrow$ Coroner
	Autopsies on conjoined twins and suspects/victims of witchcraft
Mid-19th Century	Increased demands for more scientific approaches to death investigation
1863	National Academy of Sciences
1874	First case of child abuse prosecuted under the American Society for the Protection of Cruelty to Animals $\Rightarrow$
	New York Society for the Prevention of Cruelty to Children
1877	Massachusetts became the first medical examiner state
1915	National Association of Medical Examiners
1943	National Association of Coroners and Medical Examiners
1949	American Academy of Forensic Sciences
1954	Model Post-Mortem Examination Act
1974	Canada hires nurses to perform death investigations
1978	Individual child death review teams begin
1984	National Organ Transplantation Act
1988	National Aging Resource Center $\Rightarrow$
	Renamed National Center on Elder Abuse (1992)
1990	National Fetal and Infant Mortality Review
1992	International Association of Forensic Nurses
1998	Sudden Unexplained Infant Death Investigation
1999	*Death Investigation for the Scene Investigator*
	by National Institute of Justice
2002	National Center for Child Death Review $\Rightarrow$
	Renamed National Center for the Review and Prevention of Child Deaths (2011)
2005	American Board of MDIs
2009	*Forensic Nurse Death Investigator Guidelines* by International Association of Forensic Nurses
2011	Scientific Working Group for MDIs
2009	National Academy of Forensic Science Report

(Bader & Gabriel, 2010; Hanzlick, 1997; National Institute of Justice, 2009; O'Hear, 2013; International Association of Forensic Nurses, 2014; Iserson, 2003)

INTERSECTING SYSTEMS AND SERVICES

Under the holistic umbrella of public health, the medicolegal death investigation involves multiple systems and agencies that interact during such investigations. It is imperative that the intersecting disciplines follow local, state, and federal jurisdictional statutes and guidelines, as well as approved and recognized national standards of practice.

During a death investigation, the systems and services which may be involved include, but are not limited to, the following:

- Emergency Medical Services
  - first responders;
  - emergency telephone number (9-1-1) recording; and
  - initial information pertaining to the circumstances of the death, including the witnesses, bystanders, location, and circumstances.
- For law enforcement, including local, state, provincial, federal, tribal, military, or applicable jurisdictional authority/agencies, the tasks are to:
  - First render aid, then protect lives and property.
  - Secure the scene, provide scene safety, and control access to the scene.
  - Investigate the circumstances surrounding the death, including interviewing witnesses/suspects, and documenting the death scene.

- In the event a crime has occurred, be responsible for identifying potential suspect(s) and charging those individuals.
- If necessary, be supplemented by a crime scene investigator or a death scene investigator whose role may include photodocumenting and/or video recording the death scene; documenting the scene with diagrams; collecting evidence; and testifying in court as required.
- Be responsible for notifying the legal next-of-kin, which can be carried out by a law enforcement officer and/or a police chaplain.
- Coroner:
  - Within the United States, the role of coroner is defined by statutory authority, which varies between states and jurisdictions.
  - Elected or appointed official: In the majority of US states, elected coroners serve a 4-year term; some terms run on the presidential cycle, while others may run on the gubernatorial cycle.
  - Qualifications include being of minimum age (18 to 25 years), a registered voter with no felony convictions, and may or may not include medical training (which varies in length and content).
  - Authorized to determine the COD and MOD; may order that a forensic autopsy be completed by a forensic pathologist; may identify the decedent; may notify the next-of-kin; and may sign the death certificate (Bader & Gabriel, 2010).
- Medical Examiner (ME):
  - Term is more consistently defined globally (vs. the purposes/duties of the coroner).
  - Usually a medical doctor with additional training in anatomical pathology as well as subspecialty training in forensic pathology.
  - Some states have MEs who are medical doctors with no specialized forensic training and who do not perform autopsies (e.g., *dentists*, family practice physicians).
  - Still other jurisdictions have MEs who are not physicians of any type.
- Nurse Coroner:
  - A nurse who resides in a jurisdiction with a Coroner System, and is interested in forensic death investigation and serving the residents of his or her community, may consider seeking the elective office of coroner. The nurse may initially seek experience working for the elected coroner as an assistant/deputy coroner.
  - Jurisdictional statutes; the Nurse Practice Act; and the country, province, or state's Board of Nursing Rules and Regulations Practice dictate the responsibilities of the role.
  - A nurse who is interested in running for elective office should review his or her jurisdiction's statutes and contact the Election Commission within the local jurisdiction for additional information. In areas where coroners are appointed to office, the nurse should review and follow the jurisdictional process for appointment.
- Forensic Nurse Death Investigator (FNDI):
  - An FNDI is a registered nurse who has specialized training in forensic science and medicolegal death investigation.
  - The FNDI practices according to jurisdictional statutes, the Board of Nursing Rules and Regulations (or regulator of nursing practice), and the Nurse Practice Act (or other applicable acts within the area of practice).
  - No formal credentialing process exists for the FNDI; however, the International Association of Forensic Nurses (IAFN) has published the *Forensic Nurse Death Investigator Education Guidelines* (2009) to provide a foundation for nurses pursuing practice as an FNDI (International Association of Forensic Nurses, 2014).
  - Upon completing the recommended 40-hour didactic content, the nurse completes a preceptored clinical experience. Didactic and clinical content is listed in Table 3.2.
  - The *FNDI Education Guidelines* (2009) address recommendations for FNDI faculty and preceptors.
  - When the nurse completes the didactic and clinical requirements, he or she should be equipped to provide basic training and education to multidisciplinary partners, the community, and the media in the following areas:
    - forensic evaluation;
    - DSI;

TABLE 3.2 IAFN Education Guidelines

Didactic Content	Clinical Preceptorship Content
Forensic nursing science	Death scene investigation
Multidisciplinary team concepts	Physical examination of the deceased
Roles and responsibilities of the FNDI	Collection of physical evidence
Death investigation systems	Documentation
Medical/forensic evaluation	Autopsy examination
Evidence management and evaluation	Research
Nursing management	
Criminal justice system	
Ethics	
Evaluation	

(International Association of Forensic Nurses, 2014)

- courtroom practices; and
- multidisciplinary team processes and responses.
- The FNDI should strive to build an expansive network of professional relationships through collaboration and coordination of DSIs and fatality review teams, creating guidelines based on best practices and conducting relevant research (International Association of Forensic Nurses, 2014).
- Medicolegal Death Investigator (MDI):
  - Every jurisdiction has a person/discipline that is responsible for medicolegal death investigations with varying job descriptions, practices, and responsibilities depending on the type of death investigation system and jurisdictional statutes.
  - Assists in the investigation of sudden, unnatural, suspicious, or violent deaths.
  - Acts as a liaison between the medical examiner's office, the coroner's office, law enforcement agencies, other investigative agencies, families of decedents, and the general public as determined by each jurisdiction.
  - The title bestowed upon individuals who practice in this capacity may have different designations, including MDI, ME, FNDI, Coroner, Deputy Coroner, Nurse Coroner, and Justice of the Peace.
- Forensic Science Specialists:
  - The type of specialist may be needed depending upon the circumstances surrounding the death investigation; not all forensic services are available or required for each case.
  - The more common specialties used during death investigations include toxicology; genetics (such as DNA); anthropology; odontology; fingerprints; entomology; digital evidence; pathology; trace evidence; questioned documents; ballistics; and patterned evidence (James & Nordby, 2005).
- Protective Service Agencies:
  - The role of protective service agencies is to prevent, investigate, and provide care to individuals who may be victims of abuse and neglect.
  - Child Protective Services (CPS) or other comparable agencies are responsible for civil investigations to identify child abuse and neglect, and to ensure the safety of children within their care.
  - Adult Protective Services (APS) or other comparable agencies are responsible for the safety and welfare of adults (generally 18 years and older, but the ages vary between jurisdictions) who lack the ability to comprehend and negotiate for themselves cognitively and/or physically. The majority of APS reports pertain to the older adult population.
- Public Health Agencies:
  These agencies include the:
  - Centers for Disease Control and Injury Prevention (CDC) (US)
  - Health departments
  - Injury prevention centers

- Hospitals, Hospices, and Nursing Homes
- Judicial System:
  - Applies the law to prosecute individuals who have been charged with a criminal act.
  - Provides mechanisms for the resolution of civil disputes that may arise in conjunction with a death.

POPULATIONS AT RISK

Every living person is at risk for premature death from nonnatural, sudden, and unexpected events. Populations at risk can be categorized by age; socioeconomic status; geographic location; and violent lifestyles.

- Age groups that have an increased risk of premature death include:
(1) Infants
  - Neonatal deaths
    - Death occurs prior to 28 days of age.
    - Increased risk for natural disease process related to pregnancy; delivery; prematurity; infection; and congenital abnormalities.
    - Increased risk for accidental and/or intentional suffocation.
  - Postneonatal deaths
    - Death occurs after 28 days of life and prior to the first birthday.
    - Injuries occur secondary to mobility.
    - Unable to protect themselves from unintentional injuries.
    - Vulnerable airway, which they are unable to protect, thereby increases the risk for accidental or intentional suffocation. Accidental suffocation is most often due to an unsafe sleep environment and/or bed sharing.
    - Increasing mobility increases the risk of drowning, falls, and poisoning.
    - Increased risk of abuse and/or neglect is secondary to dependency on parents and caregivers. Abusive head trauma (previously referred to as shaken baby syndrome) is most prevalent in this age group.
(2) Children
  - Toddler: Age 1 to 3 years
    - Increased risk is secondary to physical activity and mobility.
    - Increased risk of falls, drowning, and poisoning as toddlers have the ability to access situations from which they may be unable to recover.
    - Greater risk for asphyxiation is secondary to choking and strangulation.
    - Risks for abuse and neglect deaths in this age group are secondary to vocalization and toilet training issues (Lynch & Duval, 2011).
  - Child: Age 4 to 10 years
    - Increased risk related to transportation (motor vehicle collisions [MVCs], all-terrain vehicles [ATVs], bicycles, skateboards).
    - Increased risk for drowning and gunshot injuries, secondary to an inability to comprehend the scope and consequences of water and weapons.
    - Increased risk of death due to fire, secondary to experimentation.
    - Risk of abuse and neglect deaths, secondary to dependency on caregivers.
  - Preadolescent and Adolescent: Age 11 to 19 years
    - Risk for death due to impulsivity resulting in self-inflicted injuries/suicide and accidental deaths due to experimentation with drugs/alcohol.
    - Inexperience and distracted driving (MVCs, ATVs).
    - Gang violence.
    - Parental supervision generally declines with this age group (Centers for Disease Control and Prevention, 2013b, 2014a).
    - Figure 3.1 shows the top ten leading causes of death by age.

	Age Groups										
Rank	≤1	1-4	5-9	10-14	15-24	25-34	35-44	45-54	55-64	65+	All Ages
1	Congenital Anomalies 5,107	Unintentional Injury 1,394	Unintentional Injury 758	Unintentional Injury 885	Unintentional Injury 12,341	Unintentional Injury 14,573	Unintentional Injury 14,792	Malignant Neoplasms 50,211	Malignant Neoplasms 109,501	Heart Disease 477,338	Heart Disease 597,689
2	Short Gestation 4,148	Congenital Anomalies 507	Malignant Neoplasms 439	Malignant Neoplasms 477	Homicide 4,678	Suicide 5,735	Malignant Neoplasms 11,809	Heart Disease 36,729	Heart Disease 68,077	Malignant Neoplasms 396,670	Malignant Neoplasms 574,743
3	SIDS 2,063	Homicide 385	Congenital Anomalies 163	Suicide 267	Suicide 4,600	Homicide 4,258	Heart Disease 10,594	Unintentional Injury 19,667	Chronic Low. Respiratory Disease 14,242	Chronic Low. Respiratory Disease 118,031	Chronic Low. Respiratory Disease 138,080
4	Maternal Pregnancy Comp. 1,561	Malignant Neoplasms 346	Homicide 111	Homicide 150	Malignant Neoplasms 1,604	Malignant Neoplasms 3,619	Suicide 6,571	Suicide 8,799	Unintentional Injury 14,023	Cerebro vascular 109,990	Cerebro vascular 129,476
5	Unintentional Injury 1,110	Heart Disease 159	Heart Disease 68	Congenital Anomalies 135	Heart Disease 1,028	Heart Disease 3,222	Homicide 2,473	Liver Disease 8,651	Diabetes Mellitus 11,677	Alzheimer's Disease 82,616	Unintentional Injury 120,859
6	Placenta Cord Membranes 1,030	Influenza & Pneumonia 91	Chronic Low. Respiratory Disease 60	Heart Disease 117	Congenital Anomalies 412	HIV 741	Liver Disease 2,423	Cerebro-vascular 5,910	Cerebro-vascular 10,693	Diabetes Mellitus 49,191	Alzheimer's Disease 83,494
7	Bacterial Sepsis 583	Septicemia 62	Cerebro-vascular 47	Chronic Low. Respiratory Disease 73	Cerebro-vascular 190	Diabetes Mellitus 606	Cerebro-vascular 1,904	Diabetes Mellitus 5,6104	Liver Disease 9,764	Influenza & Pneumonia 42,846	Diabetes Mellitus 69,071
8	Respiratory Distress 514	Benign Neoplasms 59	Benign Neoplasms 37	Benign Neoplasms 45	Influenza & Pneumonia 181	Cerebro-vascular 517	HIV 1,898	Chronic Low. Respiratory Disease 4,452	Suicide 6,384	Nephritis 41,994	Nephritis 50,476
9	Circulatory System Disease 507	Perinatal Period 52	Influenza & Pneumonia 37	Cerebro-vascular 43	Diabetes Mellitus 165	Liver Disease 487	Diabetes Mellitus 1,789	HIV 3,123	Nephritis 5,082	Unintentional Injury 41,300	Influenza & Pneumonia 50,097
10	Necrotizing Enterocolitis 472	Chronic Low. Respiratory Disease 51	Septicemia 32	Septicemia 35	Complicated Pregnancy 163	Congenital Anomalies 397	Influenza & Pneumonia 773	Viral Hepatitis 2,376	Septicemia 4,604	Septicemia 26,310	Suicide 38,364

(Centers for Disease Control and Prevention WISQARS Database 2014)

FIGURE 3.1 Top ten leading causes of death by age, 2010.

Other issues that can contribute to premature death include:
- Socioeconomic Status
  - Persons who are homeless have an increased risk of hypo/hyperthermia, substance abuse, and trauma (National Coalition for Homeless, 2012).
  - Lower socioeconomic status increases the risk of death due to a lack of medical care.
  - A higher socioeconomic status may provide the monetary means to obtain drugs in larger quantities and higher priced designer drugs.

- Geographic Location
  - Coastline deaths are secondary to hurricanes and flooding.
  - Areas prone to wildfires create the risk for fire and smoke inhalation deaths.
  - Other geographic locations are prone to tornados, avalanches, mudslides, or earthquakes.
  - Populations that reside in war-torn regions.
  - Areas with gang violence.
- Violent Lifestyles
  - Intimate partner violence (IPV)
    - Is defined as violence between two persons in which a relationship exists or has existed.
    - Approximately 33% of females and 3% of males over the age of 12 who are victims of homicides are killed by an intimate partner (New York State Office for the Prevention of Domestic Violence, 2011).
    - Is a leading cause of homicides for pregnant women (New York State Office for the Prevention of Domestic Violence, 2011).
  - Domestic violence (DV) is an umbrella term that encompasses any violence within a household – including IPV, child abuse, and/or elder abuse – which increases the risk of premature death.
  - Gang violence includes weapons, drugs, and remorseless violence against others.

PRACTICE AND PREVENTION

The goal of the medicolegal death investigation is to determine COD and MOD. The MDI's practice should encompass multiple areas, including recognition of impending death; postmortem physical examination; DSI and documentation; forensic interviews; and records review. In addition, knowledge about applicable laws and participation in fatality review teams are also part of practice and prevention.

Signs of impending death should be understood since providers are often called prior to death, especially in cases of family anxiety or fear (See Table 3.3).

- Postmortem Physical Assessment
  - General appearance of the decedent includes a head-to-toe assessment, including the individual's height, weight, nutritional status, temperature, color, cleanliness, medical interventions, postmortem changes, and clothing/jewelry.

TABLE 3.3 Signs of Impending Death

System	Signs
Integumentary	Mottled and discolored
Respirations	Dyspnea and Cheyne–Stokes respirations
Cardiac	Decreased blood and cerebral perfusion; decreased cardiac output
Neurological	Disoriented
Nutrition	Decreased interest in fluids and food; swallowing difficulties
Urinary	Decreased output
Metabolic	Basal metabolic rate slows, secondary to decreased respiratory rate and caloric intake
Generalized	Fatigue; malaise; attempting to talk to persons who are already deceased

(Libow & Neufeld, 2008; Stanford Medical School, 2006)

TABLE 3.4 Mechanisms of Injuries Affecting the Skin

Blunt force injuries	Abrasion, laceration, contusion, petechiae, and ecchymosis
Sharp force injuries	Incision and stab wounds
Gunshot	Contact, close, medium- and long-distance gunshot wounds; entrance and exit wounds
Bite marks	May be caused by human, animal, or insect Human bites strongly correlate with physical, sexual, and child abuse
Strangulation/ Ligature marks	A furrow mark may be located around the neck indicating use of a ligature or hands. Associated findings: Petechiae, torn frenulum, abrasions, and/or contusions
Burns	Fire, electrocution, lightning strikes, cigarette burns, water, chemical or radiological; May be caused intentionally or unintentionally

(Skopp, 2010)

- Integumentary/Wound Assessment
  - Integumentary and wound assessment can provide vital information about the mechanism, COD, and/or MOD. Injuries that affect the integumentary system may additionally impact internal structures, such as organs and bones.
  - Trauma assessment includes (but is not limited to) contusions, abrasions, lacerations, burns, petechiae, gunshot wounds, bite and ligature marks, and other patterned injuries (Skopp, 2010).
  - Signs of insect and/or animal activity.
  - Birthmarks, tattoos, piercings, and scars.
  - The MDI should document his or her findings and describe what was assessed; however, the MDI should refrain from interpreting the findings until all relevant information has been ascertained (See Tables 3.4 and 3.5).
  - Abnormal skin changes can provide vital clues in determining the COD and/or the MOD (Skopp, 2010).
- Time of Death and Postmortem Changes

The body undergoes predictable, sequential changes that begin at the time of death (TOD). These postmortem body changes can be used to help estimate the TOD (American Board of Medicolegal Death Investigators, 2015; Hammer, Moynihan, & Pagliaro, 2013). Immediate postmortem changes beginning within the first 24 hours are discussed in Table 3.6 (Skopp, 2010).

Multiple factors that impact the rate of postmortem changes include:

(1) ambient temperature;
(2) body temperature (fever, hypothermia, or hyperthermia) at the TOD;

TABLE 3.5 Abnormal Skin Changes

Skin Color	Possible Cause
Light red to cherry red	Carbon monoxide
Bright pink	Cyanide
Greyish to brownish	Nitrate, nitrite, or aniline
Atrophic scarring, abscess, ulcerations, or puncture marks	Intravenous drug use
Perforated nasal septum	Intranasal drug use

(Skopp, 2010)

TABLE 3.6 Postmortem Changes Beginning within the First 24 Hours

Stage	Findings	Postmortem Time Factors
Pallor Mortis	Paling of the body	Onset: 15–20 min
Algor Mortis	Cooling of the body due to environmental temperatures	General rule is that body temperature will decrease ~1.5°C/hr during the first 8 hrs*
Rigor Mortis	State of acidosis causing muscles to *temporarily* stiffen	Onset: 1–2 hrs
		Resolution: 24–36 hrs
	Cadaveric spasm	Starts in the smaller muscles of the face and jaws; increases over time and then decreases until completely dissipated
		Instantaneous rigor, quicker onset, and resolution then full rigor; secondary to intense muscle activity; rarely seen
Livor Mortis (Lividity)	Circulation ceases and red blood cells settle into dependent body surfaces, causing a bluish purple area[†]	Onset: within minutes
		Fixed and nonblanchable: ~12 hrs
	Dark red lividity[‡]	
	Assists in determining postmortem body position and/or postmortem movement	
Putrefaction	Caused by autolysis of enzymes and microorganisms	Time is variable based on environmental factors, but usually begins within the first 24 hrs postmortem
	Begins in the colon and large intestines as a greenish discoloration in the right lower quadrant (over the cecum)	

*A multitude of factors can affect body temperature changes, including ambient air temperature, clothing worn by the deceased, and if the body is wet.
[†]Except in areas that are directly exposed to pressure (such as a diaper) and appear blanched
[‡]Dark red lividity (as opposed to the typical bluish-purple lividity) may indicate carbon monoxide poisoning, hypothermia, or cyanide poisoning.
(Hanzlick, 1997; James & Nordby, 2005; Lynch & Duval, 2011)

(3) size/weight of the decedent;
(4) geographic factors (e.g., submersion in water, humidity);
(5) muscle usage prior to death (e.g., extreme exercise or electrocution);
(6) trauma at the TOD;
(7) amount of clothing or cover on the decedent; and
(8) drug use prior to death (Hammer, Moynihan, & Pagliaro, 2013; Saint Louis University School of Medicine, 2015).

Early decompensation includes putrefaction, bloating, and skin slippage (See Table 3.7).

TABLE 3.7 Early Decomposition

Putrefaction	Caused by autolysis of enzymes and microorganisms; begins in early decomposition and proceeds through advanced decomposition
Bloating	Abdomen becomes distended and a generalized swelling of the body occurs
Skin-slippage	Skin appears as a purplish/greenish/brown marbling and the skin progressively loosens and slips off

(Hammer, Moynihan, & Pagliaro, 2013; Saint Louis University School of Medicine, 2015)

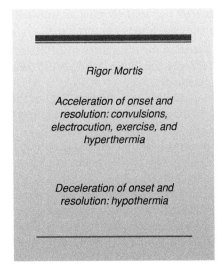

Rigor Mortis

Acceleration of onset and resolution: convulsions, electrocution, exercise, and hyperthermia

Deceleration of onset and resolution: hypothermia

FIGURE 3.2 Rigor mortis.

Depending on environmental factors, these changes usually begin within 24 to 48 hours of death (Hammer, Moynihan, & Pagliaro, 2013; Saint Louis University School of Medicine, 2015).

Advanced Decomposition

(1) bloating resolves;
(2) soft tissues continue to break down;
(3) facial bones become skeletonized (Hammer, Moynihan, & Pagliaro, 2013; Saint Louis University School of Medicine, 2015)
(4) skeletonization of the body and mummification:
 • soft tissue and organs have lost hydration and are shriveled and decayed;
 • skin surface becomes hardened and leathery; and
 • putrefactive process continues until all that remains are the skeleton, bone, or bone fragments (Bader & Gabriel, 2010) (See Table 3.8).

Estimating the Date of Death (DOD) and the Time of Death (TOD)

(1) TOD can be precise only if the death is witnessed.
(2) An MDI must consider the decedent's health history, postmortem changes, and environmental factors at the scene.

TABLE 3.8 Advanced Decompensation

Stage	Findings
Putrefaction	Begins in early decomposition and progresses through advanced decompensation; soft tissues of the body are converted to liquid and gases and may be foul-smelling
Decomposition	Organic tissue completely breaks down
Mummification	Body dries and shrivels
Skeletonization	Skeletal bones or fragments are partially or completely revealed

(Hammer, Moynihan, & Pagliaro, 2013; Saint Louis University School of Medicine, 2015)

(3) The most accurate way to determine an unwitnessed TOD, where decomposition is present, is through analysis of forensic entomology.

Calculations based on the lifecycle of blowflies may assist in determining approximately how much time has lapsed since death (Byrd, 2013). Use of this method requires knowledge about ambient air temperatures.

Temperature-based models to estimate TOD or the postmortem interval (PMI) vary. However, the most widely used method is the Rule of Thumb Model, which is calculated in the following manner:

PMI = 98.6 minus the Fahrenheit rectal temperature divided by 1.5, equaling the approximate hours since death. This method does not account for thermodynamics and is inaccurate in estimating extended periods of death (Marshall & Hoare, 1962).

Other physical findings, if properly assessed, may assist in estimating a TOD or DOD, including the emptying of the gastrointestinal tract and the urinary bladder, and the biochemical changes noted in the analysis of the vitreous humor of the eye (i.e., postmortem rise). Postmortem rise is accurate in the first 9 hours after death and must be performed in a laboratory (Palmiere & Mangin, 2012).

Death Scene Investigation and Documentation

The death scene investigation is critical in determining the COD, MOD, TOD, DOD, and extenuating circumstances surrounding the occurrence. Guidelines vary between jurisdictions; however, basic steps should be included in policies and procedures, such as the following.

Scene Response. The response of an MDI to a death scene depends on the jurisdiction in which the death occurred. Each jurisdiction has its own statutes, guidelines, policies, and procedures for how MDIs are notified of a death, the types of death to which they respond, and their role once they arrive on scene.

Approach. Upon arrival at the death scene, an MDI should take the initiative to introduce him/herself to other essential personnel on the scene and determine scene safety (National Guidelines for Death Investigators, 1997).

Scene Safety

(1) Prior to entering a death scene, the safety of the area must be assessed and established. Scene safety should take into account ongoing or unresolved criminal activity; environmental and physical risks, including unsafe structures, moving traffic, chemical threats; and any threat from onlookers/crowds.
(2) The MDI should assess his or her own safety, discuss safety risks with the incident commander on-scene if applicable, obtain clearance from the individual who is responsible for scene safety (e.g., incident commander or safety risk officer), and wear protective gear.

Maintaining the Scene

(1) In most jurisdictions, the law enforcement agency with jurisdictional authority over the incident location is responsible for securing the entrance into a death scene and for documenting who and what time persons enter and exit the scene. This process ensures scene integrity, safety, and supports the chain of custody.
(2) Prior to entering the scene, the MDI should coordinate with other participating agencies for a scene briefing to determine the scene entry point, establish the current scope of the investigation, and review the established facts of the situation. This briefing allows for an informational exchange prior to entering the scene and beginning the scene assessment.

Scene Assessment

(1) After the scene briefing, investigators may conduct an initial scene assessment and scene walkthrough, which will provide an overview of the macro- and micro-facets of the death scene.

(2) The walk-through is a valuable investigative tool; investigators have their first opportunity to evaluate the scene, locate human remains, look for evidence, and determine an investigative strategy.

(3) Both the MDI and law enforcement personnel need to accomplish scene processing, and evidence identification and collection. The crime scene for the MDI is the body or human remains and the scene adjacent to and directly associated with the body.

(4) Locard's Principle of Exchange: Every time one makes physical contact with another person, place, or thing, an exchange or transfer of physical materials occurs. The more violent the actions surrounding the death, the higher the likelihood of obtaining trace evidence. This principle connects victim, perpetrator, and scene, based on the transfer of evidence (Hammer, Moynihan, & Pagliaro, 2013).

(5) The initial walk-through should be conducted by a minimum number of individuals so as to minimize scene disturbance and prevent the loss and/or contamination of evidence (National Guidelines for Death Investigators, 1997).

Videography. Some jurisdictions with access to videography may use a video recording during the initial walk-through. This recording creates a permanent record of the actions of investigators who first enter the scene and provides documentation of the scene prior to closer photographic documentation.

Forensic Photography

(1) Photographic documentation of the scene and body creates a permanent record.

(2) Photographs should be taken of the macro- and micro-environments at the scene.

(3) The macro-environment includes the broad, large-scale description of the death scene, creating an overview. For example, the macro-environment may include the house and the decedent's bedroom where the decedent was found on the floor.

(4) The micro-environment consists of smaller areas within the macro-environment, which may be relevant to the death. The micro-environment photographs may include close-up photographs of items on the nightstand (i.e., ashtray, medication bottles, suicide note, etc.) or markings on the body.

(5) Additional training in forensic photography beyond basic crime scene investigation is prudent. Forensic photography should cover distant, intermediate, and close-up photographs; measuring scales; identification photographs; and alternate light sources.

Evidence/Property Management

(1) The MDI needs to recognize, document, and collect evidence from the body. It is imperative to properly collect, inventory, and safeguard evidence, as well as adhere to chain of custody procedures.

(2) For information pertaining to evidence identification, preservation, collection, and chain of custody in the United States, refer to the Preservation of Evidence Act (Preservation of Evidence Act, Title 17, Chapter 28 of the South Carolina Code of Laws, 2013) and applicable local/agency Rules of Evidentiary Procedure (or jurisdictional, applicable laws).

Death Scene Documentation

Accurate documentation during a death investigation of findings at the scene and on the body are essential to comprehending the totality of the event. Methods include written reports, scene and body diagrams, audio recordings, videography, and photography.

(1) Written Reports
- Written notes may be informal or formal in nature. Informal notes are those that investigators write while in the field as they document their findings.
- Depending on agency guidelines and policies, these informal written notes may be transferred or transcribed into a more formal format.
- The MDI should follow his or her agency's policies regarding written notes and how the notes are secured and possibly released under subpoena the Freedom of Information Act

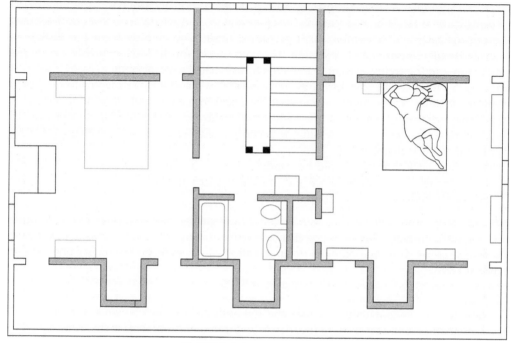

FIGURE 3.3   Scene diagram.

(FOIA) requests in the United States (or the corresponding/similar jurisdictional laws/acts in other regions), and court orders/proceedings.

(2) Scene Diagrams

Death scene diagrams are documents that provide visual and written documentation depicting the death scene as it looked when investigators/witnesses first observed it. These diagrams often include written details, a layout of the surrounding area, and the location of the decedent or other individuals present. An investigator may also ask a witness to draw a diagram based on his or her recollection of the incident location (See Figure 3.3).

(3) Body Diagrams

• Body diagrams may be used to document physical findings on the body either at the incident scene, the death location (i.e., emergency department), and/or in the autopsy suite.

• Areas of lividity should be included since they help determine whether a body was moved from the initial death scene to a secondary location (See Figures 3.4 and 3.5).

(4) Audio Recording

• Some agencies use audio recordings in lieu of or in addition to written documentation of an interview with individuals who may have witnessed or been involed in the incident or who may have information that benefits the death investigation.

• The MDI should follow his or her agency guidelines and policies as well as any applicable laws regarding the audio recording of individuals with or without their knowledge and/or consent.

Death Scene Reenactment/Reconstruction

(1) Death scene reenactment and reconstruction are useful tools to recreate actions surrounding the death and the death scene.

(2) The death scene reconstruction may consist of drawings of the scene, and the use of mannequins, photography and/or videography, investigative reports, and witness accounts.

(3) The death scene reenactment is at the core of investigation regarding sudden, unexpected death and includes the death scene and persons at the scene.

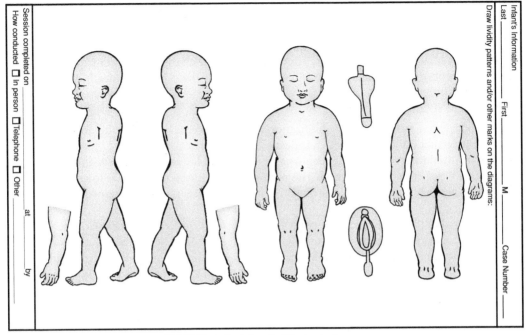

FIGURE 3.4   Infant/toddler body diagram.

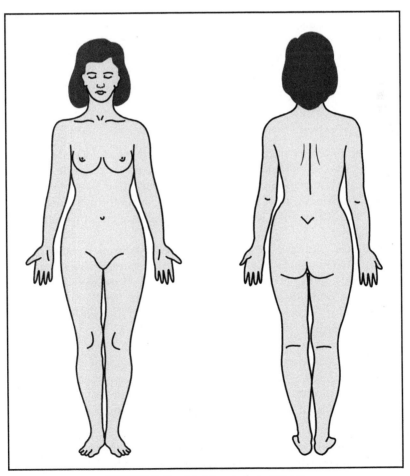

FIGURE 3.5   Adult female body diagram.

(4) The reenactment should be videographed, or photographed and/or videotaped. This provides investigators with a way to depict the known facts of the death scene and provide information to corroborate witness statements.

Forensic Interviews. Interviews are conversations in which the interviewer tries to elicit specific information from the interviewee (O'Neal, 2007). For the purpose of death investigations, four types of interviews may be used: an initial interview, a clarification interview, a follow-up interview, and an interrogation.

(1) The first two – the initial and clarification – are nonaccusatory in nature and designed to acquire factual information, which is needed to investigate a death.

- The initial interview may be lengthy and emotional for some witnesses and should take place early in the investigation. The purpose of the initial interview is to gather as much information as possible regarding the decedent and the circumstances surrounding the death.
- The goal of the clarification interview is to resolve any misunderstanding or miscommunication that may have occurred during the initial interview. This interview provides a nonconfrontational means to explain discrepancies, which may occur during the course of an investigation. The clarification interview may take place shortly after the initial interview or days or weeks later.
- During these interviews, investigators should be cognizant of the plausibility of the interviewee's account of events and note any disparities between other witness accounts, professional reports, and physical findings from the body and scene.
- A follow-up interview may be used to relay forensic and autopsy findings to the next-of-kin, answer questions that witnesses/family members may have regarding the investigation, and offer referrals for support.
- An interrogation is a more formal, controlled questioning that is conducted by law enforcement officials (LEOs) of a suspect believed to have committed a crime. During an interrogation, the LEO is not seeking information that was elicited in the initial interview. Instead, the LEO is leading the process with the goal of obtaining a truthful admission or confession (Tousignant, 1991).

Autopsy Examination

An autopsy is a postmortem examination performed by a medical doctor to aid in the determination of COD and MOD. In addition, an autopsy may be used to provide training and expand medical knowledge. An autopsy examination can be conducted for forensic or medical purposes. Each type requires a different type of authorization, autopsy protocol, and follow-up procedures (Bader & Gabriel, 2010; Bailey, 2014; Iserson, 2003). Protocols and routine laboratory testing may vary between jurisdictions.

In the United States, a forensic autopsy is a complete postmortem examination conducted by a forensic pathologist who is board-certified by the American Board of Pathology pursuant to state statutes. Other jurisdictions define "forensic pathologist" pursuant to their interpretation, needs, and structure of forensic autopsies. This autopsy is conducted for medicolegal purposes at the discretion of an ME or coroner, in order to determine the COD and MOD. In most jurisdictions, either the coroner or ME can authorize a forensic autopsy, regardless of the circumstances surrounding the death, if a forensic autopsy is needed to determine COD/MOD or if deemed necessary to legally document the physical findings and injuries (American Board of Pathology, n.d.). Forensic autopsies in certain circumstances are required by law (i.e., unexplained child deaths, deaths in custody); are usually funded by the jurisdiction indicated by statute; and may be performed regardless of the family's wishes.

(1) A forensic autopsy includes an external head-to-toe examination and an examination of internal organ systems, which are grossly and microscopically examined.

(2) The forensic autopsy may also include radiology, toxicology, and additional case-specific tests and screenings that may be needed to accurately determine the COD and MOD.

(3) In addition, during the forensic autopsy, hair and fingernails are closely examined for transfer of evidence.

(4) Gunshot wounds are examined for bullets, bullet fragments, the trajectory, and the positional relationship between the shooter(s) and the deceased.

(5) Stab wounds are examined and evaluated to assist in determining the type and size of the weapon, as well as the positional relationship between the assailant(s) and the deceased.

(6) Photographs should be taken during the autopsy to supplement written material.

(7) The National Association of Medical Examiners (NAME) has developed forensic autopsy protocols to provide basic standards of practice for forensic pathologists for a variety of different death investigation scenarios. Other agencies have also developed a variety of forensic autopsy/toxicology protocols to ensure that during specific, varying circumstances, the correct evidence is obtained (National Association of Medical Examiners, n.d).

- The US Fire Administration (UFA) has developed a Firefighter Autopsy Protocol to be followed when a firefighter dies in the line of duty (U.S. Fire Administration, Federal Emergency Management Administration, 1994).
- The National Transportation Safety Board (NTSB) has toxicology protocols that are to be followed during the autopsy of a pilot who dies in a crash, regardless of aircraft (Federal Emergency Management Administration, 2015).

A medical autopsy is a postmortem examination that is performed, usually in a hospital, to evaluate and identify the extent of a decedent's medical condition that caused or contributed to the person's death. Sometimes referred to as a clinical or academic autopsy, the results can also be used for research and teaching purposes.

(1) A medical autopsy may focus on only one organ system or on multiple organ systems.

(2) The legal next-of-kin must provide consent for a medical autopsy to be performed.

(3) A medical autopsy may be conducted by a medical doctor (MD), pathologist, or a forensic pathologist.

(4) The hospital or the next-of-kin who request the autopsy will cover the cost of the medical autopsy.

In some circumstances, an external examination may also be used to document external injuries in the absence of a forensic autopsy. An external examination may be completed along with toxicology testing and a review of the medical records.

Virtual Autopsy

(1) Autopsy methods used by departments of pathology worldwide have not evolved much during the past century. However, new postmortem examination techniques that compliment traditional autopsies are being used, including computed tomography (CT) and magnetic resonance imaging (MRI). Used in conjunction with traditional autopsy, the use of CT and MRI enhances the diagnostic quality of the postmortem examination and report. In addition, CT and MRI can assist in ruling out occult injury and thereby reduce the number of autopsies to be performed. Records can be stored for educational and training purposes (National Research Council of the National Academy of Sciences, 2009; Westphal, Apitzsch, Penzkofer, Mahnken, & Knüchel, 2012).

(2) Advantages of virtual autopsy, or virtopsy, include:

- noninvasive (especially useful when religious objections to autopsy are raised);
- visualization of skeletal and soft tissue injuries; and
- potential detection of internal bleeding; missile paths; bone and missile fragments; fracture patterns; brain contusion; occult fractures; and gas embolisms (National Research Council of the National Academy of Sciences, 2009).

Toxicology

(1) Results from toxicological analyses in death investigations are used to determine if ingested, inhaled, or injected substances were a cause or contributory factor (such as impairment) in the death.

(2) The purpose of sampling is to provide a representation of the whole so that analysis can be targeted and to provide context for the interpretation of the results.

(3) The depth of sampling is case-dependent.

(4) Drug concentrations change during the pre-terminal stage of death because of pharmacokinetics used during resuscitation and in the intensive care unit, drug degradation, formation or artifacts, and postmortem distribution. Formation of new entities and degradation of drugs may occur, especially in a putrefied corpse.

(5) Fluids and tissues may be severely affected by autolysis, decomposition, and embalming (International Association of Forensic Nurses, 2014). The integrity of toxicology specimens is optimally obtained if:
- the body is refrigerated;
- the collection of specimens occurs as close as possible to the TOD;
- the sample size is sufficient;
- the proper specimen is obtained (e.g., stomach contents; vomitus; urine; and blood, organ, and tissue specimens); and
- cross-contamination is avoided (Hammer, Moynihan & Pagliaro, 2013; James & Nordby, 2005; Lynch & Duval, 2011; Skopp, 2010).

(6) Evidential quality is assured through:
- labeling, storing, refrigerating, or freezing specimens, as appropriately defined in policies.
- maintaining verification of the identity and the integrity of samples from collection through reporting.

(7) Relevant information is provided with the samples (e.g., circumstances surrounding death). Chain of custody is maintained and documented from collection through submission, analysis, reporting, storing, and/or disposal of the specimens.

(8) Toxicology can identify varying intoxicants, drugs, and poisons.

(9) Screening may detect unsuspected homicides, suicides, and child/elder abuse and/or neglect (National Research Council of the National Academy of Sciences, 2009).

(10) Biochemistry of blood, cerebrospinal fluid, urine, and vitreous humor can provide information that is significant in determining the COD and providing clarity in forensic cases.
- Postmortem biochemistry is essential when pathophysiological changes (e.g., diabetes mellitus, ketoacidosis, and electrolyte imbalance) are not detectable during autopsy.
- Biochemistry can also provide critical information in cases of anaphylaxis, hypothermia, sepsis, and hormonal disturbances.

Blood

The blood specimen is usually tested in two stages: screening and confirmatory. After completion of both tests, the quantity of a substance and/or its major metabolite(s) is determined (Skopp, 2010).

Hair

(1) Hair can be classified as similar; dissimilar; or inconclusive.

(2) Hair samples cannot positively identify an individual.

(3) A hair sample can be used to detect drugs that have been ingested within the past 90 days (depending on the rate of hair growth); however, these tests are often cost-prohibitive.

Records Review

(1) A complete autopsy investigation should include a review of all relevant and applicable records and documents, which may assist in determination of the COD/MOD.

(2) Records may be available from a variety of sources, including EMS records, a 9-1-1 recording and/or transcript, medical records, pharmacy records, social service records, criminal history records, employment records, surveillance videos, photographs, phone records, and agency-specific records. The process to obtain the required materials depends upon jurisdictional statutes.

(3) Emergency Medical Service (EMS) Records
- Provide valuable information regarding dispatch and arrival times, names of providers who responded to the incident, and their documented observations.
- Integumentary/Wound Assessment: It may be beneficial to obtain prior EMS records on a decedent to determine how often and for what purpose he or she may have contacted EMS prior to death, what services were provided, to which facilities the decedent may have requested to be transported, and the EMS provider's observations during those responses.

(4) Emergency Telephone Number Recording (9-1-1)
- The recording, if applicable, provides information regarding the 9-1-1 caller, his or her description of events, the instructions provided by dispatchers, and information regarding the affect and response of the caller and others who may have been present at the time of the incident.
- The 9-1-1 call may capture the first utterances by a witness and subsequently help determine the COD/MOD.

(5) Medical Records
- May be extremely valuable during a death investigation in determining prior medical treatment, medical diagnoses, radiology reports, laboratory results, and prescribed medications. The data contained in those records will provide dates of treatment, names of treatment providers, and information regarding adherence to medical treatment.
- Investigators may consider reviewing records from hospitals, health clinics, physician offices, mental health counselors, psychiatric providers, drug and alcohol treatment centers, and nursing homes.

(6) Pharmacy Records
- Important when trying to determine the medication prescribed to an individual, how often the prescription had been filled, and the number of pills that were dispensed each time.
- These records may help determine if a discrepancy exists between the amount of medication expected to be found at a death scene, the amount located at the scene, and the toxicology results.

(7) Social Service Records
- Notes from social workers and protective service agencies may assist in understanding the decedent's social history and dynamics, and his or her family, social group, and/or religious affiliations.
- This history may include drug and alcohol use, history of violence, information on living conditions, and any prior social service needs of the decedent.

(8) Background Check and Criminal History
- Records may be helpful during some death investigations to provide insight into the decedent and/or family's history with the legal system.
- A general background check can provide: references; school records and transcripts; credit rating; former addresses; social service records; people living in the home; relatives; and employment history, for instance.
- During child death investigations, it is also helpful to obtain the criminal history on all caretakers and adults who were in the home at the time of the child's death. This information may provide evidence of prior accusations and/or substantiated cases of child abuse.

(9) Employment Records

Employment records may provide information on work schedule, arrival and departure times, safety training, and other work-related conditions that may have impacted the COD and/or MOD. In addition, the records may assist in determining whether the death was or was not work-related.

(10) Surveillance Videos

Recovered video from private homes, businesses, dash cams, or other sources should be secured and reviewed, as applicable, during the investigation. This information may provide a video/audio recording of the circumstances surrounding the death.

(11) Phone Records

- Information on a phone found at a death scene and phone records that the phone service provider may release may provide valuable data.
- Information such as the last known date and time of received and sent message/calls may provide information as to the approximate date and TOD. In addition, this information may reveal that the person was texting or accessing the Internet while driving a vehicle or watercraft or piloting a plane.
- The phone may provide information regarding the last persons contacted and potential emergency contacts.

(12) Other Information

An unlimited number of agencies may have information that is potentially important for a death investigation. As the case unfolds, the investigator should consider requesting any and all records that may assist in the determination of the COD/MOD.

Participation in Fatality Review Teams

Deaths are sentinel events and an indicator of the health and well-being of a community and nation. Factors associated with death are multidimensional and are best understood by multidisciplinary teams (MDTs) that serve the population under review. Participation in a review process creates synergy between the MDT members and enhances recommendations for improvement in DSIs (Michigan Public Health Institute, 2013).

Child Fatality Review Teams

(1) MDT members are professionals who are involved in the health, safety, and welfare of the population being reviewed. Prosecuting attorneys, law enforcement officials, Department of Children Services professionals, hotline workers, social workers, medical personnel, advocates, EMS staff, Department of Human Services workers, health department personnel, and coroners/MEs are essential participants.

(2) The goals of the review team must be established to determine the participants, the allotted timeframe in which the death will be reviewed, the flow and organization of the review, and the dissemination of outcomes.

(3) The reviews are either investigative or retrospective in nature.
- In investigative reviews, the teams review cases that are still undergoing investigation; participants provide information to assist with the ongoing death investigation.
- Retrospective reviews occur after cases have been closed (and in some jurisdictions, adjudicated) and focus on prevention so as to decrease risk factors and increase protective factors (Michigan Public Health Institute, 2013) (See Table 3.9).

(4) Reviews may include the evaluation of policies, procedures, laws, and systems in order to make recommendations for improvements in child health, safety, protection, and welfare, as well as the investigative process.

(5) Examples of fatality review teams include, but are not limited to:
- Child Fatality Review (CFR) or Child Death Review (CDR) Teams
  - As of 2014, 49 states had CFRs at the local, state, or combination of local and state level. Each state, based on its state statutes determines (at a minimum) which types of deaths

TABLE 3.9 Child Death Reviews

Type	Investigative	Retrospective
Organization	Local or state level	Community, regional, or state level
Participants	Professionals who were involved in investigating the specific child's death	Participants are individuals who represent an interested entity or agency, but who may not have individual knowledge of the child's death that was investigated
Purpose	Identify further investigative actions, which may be necessary to make a final determination of COD and MOD, advance the investigation, and/or identify individuals who may have played a role in the death	Focus on identifying trends to determine areas for prevention initiatives and to identify inadequacies in policies, procedures, agencies, and systems

(Michigan Public Health Insitute, 2013)

are to be reviewed. Other countries also utilize child death review, although the process and team members may differ.

- Coroners and MEs at the local level may choose to review additional deaths, which may not be required by state law.
- States may choose to enter case information into an online database that the Michigan Public Health Institute maintains (Michigan Public Health Institute, 2013).
- Fetal/Infant Mortality Review (FIMR)
  - FIMRs are occasionally conducted in conjunction with CDRs and/or maternal mortality reviews.
  - The major differences between CDRs and FIMRs are (1) the ages of the population reviewed and (2) the FIMR relies heavily on participation of neonatologists and obstetricians.
  - The National Fetal/Infant Mortality Review (NFIMR) Program is a collaboration between the federal Maternal and Child Health Bureau and the American College of Obstetricians and Gynecologists. Australia and New Zealand have jointly developed the Australia and New Zealand Stillbirth Alliance (ANZSA) to review and understand factors that contribute to stillbirths.
- Maternal Mortality Review
  - According to the World Health Organization (2015), maternal mortality is defined as the death of a woman during pregnancy or within 42 days of the end of the pregnancy (be it through delivery, abortion, or miscarriage); from a pregnancy-related cause (such as eclampsia); or an aggravation of a pre-existing condition (such as diabetes).
  - These cases do not include accidental or incidental causes.
  - Other maternal mortality reviews include death within 1 year of the end of pregnancy and/or accidental causes.
  - Obstetricians play a vital role on these review teams.
- Domestic Violence (DV) or Intimate Partner Violence Fatality Reviews
  These reviews are often combined with CDR, FIMR, and/or maternal mortality reviews. These reviews should engage additional representatives from shelters, unwed mothers' services, and advocates.
- Elder Fatality Review
  - The American Bar Association and the Office for Victims of Crime have published *Elder Abuse Fatality Review Teams: A Replication Manual*, which can be obtained through the American Bar Association, Office for Victims of Crime.
  - This team should include a gerontologist and a nursing home representative.

Other Required Legal Considerations/Documents

Protected Health Information

(1) Protected health information (PHI) refers to identifiable, individual health information and data that is regulated by the Health Insurance Portability and Accountability Act of 1996 (HIPAA) within the United States. Canada has the Personal Information Protection and Electronic Documents Act (PIPEDA or the PIPED Act). Japan's law governing individual health information is Japan's Law Concerning the Protection of Personal Information ("Privacy Law"), which took effect in 2005.

(2) HIPAA permits the release and disclosure of PHI to coroners and MEs, some jurisdictions require a court order, a court-ordered warrant, subpoena, summons by a judicial officer, grand jury subpoena, or a written administrative request that must be provided to the agency that houses the specific PHI that is being sought.

(3) HIPAA provides that PHI may be disclosed "to coroners or MEs to identify a deceased person, determine the COD or to perform other functions authorized by law." In addition, PHI may be disclosed to "facilitate the donation of transplantation of cadaveric organs, eyes and tissue" or for public health surveillance without the individual's written permission (U.S. Department of Health and Human Services, 2005, 2013).

Burial–Removal Transit Permit

(1) Many jurisdictions require the completion of some type of Burial–Removal Transit Permit and/or Death Notification Permit, which is issued by the facility in which the death occurred.

(2) The coroner or the ME may issue these permits; the ME is designated to issue the permit if the death occurred outside a facility.

Death Certificate

(1) The United States uses the Standard Death Certificate, which is issued by the CDC's National Center for Health Statistics.

(2) Non-US death certificates (DCs) may be obtained through the nearest consulate or embassy. Other jurisdictions may use similar (although jurisdictionally specific) forms.

(3) The DC serves as a surveillance tool for public health and contains valuable demographic information that provides state and national statistics regarding mortality rates and causes of death.

(4) Two of the most important pieces of information on a DC are the COD and the MOD.

(5) The system by which deaths and diseases are classified is the International Statistical Classification of Disease and Related Health Problems (ICD), which is established and maintained by the World Health Organization (WHO).
   - This coding allows for mortality rates to be compared between states and regions, as well as nationally and internationally.
   - The manual provides codes to classify diseases, signs and symptoms, abnormal findings, complaints, social circumstances, and external causes of injury or disease.

(6) In cases of nonnatural deaths, the DC also requires injury information regarding the circumstances of the death. Injury information will contain demographic data, including the location of injury; a determination if the injury was work-related; whether the injury is transportation-related and if the decedent was a driver, passenger, or pedestrian; and a description of how the injury occurred.

(7) Professionals who may sign a DC vary between jurisdictions (coroner, ME, licensed medical physician, advanced registered nurse practitioner, Justice of the Peace, etc.). According to the CDC, MEs sign approximately 20% of the death certificates annually (Centers for Disease Control and Prevention, 2012).

(8) In 2003, the CDC published the *Medical Examiners' and Coroners' Handbook on Death Registration and Fetal Death Reporting* to provide instruction on the proper way to complete and file a DC (Centers for Disease Control and Prevention, 2003).

(9) The DC provides a section for the signature of the person pronouncing death and a section for the signature of the individual who certifies the death.
- The pronouncing individual is the individual, who by state statute or other guidelines, is authorized to pronounce/verify that the person is deceased.
- The certifier is the authorized individual who attests to the cause and manner of the death for that individual. The certifier may or may not have been present at the TOD.

(10) The DC is used for a variety of purposes, including:
- to evaluate population-wide health status;
- to identify the prevalence of medical and trauma issues among specific populations;
- to provide data to allocate money and resources for research, prevention, grants, and health services; and
- to provide official information for the family and assist in allowing the decedent's estate and affairs to be put in order.

(11) A signed DC (completed or pending) is required in most locales to be completed:
- within a specified time after the death (i.e., 72 hours);
- prior to burial and/or cremation;
- in order to settle insurance issues;
- to stop benefit payments from social security, disability, and/or retirement programs; and
- so representatives may access financial documents (i.e., bank accounts), and prior to the opening of estates for Probate Court.
- Some locales impose civil and/or criminal penalties for failure to complete the DC within the allocated time frame.

(12) A supplemental or amended DC must be completed when the initial DC lists the COD as pending.

   The COD/MOD may be initially certified as pending when the certifying entity is awaiting complete autopsy or toxicology results, or further investigation is required.

(13) A certified DC is a fully completed certificate that has been signed by the certifying individual and has been submitted to the appropriate vital records office for registration.

(14) Basic guidelines for completion of the DC vary; however, some commonalities are universal:
- verification of the correct spelling of the decedent's name;
- personal signing of the DC, including electronic signature (i.e., no stamps or faxes);
- completion of all required fields (may need to note "unknown" or "pending");
- no use of abbreviations;
- the month is written out (vs. using a number);
- times are noted in military format (using a 24-hour clock);
- no alteration of the document (erasure or modification of the text is prohibited); and
- documentation is printed (not cursive) (Prentice & Arnold, 2006) (See Figure 3.6).

(15) Cause of Death
- According to the CDC, the COD section on the DC is for: reporting a chain of events leading directly to death, with the immediate COD (the final disease, injury, or complication directly causing death) and the underlying COD (the disease or injury that initiated the chain of morbid events that led directly and inevitably to death) on the lowest used line (Centers for Disease Control and Prevention, 2004).
- The most immediate (or principal) COD is listed on line "A" and the underlying (or antecedent) causes are listed on subsequent lines ("B," "C," etc.).
- The time elapsing between events must be documented (unknown, approximately, minutes, hours, or days) (Prentice & Arnold, 2006).
- The underlying, antecedent, or proximate COD is the triggering event that initiates a continuous unbroken sequence of events that produces the fatality.
- The immediate COD is the complication of the underlying or proximal cause.
- Injuries take precedence over medical causes of deaths. That is, a person may have a preexisting condition that was the terminal event (multisystem organ failure or cardiac arrest);

DHEC
PROMOTE PROTECT PROSPER

Supplemental Report of Medical Certification of Death
Public Health Statistics and Information Services

Death Certificate No.: ____________
(State Office Use Only)

Name of Deceased: ______________________ Age: ______
Date of Death: ____________ County of Death: ____________ Sex: _____ Race: _____

Reason for supplemental information:

_____ Autopsy Findings.
_____ Additional information for Classifying Cause of Death.
_____ Other, specify: ____________
_____ Cause of Death Pending on Original Certificate.
_____ Requested by physician/coroner/medical examiner.
_____ Manner of death and/or accident information.

CAUSE OF DEATH

ITEMS 24-28 MUST BE COMPLETED BY PERSON WHO PRONOUNCES OR CERTIFIES DEATH	24. DATE PRONOUNCED DEAD (MM/DD/YYYY)	25. TIME PRONOUNCED DEAD
26. SIGNATURE OF PERSON PRONOUNCING DEATH (Only when applicable)	27. LICENSE NUMBER	28. DATE SIGNED (MM/DD/YYYY)
29. ACTUAL OR PRESUMED DATE OF DEATH (MM/DD/YYYY)	30. ACTUAL OR PRESUMED TIME OF DEATH	31. WAS CORONER OR MEDICAL EXAMINER CONTACTED? ☐ Yes ☐ No

CAUSE OF DEATH (See instructions and examples)

32. PART I. Enter the chain of events-disease, injuries, or complications-that directly caused the death. DO NOT enter terminal events such as cardiac arrest, respiratory arrest, or ventricular fibrillation without showing the etiology. DO NOT ABBREVIATE. Enter only one cause on a line. Add additional lines if necessary.

Approximate interval: Onset to death

IMMEDIATE CAUSE (Final disease or condition resulting in death) a. ____________ ______
Due to (or as a consequence of):
Sequentially list conditions, if any, leading to the cause listed on line a. Enter the UNDERLYING CAUSE (disease or injury that initiated the events resulting in death) LAST
b. ____________ ______
Due to (or as a consequence of):
c. ____________ ______
Due to (or as a consequence of):
d. ____________ ______

To Be Completed By: MEDICAL CERTIFIER

PART II. Enter other significant conditions contributing to death but not resulting in the underlying cause given in PART I.

33. WAS AN AUTOPSY PERFORMED? ☐ Yes ☐ No

34. WERE AUTOPSY FINDINGS AVAILABLE TO COMPLETE THE CAUSE OF DEATH? ☐ Yes ☐ No

35. DID TOBACCO USE CONTRIBUTE TO DEATH?
☐ Yes ☐ Probably
☐ No ☐ Unknown

36. IF FEMALE:
☐ Not pregnant within past year
☐ Pregnant at time of death
☐ Not pregnant, but pregnant within 42 days of death
☐ Not pregnant, but pregnant 43 days to one year before death
☐ Unknown if pregnant within the past year

37. MANNER OF DEATH
☐ Natural ☐ Homicide
☐ Accident ☐ Pending investigation
☐ Suicide ☐ Could not be determined

38. DATE OF INJURY (MM/DD/YYYY)	39. TIME OF INJURY	40. PLACE OF INJURY (e.g., Decedant's construction site, restaurant, wooded area)	41. INJURY AT WORK? ☐ Yes ☐ No

42. LOCATION OF INJURY: State: City or Town: County:
Street & Number: Apartment Number: Zip Code:

43. DESCRIBE HOW INJURY OCCURRED:

44. IF TRANSPORTATION INJURY, SPECIFY:
☐ Driver/Operator ☐ Pedestrian
☐ Passenger ☐ Other (Specify) ______

*Additional information requested:

After the completion of the autopsy, toxicology and investigation, complete the Cause of Death and items 33 - 37 above. If this is a traumatic death, then you MUST complete items 38 -44 above.

______________________ / ____________
Signature and Title of Certifying Officer Date Signed

(State Office Use Only)
Death certificate updated pursuant to SC Reg. 61-19.
Section 18(f) ____________ ______
____
(Nosologist)

DHEC 627 (03/2009)

FIGURE 3.6 Supplemental death certificate information – Medical examiner.

however, in the case of trauma, the documentation may state, "Had it not been for the traumatic event," this death would not have occurred at this time.

- Examples of COD section:
  - Exsanguination due to multiple stab wounds
  - Liver failure due to complications of sepsis, secondary to blunt force trauma

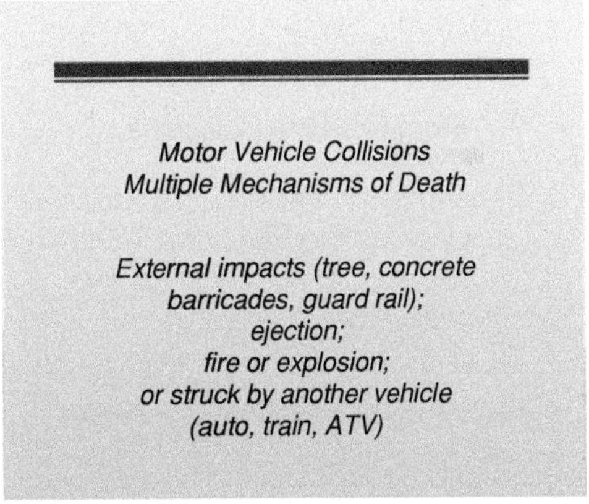

Motor Vehicle Collisions
Multiple Mechanisms of Death

External impacts (tree, concrete
barricades, guard rail);
ejection;
fire or explosion;
or struck by another vehicle
(auto, train, ATV)

FIGURE 3.7   Point to ponder: Motor vehicle collisions with multiple mechanisms of death resulting in multiple COD options.

(16) Mechanism of Death: The mechanism of death is the changes in physiology and biochemistry or the agent used to cause death. A particular mechanism can result in a variety of CODs. For example, a knife (mechanism) can cause exsanguination, a pneumothorax, or result in sepsis (See Figure 3.7).

(17) Manner of Death
   • A system used to classify the condition that resulted in the death, which explains how the COD arose through determining factors that set the circumstances into motion.
   • The five categories for MOD are: natural, accident, suicide, homicide, and undetermined (American Board of Medicolegal Death Investigators, 2015; Hammer, Moynihan & Pagliaro, 2013) (See Table 3.10).

(18) The medicolegal opinion about a COD/MOD should account for information such as medical history, circumstances surrounding the death, the crime scene investigation, the postmortem examination, tissue/organ analysis, laboratory analysis (i.e., blood, vitreous humor, cerebrospinal fluid, etc.), and interviews (Bader & Gabriel, 2010) (See Figures 3.8, 3.9, and 3.10).

Fetal Death Investigation

(1) Fetal death investigation and the role of the medicolegal death investigation system vary from state to state.

(2) Some jurisdictions do not consider a nonviable fetus to be a human, and thus, do not require any type of investigation surrounding a fetal demise.

(3) Other jurisdictions may set parameters by which fetal deaths must be investigated, such as gestation and/or weight of the fetus at the time of the demise.

TABLE 3.10 Manners of Death

Natural	Due to disease and/or the aging process
Homicide	Caused by the purposeful act of another; but is not necessarily "criminal"
Suicide	Caused by the purposeful act of self; may appear to be obvious, but can be difficult to differentiate between suicide and accidental
Accidental	Due to an injury in which the causes are not attributed to a purposeful act; may be associated with an act of omission or commission
Undetermined	Cannot be attributed to a specific manner of death to the exclusion of all other possible manners

(American Board of Medicolegal Death Investigators, 2015; Hammer, Moynihan, & Pagliaro, 2013)

Motor Vehicle Collisions

Depending on the circumstances surrounding the MVC, the MOD can be ruled an accident, suicide, homicide, or undetermined.

FIGURE 3.8   Motor vehicle collisions and manners of death.

(4) Some jurisdictions require that a representative of the healthcare facility in which the death occurred complete a Fetal Death Report.

(5) Fetal deaths, if within the statutory reporting guidelines, are then referred to the appropriate investigating agency.

(6) An MDI may be required to conduct a complete death investigation to determine if the cause of a fetal demise was the result of nonnatural circumstances, such as drug and/or alcohol consumption by the mother or assault on the mother that resulted in the fetal death.

(7) The MOD in fetal deaths due to nonnatural events may be classified as an accident, homicide, or undetermined. The consequences related to those determinations vary (American College of Obstetricians and Gynecologists, 2015; Centers for Disease Control and Prevention, 2013b).

Infant Death Investigation

(1) In 1992, the US Senate and the US House of Representatives recommended that a standard protocol be developed to investigate sudden unexplained infant deaths (SUID).

(2) The Sudden Unexplained Infant Death Investigation (SUIDI) Report Form was released in 1996 in the United States; other jurisdictions use similar (although jurisdictionally specific) forms.

(3) In 2003, the CDC convened a national workgroup to revise that form and develop training materials to be released nationally. The information put forth by the workgroup and the independent work of investigators around the country provides a detailed framework

Point to Ponder

Homicide is not necessarily illegal.
For example, a police officer who fatally shoots an offender during the commission of a crime has committed homicide, which may be deemed justifiable homicide after an investigation.

FIGURE 3.9   Point to ponder: Homicide.

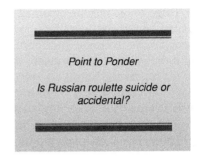

Point to Ponder

Is Russian roulette suicide or accidental?

FIGURE 3.10 Point to ponder: Manner of death.

for an MDI who investigates infant deaths (Centers for Disease Control and Prevention, 2014b).

Skeletal Remains

(1) Discovered bones, in most locales, are referred to the coroner or ME within the jurisdiction where the bones are recovered.
(2) The first step is to differentiate bone from nonbone.
(3) After determining that the item is bone, it must be ascertained if the bone is human or non-human.
(4) The case may need to be submitted to a forensic anthropologist to make a final determination.
(5) Once the remains are determined to be human, the coroner or the ME is responsible for trying to identify the individual.
(6) Skeletal remains that are unidentified should be evaluated to determine if a DNA sample may be obtained from the remains. This may be accomplished by submitting a sample to a forensic DNA laboratory that specializes in recovering DNA from skeletal remains (American College of Obstetricians and Gynecologists, 2015). Once a DNA profile is obtained, agencies will enter the profile information directly into the Federal Bureau of Investigations' (FBI) Combined DNA Index System plus Mito (CODIS+mito) database for comparison to antemortem data that may have been submitted to the National Crime Information Center (NCIC) (University of North Texas, 2007).

Identification of the Deceased

(1) Circumstantial/presumed identification
Visual identification may be performed by a family member or close friend who directly views the deceased or a photograph of the deceased. Other circumstantial identification used to narrow the search can be done with a physical description, including tattoos, scars, moles, piercings, physical deformities, and clothing/jewelry. In addition, personal identification found on the deceased may be used (Lynch & Duval, 2011).
(2) Scientific/positive identification
• A DNA sample may be obtained from an unidentified decedent for future comparison and determination of positive identification. A decedent's DNA may be compared to DNA samples from parents, siblings, and children. The samples may also be compared to other known DNA samples that belonged to a decedent (i.e., toothbrush, hairbrush). A DNA sample may be sent for analysis and comparison to the FBI's Combined DNA Index System (CODIS) or the National DNA Data Bank of Canada. To confirm identification, a specimen matching the deceased's DNA must already be in the DNA databank for a match to occur (Lynch & Duval, 2011). Many other jurisdictions within developed countries have access to similar systems. Currently, the International Criminal Police Organization (INTERPOL) is developing a missing and unidentified persons' registry, using information from police reports (Interpol, 2014).
• Fingerprints

Fingerprints may be obtained from a decedent and entered into the Integrated Automated Fingerprint Identification System (IAFIS) for comparison identification. No two people have the same fingerprints. Therefore, if the decedent's fingerprints were entered into the system prior to death, then making a positive identification from those fingerprints is possible. This is a relatively common and timely method for scientific identification, especially since it is not cost-prohibitive. Latent, visible, or molded fingerprints can also be used. This is the only scientific method that does not require a presumptive identification to execute. However, if no fingerprints are on file and a presumptive identification has been made, then latent prints can be lifted off personal items and compared to the deceased (Clark, Ernst, Hughlund, & Jentzen, 1996).

- Radiological Comparisons

  This requires ante- and postmortem records for comparison and confirmation of identification (Lynch & Duval, 2011). A radiologist or anthropologist may be required to confirm that the antemortem radiographs match the postmortem radiographs.

- Implanted Device

  Implanted medical devices, such as a pacemaker, breast implants, hip replacements, and so forth, contain identifying information on the device. Such information may be an identification number or a barcode that can then be compared to antemortem medical records and/or information provided by the company that manufactures the device.

- Dental Comparison

  Dental comparison requires ante- and postmortem records for comparison and confirmation of identification (Lynch & Duval, 2011). A forensic odontologist or anthropologist should conduct this type of comparison. Teeth last longer than any other body structures as they do not decompose and resist fire (Clark, Ernst, Hughlund, & Jentzen, 1996). As a result, dental comparison for identification may be the preferred method of identification for many types of deaths.

- Unidentified Persons

  If a decedent remains unidentified, investigators should consider entering the person's information into the National Missing and Unidentified Persons System (NamUS), the National DNA Data Bank of Canada, and/or INTERPOL, which are reporting and searching databases to assist in locating missing persons and identifying human remains (U.S. Department of Justice, Office of Justice Programs, n.d.).

Mass Fatality

The FNDI and other MDIs should be active participants in mass fatality planning and management.

(1) A mass fatality is defined as any incident that stresses the resources of a local community.

(2) Each community must evaluate its resources and develop a memorandum of agreement (MOA) with adjacent communities to establish protocols in the event that an incident occurs within a jurisdiction and depletes its resources.

(3) The Federal Emergency Management Administration (FEMA) developed the National Incident Management System (NIMS) to provide written guidelines for communities to ensure consistent communication (Federal Emergency Management Administration, 2015).

Disaster Mortuary Operational Response Team (DMORT)

(1) DMORT is a section of the Office of Preparedness and Operations that provides victim identification and mortuary services in response to mass fatality incidents where it has been requested and dispatched.

(2) These responsibilities may include:
- temporary morgue facilities;
- victim identification;
- forensic dental pathology;

- forensic anthropology methods;
- processing;
- preparation; and
- disposition of remains (U.S. Department of Health and Human Services, 2014).

Terrorism

(1) Force or violence used to coerce governments or populations with regard to political, social, or economic objectives.
(2) Usually carried out with the use of explosives; however, weapons of mass destruction (chemical, biological, or radiological devices) remain a global threat (Hammer, Moynihan, & Pagliaro, 2013).

Domestic Terrorism

Domestic terrorism involves violence that is directed toward citizens of a country or that country's infrastructure, often by persons who are citizens of or reside within that country. According to US code 18 U.S.C. §2331, "domestic terrorism" means activities with the following three characteristics:

- Involve acts dangerous to human life that violate federal or state law;
- Appear intended (i) to intimidate or coerce a civilian population; (ii) to influence the policy of a government by intimidation or coercion; or (iii) to affect the conduct of a government by mass destruction, assassination. or kidnapping; and
- Occur primarily within the territorial jurisdiction of the United States.

Regardless of country or jurisdiction, domestic terrorism is universal. Those terrorists who are not a part of a larger organization are referred to as lone wolves, stray dogs, or homegrown violent extremists.

Traumatic Deaths

(1) Traumatic deaths are sudden and can be violent, mutilating, or destructive and caused by multiple factors as shown in Table 3.11.
(2) Asphyxia is any factor that restricts blood flow or alters hemodynamics through inadequate delivery, uptake, and/or utilization of oxygen with carbon dioxide retention that may result in death.
    - Examples include, but are not limited to, drowning, hanging, strangulation, suffocation (including cosleeping with an infant [in some jurisdictions]), choking, positional, autoerotic, burking, throttling, the choking game, or compression asphyxia.
(3) History that increases the incidence of violent death includes:
    - child abuse and neglect;
    - poverty or living in overcrowded conditions;
    - unemployment and financial issues;
    - parent or caretaker has a history of being a victim of abuse;
    - IPV;
    - inability to care for self (physically and/or cognitively);
    - substance abuse (alcohol and/or drugs);
    - depression and mental health issues of the decedent, parent, or caretaker;
    - criminal behavior/record;
    - isolation and/or lack of support;
    - inability to handle stress or feeling overburdened;
    - gang affiliation;
    - extremist or terrorist affiliation; or
    - risk-taking behaviors (James & Nordby, 2005; Lynch & Duval, 2011).

TABLE 3.11 Traumatic Deaths

Mechanical	Sharp	Stabbing, sword, knife
	Blunt	Motor vehicle collision, baseball bat, gunshot
Chemical	Overdose	Drugs or alcohol
	Poison	Cyanide
	Carbon monoxide	
Electrical	Electrocution	Malfunctioning electrical circuits or wiring
	Electrical burns	Lighting
	Lightning strike	
Thermal	Hypothermia	Common in alcohol abuse
	Hyperthermia	Infant left in an enclosed car, or elderly without air conditioning
	Thermal burns	

(James & Nordby, 2005; Lynch & Duval, 2011)

National Violent Death Reporting System

(1) The National Violent Death Reporting System (NVDRS), maintained by the CDC, gathers data on violent deaths from 18 states (Hanzlick, 2007) (See Table 3.12). As defined by NVDRS, a violent death results from intentional force used by oneself or another person(s). This includes acts of omission or neglect, if perpetrated by a parent or caretaker.

(2) The NVDRS also tracks unintentional firearm, terrorism-related, and undetermined or indeterminate MODs (if force or power was involved in the death).

(3) The NVDRS has inclusion and exclusion criteria for homicides that it tracks (Centers for Disease Control and Prevention, 2004).

CONCEPTS AND ISSUES

Concepts and issues in forensic nursing and death investigations include emerging practices in education, associations, and injury prevention programs.

Emerging Practices

(1) Education
   • Advanced Forensic Nurse-Board Certification (AFN-BC): A nurse who holds a graduate degree can obtain a certification through portfolio with a death investigation focus. The American Nurses Credentialing Center, in conjunction with content expert appraisers from

TABLE 3.12 NVDRS Homicides

Includes	Excludes
Self-defense homicide	Vehicular homicide if there is no intent (such as a distracted or inebriated driver)
Prenatal violence that results in the infant's death after birth	Fetal deaths that result from violence
Fatal heart attack occurring while person is being threatened or assaulted	War
Deaths resulting from threatening or injuring even without intent to kill	Legal executions

(Centers for Disease Control and Prevention, 2013a)

the International Association of Forensic Nurses, offers this credential (American Nurses Credentialing Center, 2014).

- MDI Training Course: Basic training and master's courses are available, based on the 29 components of the National Institutes of Justice's publication *Death Investigation: A Guide for the Scene Investigator* (Saint Louis University School of Medicine, 2015).
- American Board of Medicolegal Death Investigators: The American Board of Medicolegal Death Investigators (ABMDI) offers two certifications: basic (Registry Certification) and advanced (Board Certification). This certification is based on the 29 components of the National Institutes of Justice's publication, *Death Investigation: A Guide for the Scene Investigator* (American Board of Medicolegal Death Investigators, 2015).
- *Forensic Nurse Death Investigator Education Guidelines*: In 2009, the IAFN provided didactic and clinical preceptorship guidelines; however, the Association does not currently offer a certification in death investigation.
- As forensic science and DSIs improve and expand, educational issues arise, such as qualifications of FNDI instructors, credentialing, and/or certification.
- The IAFN has recommended an FNDI faculty requirement of 600 hours of experience and practice in medicolegal death investigations (International Association of Forensic Nurses, 2014).

(2) Associations

A nurse seeking a career within the field of death investigation needs to be familiar with the various associations and align him/herself with applicable groups to engage in networking, serve on boards and committees, intern, and/or seek office.

- International Association of Forensic Nurses (IAFN)

This association is an "international membership organization comprised of forensic nurses working around the world and other professionals who support and compliment the work of forensic nursing." Its mission is "to provide leadership in forensic nursing practices by developing, promoting, and disseminating information internationally about forensic nursing science." In conjunction with the American Nurses Association, the IAFN publishes *Forensic Nursing: Scope and Standards of Practice* (International Association of Forensic Nurses, American Nurses Association, 2009).

- International Association of Coroners and Medical Examiners

The International Association of Coroners and MEs (IAC&ME) is "committed to advancing the accurate determination of the cause and the MOD through the utilization of science, medicine and the law" (International Association of Coroners and Medical Examiners, 2013).

- American Academy of Forensic Sciences

"The American Academy of Forensic Sciences (AAFS) is a professional society dedicated to the application of science to the law and is committed to the promotion of education and the elevation of accuracy, precision, and specificity in the forensic sciences" (American Academy of Forensic Sciences, 2014).

- National Association of Medical Examiners

"The National Association of Medical Examiners (NAME) is the national professional organization of physician MEs, MDIs, and death investigation system administrators who perform the official duties of the medicolegal investigation of deaths of public interest in the United States. NAME was founded in 1966 with the dual purposes of fostering the professional growth of physician death investigators and disseminating the professional and technical information vital to the continuing improvement of the medical investigation of violent, suspicious and unusual deaths" (National Association of Medical Examiner's [NAME], 2014).

- International Association for Identification

"The International Association for Identification (IAI) is a professional membership organization comprised of individuals worldwide who work in the field of forensic identification" (International Association for Identification, 2014).

- Jurisdictional Coroner/ME Associations
  Many jurisdictions have coroner and/or ME associations whose missions are to support the coroners and/or MEs in their respective states through education and training; provide resources to assist in death investigations; develop strategies to prevent loss of life; and render support when requested to aid in the timely resolution of death investigations.

(3) Injury Prevention Programs
  - Injury Prevention Programs were developed after reviewing national statistics on morbidity and mortality.
  - Using a public health approach, the CDC established the CDC's Injury Center, which is devoted to injury and violence prevention.
  - In the United States, a person dies every 3 minutes due to injury, and countless others are injured and disabled (Centers for Disease Control and Prevention, 2014a). A global perspective on death rate cannot be accurate in light of countries that do not track this data; however, jurisdictions in developed countries should be able to access data that is relative to the area of authority. The World Health Organization also tracks death data, an example of which can be found at: http://www.who.int/whr/2004/annex/topic/en/annex_2_en.pdf?ua=1.
  - Violence and injuries are the leading causes of death for ages 1 to 44 years and cost more than $406 billion dollars annually (Centers for Disease Control and Prevention, 2014a).
  - Injury prevention programs have brought about changes, such as seatbelt laws; suicide prevention programs; sudden unexplained infant death/sudden infant death syndrome awareness and prevention through the Back-to-Sleep Campaign; and concussion, fall, and prescription overdose awareness.
  - When discussing injury prevention, deaths are categorized as intentional or unintentional.
  - Intentional injuries are those that are self-inflicted (suicide) or inflicted by another person (homicide).
  - Injury prevention efforts are aimed at eliminating or reducing the occurrence of intentional and unintentional injuries.

Ethics

Death, regardless of circumstances, affects numerous families, friends, and communities in a variety of manners. The MDI must be cognizant of ethical issues in areas such as notification of the next-of-kin; organ and tissue donations; and mandatory and voluntary reporting requirements.

(1) Ethics for nurses practicing medicolegal death investigation are guided by:
  - *Forensic Nursing: Scope and Standards of Practice;*
  - Nurse Practice Act (State Board of Nursing) or similar acts in jurisdictions across the globe;
  - Nightingale Pledge;
  - affiliations or association memberships;
  - applicable credentialing guidelines;
  - policy and practice of employers;
  - International Council of Nurses (ICN) *Code of Ethics for Nurses;* and
  - International Association of Forensic Nurses (IAFN) *Vision of Ethical Practice.*

(2) Death Notification to Next-of-Kin
  - In-person notification is the preferred method for notifying the next-of-kin of a death. Phone notification may be needed if the next-of-kin is not geographically close and/or no cross-jurisdictional support is available.
  - Identifying the next-of-kin may present obstacles, especially if the event was unwitnessed. Methods include (but are not limited to): use of databases (birth, marriage, and department of motor vehicles); an occurrence in which employment is known can involve the human resources department or checking a health insurance card and contacting the listed

physician. In addition, specific programs assist with contacting relatives, such as File of Life for the older adult population or the use of the "in case of emergency" listing on a cell phone.

- Notification should be done in a timely manner and the agency responsible for making the death notification must follow protocol and ensure that the correct individual is being notified. The order of notification varies between jurisdictions; however, the general order is spouse, children, parents, siblings, grandparents, aunts/uncles, and then cousins.
- Once the individual(s) have been notified, they should be provided with truthful information regarding the known or anticipated COD, the MOD, the investigative process, the autopsy schedule and results (if applicable), available support services, and appropriate agency contact information.
- The next-of-kin may be provided with information regarding the possibility of organ and tissue donation (National Institute of Justice, 2009).
- A death notification conducted in person also provides investigative insight and information, which may assist in a COD or MOD determination. The individual providing a death notification at the decedent's known residence may request to see the decedent's residence to gain additional investigative information.
- Whether a death investigation is ongoing or completed, the nurse should refer families to support services and resources. Family and friends may benefit from the following referrals:
  - grief counseling;
  - support groups;
  - social services;
  - faith-based support groups;
  - advocacy organizations; and
  - survivor organizations.
- Referrals can have a positive impact on prevention and increase public education campaigns directed at preventing premature death.

(3) Organ and Tissue Donation
- The Health Resources and Services Administration or other similar organizations oversee organ donations.
- Nurses must familiarize themselves with healthcare, nursing, and forensic standards; ethical codes; restrictions; and policies and procedures.
- The decedent's driver's license may list the person as a donor.
- Coroners and MEs may have the authority to deny organ donation if the donation interferes with a death investigation and/or autopsy.
- Organs must be perfused in order to transplant and must be used within 6 to 72 hours after removal.
- Skin, heart valves, corneas, ligaments, tendons, and cartilage can be donated and stored for later use.
- National Organ Transplantation Act of 1984 (Health and Resource Services Administration, 2014) or jurisdictional equivalent.

(4) Mandatory and Voluntary Reporting
- Nurses should be aware of the types of deaths that must be reported to other investigating agencies and cases in which the death should be reported for legal and professional reasons and to assist with public health and prevention efforts.
- Child Protective Services
- The National Transportation Safety Board (NTSB) is the agency to which transportation deaths related to aircraft and trains must be reported (Federal Emergency Management Administration, 2015).
- Occupational Safety and Health Administration (OSHA) or the jurisdictional equivalent is the agency to which work-related deaths must be reported (Occupational Safety and Health Administration, 2015).

- Med Watch, the FDA (Food and Drug Administration) Safety Information and Adverse Reporting System, is the voluntary reporting agency to which fatal, adverse effects of medication can be reported (U.S. Food and Drug Administration, 2014).
- Licensing boards: respective boards to which licensed professionals (physicians, nurses, and pharmacists) are reported for violations of practice acts.
- The Joint Commission (JC) or the jurisdictional equivalent is the organization to which preventable, hospital-related deaths are reported (http://www.jointcommission.org/).
- National Violent Death Reporting System (NVDRS) takes reports on deaths that meet one of the following criteria (not an exhaustive listing):
  - burns over 5% of the body (required in some jurisdictions);
  - deaths that are sudden or unexpected;
  - accidental;
  - result of violence (suicide or homicide);
  - toxic agents;
  - alcohol;
  - elder neglect/abuse deaths;
  - child neglect/abuse deaths (which may include lack of properly restraining a child in a vehicle; not providing a flotation device; lack of helmet or supervision);
  - firearm deaths;
  - person in custody of law enforcement or in a correctional facility;
  - patients in a nursing home or private institution who have not been under medical care (usually within the last 48 to 72 hours);
  - associated with malpractice or any medical procedure or treatment;
  - occupational;
  - unattended;
  - neglected;
  - stillbirth greater than 20 weeks that is unattended by medical personnel;
  - death during pregnancy and up to 6 weeks' postpartum;
  - infant and/or child without a medical condition in which death is expected;
  - some infections and contagious diseases; or
  - mass fatalities (Centers for Disease Control and Prevention, 2013a).

FUTURE ISSUES

Forensic nurses caring for the deceased need to practice nursing in a sensitive, cross-cultural manner; collaborate; and integrate issues, concepts, practices, findings, and prevention strategies internationally. As the subspecialties within the forensic sciences have expanded, so have the educational and clinical opportunities for the role as an MDI. Despite one's training and expertise, it is imperative to expand one's clinical skills, participate in continuing education, seek seasoned mentors, and stay abreast of current evidence-based practice. Nurses entering into medicolegal death investigations can further evidence-based practice and research.

As forensic nurses move into the role of the MDI, preferably as a nurse coroner, an FNDI, or a board-certified AFN, it would be prudent to develop a strategic, work, and/or business plan that highlights the ways in which nurses can uniquely contribute and lead the way in the multidisciplinary collaboration of death investigations. Plans may be comprehensive and address multiple issues, or may focus on a specific area. Examples include:

(1) Developing a curriculum to instruct coroners in basic medical principles to enhance physical assessment and examination skills;
(2) Developing evaluation and quality improvement tools;
(3) Performing translational research;
(4) Leading the standardization of medicolegal death investigations; and

(5) Developing computerized databases for epidemiological studies, public health interventions and preventions, and continued quality assurance (NAME, 2014; National Research Council of the National Academy of Sciences, 2009);

(6) Developing a certification examination for FNDIs;

(7) Serving as a mentor;

(8) Developing standardized protocols to decrease discrepancies between agencies and jurisdictions; and

(9) Collaborating on legal reforms in death investigation systems.

CASE STUDIES

CASE STUDY #1

A mother finds her 5-month-old infant unresponsive in the crib and calls 9-1-1. The EMS responds and transports the infant in full arrest to the emergency department (ED), where life-saving techniques are attempted to no avail and the infant is pronounced dead. The FNDI responds to the ED and conducts an initial postmortem assessment, finding a clean, well-nourished infant of appropriate size (length and weight) and no apparent signs of trauma. The FNDI and a detective from the local law enforcement agency interview the mother, who rode in the ambulance. The FNDI and the detective also interview the ED physician, who denies any signs of trauma and reports that the infant likely died from sudden infant death syndrome (SIDS). The detective believes that the death is due to SIDS and plans to close the case. Accompanied by a law enforcement official and the decedent's mother, the FNDI returns to the incident location to gather more information about the circumstances surrounding the death. The FNDI completes a sudden, unexpected infant death investigation (SUIDI) Reporting Form with scene reenactment photos. The incident scene investigation reveals empty bottles of methadone located in the refrigerator and an additional bottle that is located in close proximity to the infant's crib. The infant's bottle and the empty methadone bottles are taken into evidence.

The FNDI schedules the infant for autopsy, which does not reveal an anatomical or genetic cause of death. Toxicology results reveal that the infant had a toxic level of methadone. The cause of death is classified as toxic effects of methadone and the manner as homicide. The FNDI and the detective reinterview the mother and she admits to using methadone to soothe the baby and help with teething pain.

CASE STUDY #2

At 0300 hours, the FNDI is notified of a traffic-related fatality and responds to the incident location along with local law enforcement officials. The investigation reveals that the unrestrained driver was traveling west on a two-lane road when the driver lost control of the vehicle and struck a tree on the side of the road.

The decedent is a 20-year-old White male, who, according to the driver's license in his back pocket, lived in a different part of town. Blunt force trauma and what appear to be deep, extensive incisions (as opposed to lacerations) are present on the anterior lower arms. (All areas of trauma will be extensively documented and photographed during autopsy, although the FNDI should thoroughly note any observations, complete a body diagram, and ensure that scene photographs are obtained.) The scene investigation reveals no skid or tire marks. The scene, automobile, and decedent are photographed; a scene diagram is sketched, and a written report is generated. No witnesses are present to interview.

After confirming the identity of the decedent through the driver's license and the Department of Motor Vehicles, the FNDI and the law enforcement officer respond to the decedent's address to make the death notification to the next-of-kin. After briefing the family, the FNDI asks to see the decedent's bedroom. The FNDI enters the room to find a box cutter, a bloody towel, and a suicide note. The family reports that his girlfriend broke up with him the day prior and that he was "very depressed." The family members were unaware that he had left the residence until the FNDI made the death notification.

Photographs, a sketch, and the written report detailing the decedent's bedroom (box cutter, bloody towel, and suicide note), along with the suicide note are taken to the autopsy site and the chain of evidence is signed over to the forensic pathologist.

REVIEW QUESTIONS

1. To be viable for transplant, organs must be perfused and used within:
   a. 24 hours.
   b. 48 hours.
   c. 72 hours.
   d. 96 hours.

2. The Model Post-Mortem Examination Act (1954) recommends a forensic examination in all of the following types of cases except the:
   a. death of an older adult.
   b. death of a prisoner.
   c. threat to public safety.
   d. violent death.

3. Which entity is responsible for conducting a civil investigation of child abuse and neglect?
   a. Child protective services
   b. Coroner
   c. Law enforcement
   d. ME

4. A coroner can (usually) do all of the following except:
   a. conduct a death scene investigation.
   b. determine the COD/MOD.
   c. issue a subpoena.
   d. perform an autopsy.

5. Toddlers are at an increased risk of death from all of the following except:
   a. asphyxiation.
   b. falls.
   c. fire.
   d. poisoning.

6. Examples of asphyxia include all of the following except:
   a. compression.
   b. drowning.
   c. positional.
   d. sudden infant death syndrome.

7. Under specific guidelines, an autopsy can be performed without permission from the next-of-kin.
   a. True
   b. False

8. Livor mortis is:
   a. a temporary stiffening of the muscles after death.
   b. also known as lividity.
   c. fixed and nonblanchable over time.
   d. the pooling and settling of blood in dependent areas.

9. The triggering event that initiates a continuous sequence of events resulting in death is referred to as the:
   a. cause of death.
   b. manner of death.
   c. mechanism of death.
   d. proximate cause of death.

10. Which of the following is not a manner of death?
   a. Accidental
   b. Intentional
   c. Suicide
   d. Undetermined

DISCUSSION QUESTIONS

1. What are the five categories of manner of death?
2. Name and define five types of traumatic deaths.
3. Differentiate between cause of death, proximate cause of death, mechanism of death, and manner of death.
4. Differentiate between circumstantial (presumed) identification and scientific (positive) identification.
5. Describe cases that fall within the various mandatory reporting guidelines.
6. List the stages of mortis, the associated findings, and the time frame for each stage.
7. Identify skin changes at death that can indicate the cause of death.
8. Discuss how to effectively conduct a death scene investigation.
9. Describe the disciplines that interact during a death scene investigation and their roles.
10. Describe risk factors for premature death that are associated with various ages and groups.

REFERENCES

American Academy of Forensic Sciences. (2014). *About American Academy of Forensic Sciences.* Retrieved from http://aafs.org/about/about-aafs

American Bar Association, Office for Victims of Crime. (2005). *Elder abuse fatality review teams: A replication manual.* Retrieved from http://apps.americanbar.org/aging/publications/docs/fatalitymanual.pdf

American Board of Medicolegal Death Investigators. (2015). *Welcome to ABMDI.* Retrieved from http://www.abmdi.org/

American Board of Pathology. (n.d.). *Pathway.* Retrieved from http://www.abpath.org/ (password protected, must be a member).

American College of Obstetricians and Gynecologists. (2015). *National fetal infant mortality review program.* Retrieved from http://www.nfimr.org/

American Nurses Credentialing Center. (2014). *Advanced forensic nurse.* Retrieved from http://www.nursecredentialing.org/Certification/NurseSpecialties/ForensicNursingAdvanced.html

Bader, G. M., & Gabriel, S. (2010). *Forensic nursing: A concise manual.* Boca Raton, FL: Taylor & Francis CRC Press.

Bailey, R. (2014). *Biology prefixes and suffixes.* Retrieved from http://biology.about.com/od/prefixesandsuffixes1/g/prefixauto.htm

Byrd, J. H. (2013). *Forensic entomology.* Retrieved from http://www.forensicentomology.com/info.htm.

Centers for Disease Control and Prevention. (2003). *Medical examiners' and coroners' handbook on death registration and fetal death reporting: 2003 revision.* Hyattsville, MD: US Department of Health and Human Services.

Centers for Disease Control and Prevention. (2004). *Instructions for completing the cause-of- death section of the death certificate.* Hyattsville, MD: US Department of Health and Human Services. Retrieved from http://www.cdc.gov/nchs/data/dvs/blue_form.pdf

Centers for Disease Control and Prevention. (2012). *Death certificate.* Retrieved from http://www.cdc.gov/nchs/nvss/vital_certificate_revisions.htm

Centers for Disease Control and Prevention. (2013a). *National violent death reporting system.* Retrieved from http://www.cdc.gov/ViolencePrevention/NVDRS/index.html

Centers for Disease Control and Prevention. (2013b). *WISQARS database*. Retrieved from http://webappa.cdc.gov/sasweb/ncipc/leadcaus10_us.html

Centers for Disease Control and Prevention. (2014a). *Injury and violence prevention and control*. Retrieved from http://www.cdc.gov/injury/

Centers for Disease Control and Prevention. (2014b). *Sudden unexpected infant death initiative*. Atlanta, GA: Centers for Disease Control and Prevention. Retrieved from http://www.cdc.gov/sids/suidabout.htm

Clark, S. C., Ernst, M. F., Hughlund, W. D., & Jentzen, J. M. (1996). *MDI: A systematic training program for the professional death investigator*. Big Rapids, MI: Organizational Research & Assessment.

Elrouby, F. A. (2013). The medicolegal aspect of antemortem and postmortem eye examination. *J Forensic Odonto-stomatol.*, 31(suppl 1), 137.

Federal Emergency Management Administration. (2015). *National incident management system*. Retrieved from http://www.fema.gov/national-incident-management-system

Hammer, R. M., Moynihan, B., & Pagliaro, E. M. (2013). *Forensic nursing*. Sudbury, MA: Jones & Bartlett Publishers.

R. L. Hanzlick (Ed.). (1997). *Cause-of-death statements and certification of natural and unnatural deaths*. Northfield: IL: College of American Pathologists. Retrieved from https://netforum.avectra.com/temp/ClientImages/NAME/8c58e7e9-b2fa-44a9–8d1b-3085cd14bf25.pdf

Hanzlick, R. L. (2007). *Death investigation: Systems and procedures*. Boca Raton, FL: CRC Press.

Health and Resource Services Administration. (2014). *National Organ Transplantation Act of 1984*. Retrieved from http://optn.transplant.hrsa.gov/policiesAndBylaws/nota.asp

International Association of Coroners and Medical Examiners. (2013). *Home*. Retrieved from http://www.theiacme.com

International Association of Forensic Nurses, American Nurses Association. (2009). *Forensic nursing: Scope and standards of practice*. Silver Spring, MD: Nursesbooks.org. Retrieved from http://www.nursingworld.org/Homepage-Category/NursingInsider/Archive_1/2009-NI/July09NI/Co-Published-Standards-Forensic-Nursing.aspx

International Association of Forensic Nurses. (2014). *Forensic nurse investigator guidelines*. Elkridge. MD: International Association of Forensic Nurses. Retrieved from http://c.ymcdn.com/sites/www.forensicnurses.org/resource/resmgr/About/FNDI_Flyer_2014-FIN-PQ.pdf?hhSearchTerms = %22FNDI%22

International Association for Identification. (2014). *International Association for Identification mission statement*. Retrieved from http://www.theiai.org/about/index.php

Interpol. (2014). *Interpol*. Retrieved from http://www.interpol.int/INTERPOL-expertise/Forensics/DVI-Pages/Database-of-missing-persons-and-unidentified-bodies

Iserson, K. V. (2003). *Macmillan encyclopedia of death and dying*. New York, NY: Macmillan Publishing.

James, S. H., & Nordby, J. J. (2005). *Forensic science*. Boca Raton, FL: CRC Press Taylor & Francis.

Journal of Forensic Odonto-stomatology. (2014). The medicolegal aspect of antemortem and postmortem eye examination, p. 137.

Libow, L. S., & Neufeld, R. R. (2008). The autopsy and the elderly patient in the hospital and the nursing home: Enhancing the quality of life. *Geriatrics, 63*(12), 14–18.

Lynch, V. A., & Duval, J. B. (2011). *Forensic nursing*. St. Louis, MO: Elsevier/Mosby.

Marshall, T. K., & Hoare, F. E. (1962). Estimating the time of death: The rectal cooling after death and its mathematical expression. *Journal of Forensic Sciences, 7*(1), 56–81.

Michigan Public Health Institute. (2013). *National Center for the Review and Prevention of Child Deaths*. Retrieved from http://childdeathreview.org/

National Association of Medical Examiners (NAME). (2014). *About NAME*. Retrieved from http://www.thename.org

National Association of Medical Examiners. (n.d.). *National Association of Medical Examiners web site*. Retrieved from http://www.thename.org

National Coalition for Homeless. (2012). *Hate crimes against the homeless: An organizing manual for concerned citizens*. Washington, DC: National Coalition for Homeless. Retrieved from http://www.nationalhomeless.org/publications/hatecrimes/hatecrimesmanual12.pdf

National Guidelines for Death Investigators. (1997). *Research report*. Washington, DC: U.S. Department of Justice.

National Institute of Justice. (2009). *A guide to death scene investigation: Establishing and recording decedent profile information*. Retrieved from http://beta.nij.gov/topics/law-enforcement/investigations/crime-scene/guides/death-investigation/Pages/decedent-profile.aspx

National Research Council of the National Academy of Sciences. (2009). *Strengthening forensic science in the United States: A path forward*. Washington, DC: National Academies Press. Available from https://www.ncjrs.gov/pdffiles1/nij/grants/228091.pdf

New York State Office for the Prevention of Domestic Violence. (2011). *National data on intimate partner violence*. Retrieved from http://www.opdv.state.ny.us/statistics/nationaldvdata/nationaldvdata.pdf

Occupational Safety and Health Administration. (2015). *Worker fatalities reported to federal and state OSHA*. Retrieved from https://www.osha.gov/dep/fatcat/dep_fatcat.html

O'Hear, M. (2013). The troubled history of death investigation in America. [Life sentences blog]. Retrieved from http://www.lifesentenceblog.com/? = 6414

O'Neal, B. (2007). *Investigating infant deaths*. Boca Raton, FL: CRC Press.

Palmiere, C., & Mangin, P. (2012). Postmortem chemistry update, Part I. *International Journal of Legal Medicine*, *126*(2), 187–198.

Prentice, N., & Arnold, R. M. (2006). *Fast Fact and Concept #155: Completing a Death Certificate*. End of Life/Palliative Education Research Center, New York, NY. Retrieved from http://www.eperc.mcw.edu/EPERC/FastFactsIndex/ff_155.htm

Preservation of Evidence Act, Title 17, Chapter 28 of the South Carolina Code of Laws. (2013). Retrieved from http://www.scstatehouse.gov/code/t17c028.php

Saint Louis University School of Medicine. (2015). *Medicolegal death investigator training course – MLDIC*. Retrieved from http://medschool.slu.edu/mldi/

Stanford Medical School. (2006). *End of life curriculum project*. Retrieved from http://endoflife.stanford.edu/M06_last48hr/signs_imp_death.htm

Skopp, G. (2010). Postmortem toxicology. *Forensic Science, 6*(4), 314–325.

Tousignant, D. D. (1991). Why suspects confess. *FBI Law Enforcement Bulletin, 60*(3), 14–18.

University of North Texas. (2007). *Center of human identification*. Retrieved from http://www.hsc.unt.edu/departments/pathology_anatomy/dna/Forensics/Initiative/Initiativ e.cfm

U.S. Department of Health and Human Services. (2005). *Health information privacy: When does the privacy rule allow covered entities to disclose protected health information to law enforcement officials?* Retrieved from http://www.hhs.gov/ocr/privacy/hipaa/faq/disclosures_for_law_enforcement_purposes/505.html

U.S. Department of Health and Human Services. (2013). *Health information privacy: Health information of deceased individuals*. Retrieved from http://www.hhs.gov/ocr/privacy/hipaa/understanding/coveredentities/decedents.html

U.S. Department of Health and Human Services. (2014). *Disaster mortuary operation response teams (DMORTs)*. Retrieved from http://www.phe.gov/Preparedness/responders/ndms/teams/Pages/dmort.aspx

U.S. Department of Justice, Office of Justice Programs. (n.d.). *National missing and unidentified persons system*. Retrieved from http://www.namus.gov/about.htm

U.S. Fire Administration, Federal Emergency Management Administration. (1994). *Firefighter autopsy protocol*. Washington, DC: U.S. Fire Administration. Retrieved from http://www.usfa.fema.gov/downloads/pdf/publications/fa-156.pdf

U.S. Food and Drug Administration. (2014). *MedWatch: The FDA safety information and adverse event reporting program*. Retrieved from http://www.fda.gov/Safety/MedWatch/

Venes, D., & Taber, C. W. (2013). *Taber's cyclopedic medical dictionary* (22nd ed.). Philadelphia, PA: F.A. Davis Publishing.

Westphal, S. E., Apitzsch, J., Penzkofer, T., Mahnken, A. H., & Knüchel, R. l. (2012). Virtual CT autopsy in clinical pathology: Feasibility in clinical autopsies. *Virchows Archives, 461*(2), 211–219.

World Health Organization. (2015). *Health statistics and information systems: Maternal mortality ratio (per 100 000 live births)*. Retrieved from http://www.who.int/healthinfo/statistics/indmaternalmortality/en/

CHAPTER 4

Forensic Mental Health Nursing

Norah Sullivan
Ashley Smith

OBJECTIVES

At the completion of this chapter, the learner will be able to:

- Differentiate forensic mental health nursing (FMHN) from corrections nursing and areas where practice may overlap.
- Identify key nursing and psychiatric theories used in FMHN.
- Describe specific, vulnerable populations that FMH nurses are likely to encounter in practice.
- Distinguish specific skill sets essential for FMHN practice.
- Recognize core concepts for mastery by FMH nurses.
- Discuss the unique challenges with patients and appropriate interventions for FMH nurses.
- Articulate multiple FMHN interventions.
- Recognize ethical dilemmas that FMH nurses may encounter in practice.
- Articulate gaps in research pertaining to FHMN.
- Identify developing roles and appropriate settings for FMHN practice.
- Discuss the interface with other systems required in various FMHN settings.

KEY TERMS

Countertransference: The clinician's response to the projected emotions of the patient.

Forensic mental health nursing and forensic psychiatric nursing: These terms are often used interchangeably. In this chapter, we use "forensic mental health nursing" as it applies more globally to the role.

Mental health treatment team: A cohort of multidisciplinary providers who collaborate on the development and delivery of psychiatric care. The team typically consists of a psychiatrist, nurse, social worker, and psychologist.

Therapeutic alliance: The establishment of a relationship with the patient that forms the basis of FMHN. It is patient-centered a used tool to move the patient toward disclosure, self-evaluation, process of change, and planning for the future.

Transference: The displacement of emotions from a past relationship onto the current treatment provider, erecting a barrier to the development of a functional therapeutic alliance.

INTRODUCTION

Forensic mental health nursing focuses on the treatment of individuals who are involved with the legal system and who suffer from mental illness that impacts their status and functioning within the legal system or has played a role in their commission of a crime (Mason, 2011; Mullen, 2000). Although FMHN is a unique specialty, it shares characteristics with other types of nursing, including corrections nursing and psychiatric nursing in correctional settings. Unlike those specialties, however, which focus solely on perpetrators of crime, FMHN focuses on two patient populations: perpetrators and victims of a crime. Perpetrators comprise the first and most common FMHN patient population. These individuals may or may not be detained in prisons or jails; they are typically housed in a separate psychiatric facility. The victims of crime who comprise the second patient population are usually based in the community. Regardless of the patient population, the focus of FMHN is the stabilization and treatment of psychiatric illness as it pertains to the legal system (Mason, 2011; Mullen, 2000).

A distinction must be made between registered nurses who provide medical care in a forensic facility and FMH nurses. Medical nurses in custodial settings (jails, prisons, forensic hospitals) care for the physical needs and conditions of patients. The extent of their role varies within the scope of practice for their levels of education and credentialing. To provide nursing care effectively and objectively, these nurses are typically not informed of the full nature of the crime committed. In contrast, forensic mental health nurses are aware of the details of the charges or crimes. In this sense, some crossover exists with FMH nurses and psychiatric nurses who work in corrections facilities. For FMH nurses, the differences lie in the relationship with the patient and the role of the nurse. The FMHN assessment includes investigative aspects, notably elements of mental competence, the existence of intent, and the impact of psychiatric disorders on the capacity to make decisions. In addition, the FMH nurse collaborates in the development of official legal and clinical assessments, depending on the nurse's level of credentialing and scope of practice. The nature of the relationship with the patient also differs in that the goals of treatment include exploring the nature of crime, its elements, and internal states before, during, and after the crime, as well as the consequences (Mason, 2011) (See Table 4.1).

HISTORY AND THEORY

Historical Timeline

Much of the case law resulting in alternate disposition of defendants with mental illness is relatively recent. Not until 1638 in the United States did the trial of Dorothy Talbye result in the first description of a person with a mental illness being convicted of a capital crime (Kaltman, 2013). Despite dramatic evidence of a delusional disorder, she was charged and convicted of

---

TABLE 4.1 Key Concepts in Forensic Mental Health Nursing

Clinical boundaries
Clinical supervision to guide individual development
Criminalization of the persons with mental illness
Definition of forensic mental health nursing
Nurse–patient relationship as therapeutic intervention
Therapeutic alliance
Transference/countertransference
Posttraumatic stress disorder
Violence prevention

the murder of her daughter. Almost 200 years later, the trial of William Hatfield in England resulted in the Criminal Lunatics Act. This case established hospitalization as an alternative to incarceration for crimes committed by persons with mental illness. In 1986, the case of *Ford v. Wainright* in the United States resulted in the determination that the Eighth Amendment prohibits capital punishment for persons who are declared mentally insane. A brief review of key events follows.

Prehistoric: Humoral theory of mental illness: bloodletting, sweating, exorcism, purging, sexual intercourse as treatment; evidence of lobotomy seen in archeology and art

25 BC–2146 AD: Celsus and Galen use trephining (hole in skull)

1247: First psychiatric hospital, St. Bethlehem (Bedlam), opens in London

1537: Development of triangular trephine to open the skull

1638: Trial of Dorothy Talbye, United States (US)

1800: James Hatfield case results in Criminal Lunatics Act

1845: United Kingdom (UK) Lunacy Act establishes asylum for pauper lunatics

1873: Linda Richards becomes the first professional nurse and the first US psychiatric nurse

1850–1900: Psychiatric hospitals parallel the development of medical hospitals

1900: "Moral treatment" evolves and is implemented in newly created "asylums"

1913: Johns Hopkins School of Nursing is the first to include psychiatric nursing in its curriculum

1920: Harriet Bailey authors the first psychiatric nursing textbook, *Nursing Mental Diseases*

1930s: US; More than 450,000 institutionalized patients are in 477 asylums

1930s: Transorbital lobotomy is introduced by Antonio Moniz at the University of Lisbon

1936–1951: W. Freeman expands the use of lobotomy for multiple diagnoses

1949: Antonio Muniz receives the Nobel Prize in Medicine for lobotomy

1950s: Hildegarde Peplau develops psychiatric nursing as a specialty

1953: First antipsychotic agent chlorpromazine (Thorazine) is introduced as a "chemical lobotomy"

1959: UK Mental Health Act requires judicial order for detainment after false confinement cases

1967: Haloperidol, the second antipsychotic medication, becomes available

1960s: US de-institutionalization of persons with mental illness becomes public policy

1983: William Eckert introduces the *concept* of "living forensics"

1988: New York Medical Examiner H. McNamara introduces the *practice* of "living forensics"

1989: Virginia Lynch establishes forensic nursing as a scientific discipline

1991: International Association of Forensic Nurses (IAFN) is founded and recognized by the American Academy of Forensic Sciences

1997: IAFN and the American Nurses Association publish *Scope and Standards of Forensic Nursing Practice*

Nursing Theories Pertaining to Psychiatric Nursing

Nursing theory is derived from clinical practice. It enables nurses to develop professional goals and standards as well as a professional identity. A grounding in nursing theory helps nurses to problem-solve as clinical practice evolves. Nursing theory can facilitate understanding the roles of nurses and their relationships with patients and the communities with which they interact. Many nursing theories exist, and have evolved over time. Since psychiatric nursing focuses on the intangible elements of a person (thoughts, beliefs, perception), it is easy for novices to rely upon more objective aspects of the role (medication management, patient safety). Several nursing theories mentioned below are especially useful to psychiatric nurses in keeping the focus on the relationship with the patient and can easily be implemented in a forensic setting.

Hildegard Peplau (1909–1999). Developed in the asylums of the mid-1900s, the Theory of Interpersonal Relations is specific to psychiatric nursing (Peplau, 1952). The theory focuses not on the physiological needs of the patient, but on the value of a transformative therapeutic relationship between the nurse and the patient. Peplau's work led to the development of psychiatric nursing as a specialty and her theory has been expanded to apply to all nursing care. She identified psychiatric nurses as one of four critical professions in the delivery of psychological care—along with psychiatrists, social workers, and psychologists. As the theory involves a developing, interactive process, it does not apply to individuals who cannot engage in ongoing discourse. However, it can be applied to interactions with the family members of infants, children, and individuals in an altered mental state who cannot communicate meaningfully. Therapeutic relationships with family members can enable the psychiatric nurse to develop a plan of care for an uncommunicative patient.

Martha E. Rogers (1914–1994). The Science of Unitary Human Beings is a more metaphysical theory of nursing relationships. It envisions humans and their environments as energy fields engaged in a fluid, mutual, intuitive process. These fields are unique, open patterns of energy that are in continual interaction with one another. The role of the nurse within this framework is to move patients to wellness through interaction with them and their environment. Rogers sees nursing as a creative and imaginative combination of theory and practice that is rooted in science (physics) and applied artistically. The Rogerian model encourages the use of complimentary alternative medicine (therapeutic touch, acupuncture, massage, guided imagery, aromatherapy, journaling, humor, guided reminiscence). Rather than reducing assessment to individual components (physical, mental, spiritual), Rogerian nursing observes patterns and themes within a human being and works to stabilize those patterns by letting go of the traditional limitations of identified goal, time, and space.

Jean Watson (1940–Present). The Theory of Transpersonal Caring defines ten "carative" factors that serve as the basis of the science of caring. This theory encourages nurses to move beyond the physical tasks of care to the interpersonal relationship that is therapeutic for the patient. This theory focuses on physical, mental, emotional, and spiritual aspects of care that combine to facilitate healing. By weaving elements of metaphysical and transcendent human experiences into the transpersonal caring process, this theory has much in common with Martha Roger's Science of Unitary Human Beings.

Personality and Behavioral Theories

Theories of personality and behavior are used to understand the workings of the mind and human relationships. Most nursing programs include a brief introduction to the major theories. Several are mentioned here, although many more exist. Experience with psychiatric patients will likely prompt additional exploration and use of these theories to understand the thoughts, decisions, and actions of an individual engaged in a forensic mental health setting.

Sigmund Freud (1856–1939). Psychodynamic theory provided the first real language of psychiatric theory, including personality structures, levels of consciousness, instinct, the nature of anxiety, and defense mechanisms. Mental illness is viewed as unconscious conflict from childhood that results in problematic behavior. Treatment is based on exploration of the origins of conflict within the individual and is insight-based.

Carl Jung (1875–1961). Analytical Psychology defined the concept of "persona" as the face that the personality presents to the world. Jung introduced the concept of the "collective unconscious" as a human repository of shared past and myths, including universal archetypes. The treatment goal is the discovery of one's unique identity.

Harry Stack Sullivan (1892–1949). His Interpersonal Theory focused on interactions between an individual and his or her environment. He suggested that personality is formed through interaction with significant others. Symptoms of mental illness and anxiety arise from interpersonal conflict in significant relationships. Treatment focuses on anxiety and its cause with the therapist as the participant-observer.

Erik Erikson (1902–1994). The basis of Psychosocial Theory is the context of social interaction through which responses to the individual shape the ego, personal mastery, and development through defined stages. Mental illness is viewed as conflict arising from failed mastery of a developmental stage. Psychiatric nurses assess developmental levels and identify interventions to enable the patient to master the requisite tasks of that stage.

Carl Rogers (1902–1987). His Person-Centered Theory of self-actualization uses client-centered psychotherapy. He describes personality as a dynamic process that evolved through relationships. This theory espouses acceptance of the individual and progress is achieved through close collaboration and a strong therapeutic alliance.

Abraham Maslow (1908–1970). The Self-Actualization Theory identifies a hierarchy of human needs. Satisfaction of primitive needs leads to more advanced psychological needs becoming the primary motivating factors. Thus, a cumulative progress leads to a peak experience, which produces long-lasting, beneficial effects.

Theories of Crime

A fascination with crime has long existed, along with interest in the motivation and state of mind of the criminal. Societies have sought explanations; many theories of crime have developed. Each theory reflects the social values and beliefs of the dominant culture, and acts are considered criminal based on those values and beliefs. Thus, the nature of what is considered criminal varies (Marsh, Melville, Morgan, Norris, & Cochrane, 2011). For example, shooting one's neighbor in the urban United States because of his or her political views is regarded as a crime. However, shooting a rebel soldier in the Middle East, if conducted by an American soldier on a military mission, is not. Theories of crime tend to reflect anthropological and psychological etiologies. Some derive from specific disciplines or socio-political-economic climates. Working with the legal system in developing treatment plans and modalities for psychiatric forensic patients prompts the need to understand the concepts of criminality and how they are defined. As a forensic nurse's individual practice evolves, he or she would benefit from studying theories of crime. Although this study is not appropriate for novices, any attempts to impact the legal system require knowledge of theories of crime and treatment, and the subject is appropriate for advanced practice forensic nurses.

   Some of the major theories are:

- Classical: Crime is committed after a thoughtful evaluation of the risks and benefits and deterrence is possible.
- Deterrence: If punishment is swift and harsh enough, it will serve as a deterrent.
- Biosocial: The combined effects of biology, environment, and behavior are the etiology of crime.
- Psychological: Criminal behaviors are the result of deviant personality states or psychiatric illness.
- Social learning: Defines criminal behavior as a process that is learned and reinforced through social interaction.
- Social bonding and control: Based on the concept that all individuals have a criminal drive but conform to social organization; crime occurs when social structure weakens.
- Social disintegration: The degradation of social structures leads to the development of crime within a family, community, or region.
- Consensus: The powerful majority uses the law to keep the minority powerless and crime is conformity with the norms of the minority.
- Integrative: Combines elements of other theories.

INTERSECTING SYSTEMS AND SERVICES

Forensic psychiatric patients may be perpetrators or victims, and are seen in a variety of settings, including emergency departments, inpatient psychiatric units, outpatient mental health clinics, court systems, probation departments, supervised community housing, foster homes, immigration detention settings, and more. These patients and their families benefit from services throughout the community. The impact of mental illness as well as legal entanglement has a profound impact on family members, often resulting in a loss of family support or even estrangement. When one imagines his or her own conflict in creating a therapeutic relationship and advocating for a patient who has committed heinous crimes, one can gain insight into the struggle of family members. This struggle is exacerbated when the patient is the family breadwinner or primary caregiver. The stigma associated with mental illness or addiction can increase the difficulty of reaching out for help and accessing it. Changes in laws and prosecution patterns often increase the numbers of patients being managed within the community instead of hospitals or jails. Forensic mental health patients and their families often need a broad array of services to help them succeed, including services from the dimensions listed in Figure 4.1.

- Mental health: Psychiatric facilities—inpatient and community-based, crisis clinics, addictions treatment, supervised housing agencies, forensic facilities, and mental health homecare services
- Health care: Medical hospitals and clinics, emergency services, and public health agencies

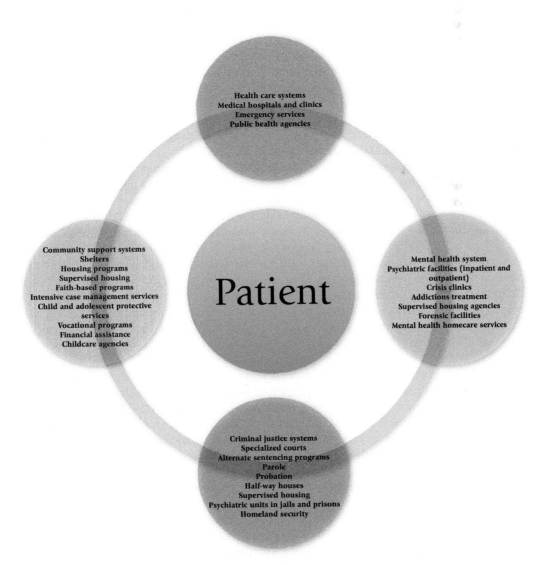

FIGURE 4.1   Intersecting systems.

- Criminal justice: Specialized courts, alternate sentencing programs, parole, probation, half-way houses, supervised housing, psychiatric units in jails and prisons, and immigration detention centers
- Community support: Shelters, housing programs, foster homes, faith-based programs, intensive case management services, child and adult protective services, vocational programs, financial assistance, and childcare agencies

PRACTICE AND PREVENTION

Assessments

Formal forensic assessments used by the courts require input from a team of clinicians, including nursing staff. Each discipline has its own theoretical base and format. A variety of evidence-based, psychometric instruments exists to utilize in assessments. However, a sound assessment combines findings from all members of the team. Assessment is the first step of the nursing process, but is truly an ongoing process. Working with the psychiatric population in a forensic setting may require persistence, assertiveness, and creativity due to the physical setting (prisons, courtrooms, seclusion rooms, hospitals, half-way houses) as well as the conditions of the patient (restrained, accompanied by guards, violent, psychotic, in withdrawal or uncooperative) (Walsh, 2001). The goal of the assessment should guide the process.

In acute care settings, nurses often initiate the process of admission. Having the first contact with the patient provides a unique opportunity to establish open, honest, and respectful communication. Any information provided by the patient about occasions of violence or the crime that has involved the person in the legal system should be carefully and thoroughly documented. Identifying the cascade of events leading to violence can guide clinicians to prevent violence. Nursing assessments routinely evaluate specific domains of risk: dangerousness, mental instability, self-harm, and vulnerability (Mason, 2011; McClelland, 2001).

The FMH nurse's assessment typically includes medical, psychiatric, substance abuse, and criminal history, but an assessment for violence toward self and others is particularly important. Entering the 21st century, rates of suicide and self-harm were higher in forensic settings than in the general population and suicide was the leading cause of death in United States prisons (White, 2001). Green, Andre, Kendall, Looman, and Polvi (1992) found that in the Canadian prison population, the first 6 months after sentencing is a very high-risk period, regardless of the length of sentence. Basic nursing education and clinical practice should result in the mastery of assessment skills for suicidality and self-harm. Many structured interviews and assessments exist to determine the risk for suicide. Risk factors include gender, age, race, family history, mental illness, substance abuse, medical comorbidity, socioeconomics, isolation, hopelessness, and access to lethal means (World Health Organization, 2014) (See Table 4.2). In the corrections settings, the additional burdens of the length of sentence and victimization by peers must be included in the assessment. Incarceration is likely to magnify the risks for self-harm and minimize the intensity of protective factors, such as family support, religious affiliation, leisure activity, as well as hope and plans for the future (Burrows, 1995). Risk assessment must be ongoing; appropriate psychiatric care and interventions must be easily accessible. Almost one million cases of suicide occur annually across the globe. The World Health Organization (WHO) has listed suicide as a priority global health issue in the WHO Mental Health Gap Program. A suicide prevention program known as SUPRE is available for professionals of all disciplines (World Health Organization, 2014).

Within institutions and agencies, multidisciplinary teams design and deliver mental health treatment. A treatment team typically includes a psychiatrist, nurse, social worker, and psychologist as well as other disciplines or staff pertinent to the setting and population. Although each discipline has a unique focus, the treatment team shares information through documentation and discussion at team meetings. Typically, the team reviews the data and the plan of care, identifying the goals of treatment and the selection of appropriate interventions (McClelland, 2001; Rasmussen, Rummans, & Richardson, 2002; Walsh, 2001). Careful and thoughtful assessment enables the treatment team to include interventions that support the treatment goals.

TABLE 4.2 Risk Factors for Suicide

Access to lethal means
Age
Family history
Hopelessness
Isolation
Length of sentence
Male gender
Medical comorbidity
Mental illness
Race
Socioeconomics
Substance abuse

The FMH nurse plays a key role within institutions of care by virtue of managing the milieu and having extensive contact with patients. Forensic mental health nurses typically see patients throughout a shift in structured (group) and unstructured settings (milieu) as well as through individual contact. In addition, observation of the patient's interaction with peers can be especially enlightening; the FMH nurse is likely the only member of the treatment team with this degree of access. The FMH nurse's assessment is unique in that it includes investigatory components from which the nurse draws clinical conclusions (Mason, 2011). These conclusions are shared with the treatment team for consideration in developing forensic assessments and treatment plans.

This information and the FMH nurse's conclusions contribute to a variety of formal assessments made by primary clinicians and treatment teams. The types of assessments to which FMH nurses contribute include: pretrial, presentence, mental status, suicidality, violence potential, and dangerous offender (McClelland, 2001). Although entry-level FMH nurses do not typically perform these forensic assessments, the information they obtain and document is incorporated into the assessment for the courts. With additional formal educational and clinical training, FMH nurses in advanced practice roles can take on a greater responsibility within the legal system. Master's and doctoral degrees, along with advanced certification, prepare nurses to complete forensic assessments for the courts and associated agencies, including assessment of competence to stand trial, capacity to determine right/wrong, as well as fitness to stand trial.

Interventions

Many therapeutic interventions are available to FMH nurses (See Table 4.3). Some are well-known to entry-level nurses, for example, medication and safety management. Other interventions – such as motivational enhancement – require specialized training. The FMH nurse can acquire skills in many of these interventions through continuing education and nonacademic training: motivational enhancement, anger management, and relaxation therapy. Various complementary alternative medicine programs offer seminars and training in guided imagery, mindfulness, loving kindness, meditation, and other nontraditional interventions. More complex interventions – such as cognitive behavioral and trauma therapies – are typically acquired through advanced education and clinical training. Forensic mental health nurses collaborate or play a supportive role in the delivery of an array of interventions, such as electroconvulsive therapy (ECT) and occupational therapy. The most commonly used, evidenced-based interventions are:

- Ancillary: Occupational, recreational, art, music, and vocational therapies
- Anger management: Helping patients identify cognitive triggers, techniques for controlling anger, and cognitive restructuring to prevent activation and distortion

TABLE 4.3 Therapeutic Interventions in Forensic Mental Health Nursing

Ancillary therapies
Anger management
Aversion
Cognitive-behavioral therapy
Exercise
Goal setting
Group therapy
Milieu management
Modeling of behavior
Motivational enhancement
Pharmacotherapy
Prevention of suicide or harm
Psychiatric rehabilitation
Psychoeducation
Relaxation therapies
Reality testing
Safety management on the unit
Setting limits
Somatic therapies
Substance abuse treatments
Trauma therapies

- Aversion: Used less frequently—provides an unpleasant sensation paired with a stimulus to induce an aversion to the stimulus
- Cognitive behavioral: Therapy techniques and models that focus on changing the patient's cognitive processes and behavioral responses
- ECT: Electroconvulsive therapy
- Exercise: Known to affect neurotransmitter functioning and sense of well-being
- Goal setting: Identification of values to determine goals, pathways, and obstacles
- Group therapy: Use of the environment and dynamics of a group as surrogates to observe and analyze a pattern of roles, reactions, and interactions with the world at-large
- Milieu management: Assessment of the number, experience, skill, availability, and anxiety of staff in relation to patient acuity, activity, and volatility; evaluating the "saturation" of the milieu by assessing the impact of challenging patients on the therapeutic status of the unit; if oversaturation occurs, the organization and therapeutic capacity of the unit collapse (Chandley, 2002)
- Modeling of behavior: Staff model appropriate techniques of communication, social interactions, therapeutic interactions, disclosure, behavioral control, expression of negative emotions and reactions, interpersonal boundaries, respect, and constructive feedback
- Motivational interviewing: Therapeutic approach that does not offer resistance, but highlights the disparity of the client's thoughts and feelings through reflection of his or her statements
- Pharmacotherapy: Use of medication to manage mood, thought, and substance abuse disorders
- Psychiatric education: Groups that focus on improving psychiatric health status and maintenance through education and skill development
- Psychiatric rehabilitation: Foster hope, increase functioning, engage family and community, and strengthen relationships with collaborative services
- Reality testing: Challenging perceptions and identifying cognitive distortion
- Relaxation: Guided imagery; mindfulness-based practices

- Safety management on the unit: Preventing suicide, violence, and self-harm; protecting vulnerable patients from aggressive or violent peers
- Setting limits: Orienting patients to the institutional routines and culture; providing immediate and appropriate feedback when those regulations are violated; using alternatives such as a low-stimulation environment
- Substance abuse treatment: Physical impact of substance use, motivational enhancement, coping skills, and pharmacological support
- Spiritual practices: Meditation, prayer, and rituals
- Trauma: Exposure therapy/acceptance and commitment therapy/eye movement/desensitization response

Two specific interventions will be described further, but FMH nurses should remain alert for opportunities to add to their skill sets through training, and mastery of these skills through practice with clinical supervision. Clinical supervision consists of a mentoring relationship with a more experienced peer who helps the novice process experiences, situations, and emotional responses that arise in relationships with clients. Clinical supervision is particularly important for novice psychiatric nurses.

Electroconvulsive Therapy

Often thought to be outdated and barbarous, ECT is still widely used in mental health, most notably for depression that is not alleviated by medication and therapy (American Psychiatric Association, 2000). It is indicated for treatment of severe depression that is unresponsive to pharmacotherapy. A brief, grand mal seizure is induced under anesthesia by applying electrical current through electrodes applied to the head. The electrode placement may be bilateral, unilateral, or bifrontal.

Typically, the course of treatment includes an initial series of 6 to 12 episodes, but weekly or bi-monthly treatment can be used as maintenance therapy. ECT's response rate of 80% or more is equal to or better than response rates to antidepressant medications. Mortality and morbidity are believed to be lower with ECT than with the administration of antidepressant medications, despite the frequent use of ECT in older adults or patients with medical complications (American Psychiatric Association, 2000; Rasmussen, Rummans, & Richardson, 2002). Potential adverse effects include cognitive impairment – most commonly, short-term memory loss (American Psychiatric Association, 2000) that may be transitory or permanent. Systemic effects, such as transient cardiac arrhythmias, myalgia, and induction of status epilepticus, are easily managed pharmacologically at the time of treatment. Although not strictly a nursing intervention, ECT requires expert nursing care before and after the procedure.

Pharmacotherapy

Pharmacotherapy is a critical component of treatment; the numbers and classes of approved agents continue to increase. During the 1960s, the development of the first antipsychotic medication, chlorpromazine (Thorazine), was the foundation of the de-institutionalization of persons with mental illness in the United States (Faria, 2013). Familiarity with the indications, effects, and potential side effects as well as methods of administration is critical for FMH nurses. Current classes of medications include:

- Abstinence-based agents: Alcohol antagonist, opioid antagonist, gaba-taurine analogue
- Alpha-blockers
- Anti-androgens
- Antidepressants: Selective serotonin reuptake inhibitors, serotonin and norepinephrine reuptake inhibitors, tricyclic antidepressants, monoamine oxidase inhibitors, atypical (a class of antidepressants, such as bupropion)
- Anti-epileptics
- Antipsychotics: Typical, atypical

- Anxiolytics: Benzodiazepines, GABAnergic agents, hypnotics, sedatives, beta-blockers
- Mood stabilizers
- Opiate agonists/opiate antagonists/mixed opiate agonists–antagonists
- Simulants

Delivery methods now include oral tablets and liquids, sublingual tablets/film, and intramuscular/depot injections and patches. The duration of action ranges from hours to months in efficacy, enhancing adherence and pharmacologic efficacy.

POPULATIONS AT RISK

- Cultural subgroups such as ethnic, racial, aboriginal, and religious minorities require attention to different values and norms held within the particular culture (Kaplan, Sadock, & Grebb, 1994; Tasman, 2013). Interventions may require extensive adaptation to accommodate the traditional roles of men and women, the positions of power within the family, and the cultural interpretation of mental illness. Strong spiritual beliefs and practices may influence the patient's locus of control, as well as the suitability of interventions. Many trafficked persons will exhibit symptoms of posttraumatic stress disorder (PTSD) that may be difficult to detect in cultures that manage and express emotions differently than one's own.
- Geriatric or older adult offenders present challenges in the physical adaptation to forensic environments and services as well as more complex issues of health care, entrenched patterns of mental illness, multiple treatment failures, and family resources (Das, Murray, Driscoll, & Nimmagadda, 2011; Stojkovic, 2007). They are likely to be more sensitive to pharmaceutical agents, and a greater danger of polypharmacy exists.
- Sexual minority (gay, lesbian, transgendered, and bisexual) adolescents have higher rates of suicidality and suicide attempts (The National Child Abuse Traumatic Stress Network, 2006; Institutes of Medicine (US) Committee on Gay, Lesbian, Bisexual and Transgender Health Issues and Research Gaps and Opportunities, 2011). As these adolescents struggle with sexual identity, the lack of acceptance often results in isolation and increased substance abuse. The absence of family and social support often leads to homelessness. In addition, these adolescents experience higher rates of interpersonal violence (Heck, Flentje, & Cochran, 2013). School bullying, interpersonal violence – especially rape – and abandonment by families or institutions increase the likelihood that these adolescents will display psychopathology (Institutes of Medicine (US) Committee on Gay, Lesbian, Bisexual and Transgender Health Issues and Research Gaps and Opportunities, 2011). They often exhibit greater hostility, affect dysregulation, and a marked inability to trust. Custodial care increases the potential for victimization: safety must be a priority in custodial placement. Assessment and treatment plans should include a history of assault as well as PTSD. Little research is available differentiating the mental health issues of adolescents from middle-aged or senior sexual minorities. Most studies include subjects across the age span. However, those few studies that are available indicate that older lesbian, bisexual, gay, transgender (LBGT) individuals have higher rates of suicide than the general public (Institutes of Medicine (US) Committee on Gay, Lesbian, Bisexual and Transgender Health Issues and Research Gaps and Opportunities, 2011). Additional research is needed to determine precipitating factors, including past trauma, current social support, substance abuse, and the degree of internalized homophobia. Within North America and Europe, the status and acceptance of sexual minorities differs greatly than the climate in which today's LBGT elders matured (Institutes of Medicine (US) Committee on Gay, Lesbian, Bisexual and Transgender Health Issues and Research Gaps and Opportunities, 2011).
- Substance abuse is global and involves a wide variety of chemical compounds, both naturally occurring and manufactured. Abuse of these agents can render an individual incapable of behavioral control and unable to make responsible decisions. However, since ingestion is voluntary, the issue of personal responsibility remains for both victims and perpetrators. It is well

established that the majority of crimes are associated with substance abuse (Substance Abuse Mental Health Services Administration, 2004). In 2008, the Justice Policy Institute reported that admission to substance abuse programs resulted in decreased crime rates in the United States (Justice Policy Institute, 2008). Since the use of drugs or alcohol seems to be simply a matter of choice, rather than the result of neurological drives and rewards, it is difficult to envision addiction as a mental illness. The commonly held disdain for individuals with substance use disorders is not felt toward persons with other chronic illnesses, such as diabetes, whose lifestyle may have resulted in multisystem failures. Addiction is a psychiatric illness that, like others, is a biopsychosocial phenomenon with genetic, biological, sociocultural, psychiatric, and economic etiologies (Buchman, Skinner, & Illes, 2010). Data published by the United Nations indicates that opiates (natural and synthetic) dominate the drug trade, followed by cocaine and amphetamine-like drugs. The existence of the "dark net" – illicit Internet sales – has complicated the prosecution of traffickers (Economist, 2014). New markets, routes, and sources of illicit drugs continuously evolve (United Nations Office on Drugs and Crimes, 2014).

- Female offenders have often been placed in higher forensic security settings than would normally be indicated by their offenses because of the severity of their behavioral disturbances (Aiyegbusi, 2002). Lifetime histories of genetic vulnerability (i.e., parental mental illness, fetal exposure to alcohol and drugs), physical neglect, and severe trauma often lead to offenses of interpersonal violence with individuals who represent the offenders attachment figures (family members). Compounding the problem is that traumatized women react strongly to the loss of control and, when incarcerated, often experience additional trauma at the hands of male corrections officers (Aiyegbusi, 2002). Many female offenders present with histories of violent physical and sexual trauma as children, reflected in severe attachment disorders. The lack of ability to trust and truly engage in the therapeutic alliance results in resistance to treatment and active sabotage of treatment modalities. Female offenders with attachment disorders are well known to "test" their providers by acting out. These tests serve to counteract expected rejection and neglect on the part of the care provider. As their traumas often occurred in key developmental phases, the women tend to recreate the internal and external conflict and abuse they have experienced in the past. Through the psychic process of transference, the cumulative anger is displaced onto the treatment provider, resulting in rejection of the provider, negative affective behaviors, and even active sabotage while craving the attention and care of the provider. Through the process of countertransference, this rejection of care is experienced as personally critical and punishing to the provider and leads the provider to feel the same way toward the offender as the original family member. Thus, the trauma is recreated and reinforced, aborting any therapeutic progress. Alternately, the offender may appear compliant and even seductive, as she is unable to recognize appropriate personal boundaries and thus protect herself from revictimization. In this scenario, the negative affective behavior is expressed more subtly and in passive ways (Aiyegbusi, 2002).

- Psychiatrically disordered offenders require that the FMH nurse balance safety, the therapeutic alliance and even custody in providing care. As safety in custodial care requires continual assessment and management, it can easily become the primary function of forensic nurses at the expense of therapeutic alliance and psychosocial interventions. Medication management, psychosocial interventions, and cognitive behavioral therapies are supported by evidence-based research. Staff education and supervision are critical as are adequate staffing levels to ensure that these patients receive the elements of effective care. Inadequate care results in prolonged stays in custodial care and failure of treatment, rendering re-offense a likely outcome (Ewers, 2002). The lack of financial resources, the stigma of mental illness, and the decreased ability to fully participate in the legal process are factors to be considered in the planning and delivery of the patient's care.

- Juvenile offenders are typically placed or incarcerated in separate settings, such as foster homes or juvenile detention facilities. However, the increasing number of juvenile perpetrators has often required incarceration within adult facilities. In addition, the physical, emotional, and intellectual developmental stages of juveniles incarcerated together vary dramatically. Juveniles are at particular risk for victimization and additional corruption by peers. Incarceration requires specific attention to their growth and developmental needs as well as health care, nutrition, activity, and education. Engaging family members is an integral part of treatment planning and re-integration (Peternelj-Taylor, 2006).

- Immigration applicants include survivors of torture, abuse, female genital mutilation (FGM), and human trafficking. These individuals have trauma histories that are likely to have resulted in PTSD. Many are culturally estranged and fearful of authorities as their torturers may have been local or national police and authority figures. Their reactions may be confounding to interpret due to cultural expression and norms.

Female genital mutilation is often thought to exist only in developing countries of the Middle East or Africa. However, it exists in industrial countries as well. In 1996, a landmark case in the United States identified FGM as a form of gender-based persecution, allowing the victims the right to apply for asylum. Shortly afterward, the Girls Protection Act outlawed FGM in the United States, but still, many young girls are returned to their countries of origin during school vacations and are forced to undergo this procedure. The Act has been amended to allow for prosecution of parents who arrange for FGM in other countries.

In the United Kingdom UK, the government has established national procedures to eliminate FGM. Its prime minister has announced that parents who fail to protect their daughters from FGM will be prosecuted as well (BBC UK, 2014). To date, France has prosecuted more than 100 cases of FGM (The Guardian, 2014).

Ethiopia and Niger have significantly reduced the rates of FGM, but Somalia and Guinea have not outlawed the practice and it flourishes. Egypt recently announced the first prosecution of the father of a child and the doctor who performed FGM after the 13-year-old victim died. Although the practice was made illegal in Egypt in 2008, this case is the first prosecution (Dale, 2014).

In 2010, the American Academy of Pediatrics issued a policy statement suggesting that pediatricians provide a clitoral nick to satisfy cultural demands for FGM without inflicting harm to the child. The uproar that followed resulted in retraction of the policy (Chen, 2010; Equality Now, n.d.; Lauden, 2010).

Only a few cases of FGM that have been performed in the United States have been prosecuted, so it is unlikely in the near future that FMH nurses will provide care to perpetrators of FGM (Equality Now, n.d.). However, should the occasion arise, the ethical conflict between religious practice and illegal acts will need to be addressed. In an expanding setting for FMH nurses, caring for victims of FGM in detention centers and in the community is a new practice opportunity. Providing nursing care for these applicants requires skill in working with issues of trauma as well as the anxiety of potentially having to return to a country where physical danger is a threat.

- Perpetrators of interpersonal violence are sometimes classified by causality: personality disordered, impulse-control disordered, and substance abusers (Corvo, Dutton, & Chen, 2008). Reviews have examined a variety of treatment programs for perpetrators of interpersonal violence; none has shown a clear efficacy for all types. Corvo, Dutton, and Chen (2008) have described the lack of evidence-based research on the variety of treatments available and the efficacy for each type of perpetrator. They suggest that a particularly thorough assessment should be used to design individual treatment plans incorporating various treatment modalities. Engaging family members is rarely difficult, but introducing new boundaries, limit setting, and changing the patterns of family and interpersonal dynamics and violence is difficult. The battered family members will need individual treatment within the community in conjunction with the patient.

- Victims of human trafficking present unique challenges, as they are usually involuntary perpetrators of a crime but often surface in the criminal system. In forensic mental health settings, these victims often suffer from undiagnosed PTSD due to the methods of coercion used to enforce compliance. They have often been kidnapped, raped, beaten, tortured, and psychologically terrorized.

Their traffickers often hold complete psychological control over the victim without the necessity of physical confinement or restraint. It is a complex and multilayered process of mentally disarming the victim, leaving them fully dependent on the trafficker, without thought or hope of escape. Separating the victim from the trafficker and providing a culturally sensitive interpreter is imperative to instill a sense of safety. The first priorities of care are safety and unmet medical needs. Forensic mental health nurses will need to coordinate with federal immigration and human service agencies to provide comprehensive services. Particularly difficult may be the "happy trafficker," which is the victim turned trafficker, typically women who are being used as recruiters (Cabelus, 2011).

CONCEPTS AND ISSUES

Therapeutic Alliance

In psychiatric nursing, the alignment of patients with nurses is critical to the patient's recovery through the process of meaningful change. This alliance has been described as the therapeutic or working alliance. This relationship requires the close collaboration between patient and staff member to support and develop individual change, responsibility, and empowerment. The process involves the nurse not as an observer or a guide, but as a companion in the journey. Kirby and Cross (2002) suggest a continuum of five stages of a therapeutic alliance:

- Survival: Focuses on the immediate crisis
- Recovery: Allows the patient to expand functioning and involvement in his or her care
- Growth: Represents a period of increasing awareness and understanding
- Reconstruction: Includes the development and implementation of new skills and approaches to living
- Reintegration: Represents the full empowerment of the patient and the realization of potential in reconfiguring relationships within the world and in managing his or her mental health

This alliance can be a particularly difficult concept to embrace, especially when the patient can be seen as not even deserving of treatment due to heinous crimes, deviant behaviors, and manipulative interactions. The FMH nurse is called upon to become an ally to rapists, child abusers, murderers, and human traffickers. However, psychiatric nursing is based on the ethical concept of respect that is universally afforded to every patient regardless of alienating qualities or behaviors. Personal feelings and experiences cannot help but color the relationship, so psychiatric care is most often provided by a team of clinicians. This ensures that appropriate alliances are created and the treatment goals guide the delivery of care. Treatment teams also exist to protect staff members from manipulation, poor personal boundaries, and secondary traumatization.

When establishing a therapeutic alliance, especially with a manipulative patient, the FMH nurse must recognize and address the need for personal and clinical boundaries. Patients with characterological disorders, such as antisocial, borderline, or narcissistic personality disorders, have lifelong patterns of maladaptive coping strategies and manipulative interactions. These patients tend to push the boundaries of relationships (and patience), making collaboration a constant challenge. Therapeutic goals and interventions delivered by the treatment team are crucial, as is clinical supervision to manage the development of transference and countertransference between patient and staff. If unattended, the conflictual interactions of the patient will be mirrored within the treatment team. The unmanaged countertransference with a difficult patient leads to failure of treatment and compassion fatigue as well as vicarious traumatization (Aiyegbusi, 2002).

Transference and Countertransference

These are emotional transactions between providers and patients, which are part of the therapeutic alliance. They occur routinely, but are most challenging when dealing with patients who have certain mental disorders. These transactions have the potential to fully derail the therapeutic alliance, so careful attention must be paid to this process.

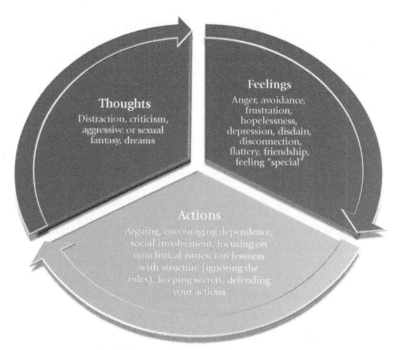

FIGURE 4.2   Signs of countertransference.

Within a therapeutic relationship, the patient often displaces the emotion associated with a significant relationship from the past onto the clinician. The transferred feelings may be rage, distrust, dependence, idealization, or erotic attraction. The process is unconscious and the patient projects a mental representation of the past relationship. Anxiety and vulnerability increase the likelihood of transference within the therapeutic alliance. In a therapeutic relationship, the transferred emotion and original relationship is explored when the patient becomes aware of the transference (Hughes & Kerr, 2000).

Countertransference is the response elicited in the clinician by the patient's projections and behavior. It includes the thoughts and feelings that emerge and is the key to identifying the role that the patient subconsciously wants the clinician to play (See Figure 4.2). When the clinician does not examine this response, he or she falls into recreating the troubled scenario the patient is constructing (Hughes & Kerr, 2000).

Transference and countertransference are likely to be more charged and more challenging when dealing with a patient who is unlikely or unable to reflect on his or her emotions and more apt to act on those feelings. Patients with rigid expectations or a distorted sense of self and others are less able to examine emotional states and articulate their needs or wants from the clinician. The most problematic and intense transference and countertransference typically occur with patients who suffer from personality disorders (Hughes & Kerr, 2000; Mason, Lovell, & Coyle, 2008).

Personality

Personality may be described as the emotional and behavioral components of an individual that drive the daily organization of self and relationship to the world (Sadock & Sadock, 2007). When those traits are imbalanced or dysfunctional and result in the inability to relate to others and the environment (within an acceptable range), the individual is considered to have a personality disorder.

Personality disorders have been difficult to define in exact measures as the traits, behaviors, and manifestations are broad and co-morbid thought or mood disorders may exist (American Psychiatric Association, 2013). Typically, individuals with personality disorders perceive and interact with the world in dysfunctional and even destructive ways. In closed environments (psychiatric hospitals and corrections facilities), these are the patients who typically break the rules and test the boundaries of the unit and the staff (Mason, Lovell, & Coyle, 2008; Schafer, 2002). In addition, they project their internal chaos onto the unit and the staff. The severity of the reactions they provoke among staff can result in the failure to develop a therapeutic alliance and distorted forms of caring. With continued exposure to this type of patient, nurses may develop the belief that personality-disordered patients cannot improve, and withdraw from them (Motiuk & Porporino, 1991; Schafer, 2002).

Conflict within the treatment team will be reflected in the environment. Conflict with patients will be reflected in the treatment team. Open communication among team members and clinical supervision enable staff members to identify splitting behaviors and dysfunctional therapeutic alliances, and remain focused on therapeutic goals. The model of primary nursing – in which one nurse attends to the needs of the personality-disordered patient – increases the likelihood of this boundary violation and is rarely used in mental health hospital settings (Schafer, 2002).

Posttraumatic Stress Disorder

Posttraumatic stress disorder PTSD is a well-known concept that has been understood beyond the limits of combat soldiers from whom the concept was originally identified and defined. The disorder is now commonly diagnosed in survivors of violent crime, child abuse, sexual assault, and interpersonal violence. In addition to patients whose previous life experiences may have resulted in PTSD, the condition is now being observed in perpetrators of crimes who were significantly impaired by mental illness or substance abuse at the time of the criminal act (Edment, 2002). After being re-stabilized through treatment, signs and symptoms of PTSD emerge, requiring an adjustment to treatment plans and goals. A history of trauma is common in patients with personality disorders or substance abuse diagnoses and cannot be ignored in treatment planning.

Ethical Issues

Autonomy versus Mandated Care. Forensic mental health nursing practice presents several ethical conundrums (See Table 4.4). One is the conflict between the goal of autonomy and the reality of compulsory care. Patients are often mandated to treatment, especially in cases of substance abuse, sex crimes, and severe mental illness. Attempting to establish a therapeutic relationship with an individual who is not a voluntary participant and is unwilling to engage is a daunting skill to master.

Another aspect of mandated care is mandatory medication administration. Normally, patients have the right to refuse medication. Cultural values and practices influence the decision to use psychoactive medications. For instance, aboriginal and Native American cultures rarely endorse pharmacological management of mental illness as it is often seen as a spiritual malady. In forensic settings, the risks of danger to self or others and the impact on the environment trump the value of autonomy. Restraint, seclusion, and involuntary medication are often used to contain violent patients when less restrictive interventions fail. However, the basis of FMHN is the personal relationships with patients; the establishment of a therapeutic alliance while providing unwanted, mandated interventions presents a unique challenge.

Restraint. Forensic mental health nurses implement a variety of methods of restraint (Stokowski, 2007). In contrast to corrections staff, FMH nurses use restraints primarily to ensure safety, not exert control (Huf, Coutinho, Adams, & TREC-SAVE Collaborative Group, 2012). Restraint

TABLE 4.4 Ethical Issues

Autonomy vs. mandated care
Use of restraints
Privacy vs. public right to know

may take the form of hands-on containment, physical restraints, chemical restraints, or seclusion. As a staff member's application of restraints on a patient seems to conflict with developing a therapeutic alliance, this topic requires additional investigation. Collins (2000) introduced the term "relational security" to describe the combined role of forensic nurses in maintaining both security and a therapeutic alliance. These seemingly opposing concepts can be blended in the complex relationship of the forensic nurse and the patient. Knowledge of the patient, stressors, patterns of coping, and the clinical relationship with the staff combine to enable the FMH nurse to maintain patient and environmental safety in the least restrictive manner using alternatives to physical restraint when possible (Stokowski, 2007). This relational security is unique to forensic nurses, as other custodial disciplines do not share a therapeutic alliance with the patients.

The power to restrain complicates the capacity for therapeutic alliance because it creates a strong power differential in the relationship. Given this complexity, the task of engaging and managing the alliance requires considerable skill. The result of this aspect of the relationship is difficult to measure; little or no evidence-based research exists on this nature of the collaboration. To establish rapport and simultaneously address the behavior and intent in the context of treatment, the FMH nurse must develop the capacity to separate or compartmentalize the patient's criminal intent and his or her behavior (Chandley, 2002; Woods, 2002).

Privacy versus Public Safety. Privacy and the public's right to know present another conflict. In the private sector, formal consent to releases of information are required to reveal aspects of care, specifically any mental health or substance abuse diagnosis and treatment. However, the forensic network of care and services requires the release of personal information to cooperating entities and the public without voluntary consent. One example is the sex offender registry, which lists the current address and degree of charge for sex offenders in the United States. This registry evolved to enable members of the community to identify the presence of sex offenders within their community and the proximity to vulnerable victims, especially children.

FUTURE ISSUES

Forensic Mental Health Nursing

Forensic mental health nursing is one of the least well-defined areas of practice. Since treatment for offenders and victims crosses multiple disciplines, domains, and settings, it is challenging to completely capture the full range of practice issues and competencies. To date, no country has articulated criteria or a specific training program for FMH nurses. Canada currently has structured preparatory programs at the baccalaureate level for psychiatric nurses. However, most mental health registered nurses complete generalist educational programs and acquire clinical skills through experience. A number of forensic programs exist in various countries, but most commonly at the graduate-degree level. Forensic mental health nurses are forging their own educational pathways by combining training and experiences in psychiatric and forensic nursing.

Treatment Matching

A lack of evidence-based research exists regarding best treatment outcomes for specific mental health/criminal offense populations (Petrila, 2004). Current practice requires highly individualized treatment programming often without the evidentiary base on which to rely (Livingston, Nijdam-Jones, & Brink, 2012; Waltz, et al., 2014).

Personality Disorders

Personality disorders remain the most difficult mental illnesses to treat. The few effective treatment options that have been identified require expensive and prolonged treatment. Patients with severe personality disorders present vexing issues and often do not benefit from established forms of treatment because the therapeutic alliance fails.

Special Courts

Many new types of special courts have evolved to address specific populations. These include county and regional courts that deal specifically with veterans, mental illness, substance abuse, and families. In addition, in the United States, several states now have specialized courts for individuals trafficked into the commercial sex trade. Never before has the United States legal system considered commercial sex trade workers as victims, rather than perpetrators. All these innovative courts offer alternatives to traditional legal adjudication and specialized treatment-based options. Some evidence-based research suggests the efficacy of special courts, but little evidence-based research guides their treatment programs (Petrila, 2006; Redlich, 2006).

Access to Mental Health Care

Access to mental health care is severely limited in many areas of industrialized countries and non-existent in many developing countries. The goal of deinstitutionalization of persons with mental illness in the United States in the 1970s was that care would be delivered in community clinics (Faria, 2013). However, the decline in healthcare dollars often is reflected in the defunding of psychiatric services. Many community agencies are overwhelmed, understaffed, or no longer exist. Thus, the lack of care for persons with a chronic mental disorder has resulted in uncontrolled illness and subsequent homelessness. The natural sequelae are often substance abuse and crime; thus, a vicious cycle is perpetuated.

In the United Kingdom, the role of the FMH nurse is more widely recognized and developed. Forensic mental health nurses are integral members of treatment teams on inpatient units and in community-based outpatient and aftercare programs. Many community programs use FMH nurses as case managers as well as clinicians. They play a key role in developing treatment plans, providing care, and evaluating patient progress (National Forensic Nurses' Research and Development Group, 2008).

Restraints

The use of restraints continues to be controversial and closely monitored. Considered as a last resort, restraint is used only for patient and staff safety within forensic mental health settings. However, ongoing research has resulted in widespread policy and practice changes for using restraint, and new guidelines and interventions are being evaluated (Huf, Coutinho, Adams, & TREC-SAVE Collaborative Group, 2012; Livingston, Nijdam-Jones, & Brink, 2012; Stokowski, 2007).

Workplace Violence

Violence has often been considered an occupational hazard in medical and psychiatric settings, especially emergency departments and correctional institutions (Finn, 2011; Park, Cho, & Hong, 2015). The full extent of workplace violence is generally unclear. Many interventions have been implemented in clinical and forensic settings to limit the possibility for violence. Working with forensic mental health clients requires attention to the safety of the patients, staff, facility, and community. As frontline staff, FMH nurses are responsible for the initial and ongoing assessment of the potential for violence and for possessing the skills to deescalate situations to prevent violence. Although individual factors vary, common patterns of cognitive distortion and escalation exist. However, violence prevention requires additional research into the nature and dynamics of violence, so more effective prevention strategies may be developed.

Career Opportunities

A variety of career options exist within the FMHN domain, with more emerging as the specialty grows. Levels of professional preparation including formal education, training, and certification open other opportunities for FMH nurses. One of the most common practice settings is the inpatient forensic mental health unit. Usually located in a psychiatric hospital, forensic mental health units may house patients who are undergoing pre-trial, court-ordered, psychiatric assessments or psychiatric patients who have a history of forensic charges. Alternately, corrections psychiatric units employ FMH nurses to care for inmates with mental illness. These inmates are normally housed separately from the general population with different programming and ongoing psychiatric care.

Community forensic psychiatric nursing is often comprised of intensive case management programs, but the role of the FMH nurse can be greatly expanded. In such programs, forensic nurses may have a caseload of psychiatric clients and work to keep them engaged in the community, and out of hospitals and jails. This work requires an array of skills and may include medication administration and management, individual therapy, and psychiatric rehabilitation.

Substance abuse treatment centers have been an untapped arena for FMH nurses. Many participants are mandated to treatment and are likely to be adjudicated by mental health or drug courts. This mandatory treatment often requires 2 full years or more of treatment with intensive, interagency cooperation with the courts, parole services, community mental health agencies, housing resources, and social services. These systems often require comprehensive legal reporting on a monthly basis. Use of pharmacologic agents to support sobriety is often well-received by the legal system and long-acting agents are particularly useful.

Immigration services present another venue for FMH nurses. The basis of application for political asylum differs among countries, but typically includes persecution, torture, human trafficking, child soldiering, and female circumcision. Applicants are sometimes confined in detention centers; others are allowed to remain in the community. Detention centers typically provide only secure containment and little, if any, medical or mental health services. However, these facilities, as well as community agencies, are suitable settings for FMH nurses. Some of the early engagement by FMH nurses in this realm includes the evaluation and documentation of the medical or mental health trauma. Some agencies require advanced practice status to ensure that the examiner qualifies as an expert witness before a judge during immigration hearings. As the number of applications by survivors of FGM increases, sexual assault nurse examiners and FMH nurses are well-positioned to fill this role and expand the settings for forensic nursing practice. The ability to assess both the physical and mental status of the applicant is an ideal use of forensic nursing skills.

As more communities realize the need for separate mental health courts, new opportunities for FMH nurses will arise. These nurses often work in a case management role. However, this role can be expanded to include to assessments, client management, and tracking.

The following list suggests current opportunities in FMHN, but new opportunities are being created as the profession advances:

- Forensic mental health homecare
- Case management agencies
- Psychiatric corrections units
- Forensic hospitals
- Special courts: Mental health, drug, veterans, and immigration hearings
- Community, psychiatric, and housing agencies
- Probation/parole programs
- Mental health professional commitment evaluations
- Community living programs
- Immigration services
- Sex offender community services, residences, and treatment programs
- Domestic violence programs
- Human trafficking services and programs

Forensic mental health nursing is a unique and evolving subspecialty of forensic nursing. It demands expanded skills of assessment, the ability to form a therapeutic alliance with some of the most odious patients, the application of well-chosen psychiatric interventions, and intense collaboration with treatment teams and community agencies. This specialty has a growing presence, largely within industrialized countries, but holds the potential for extraordinary impact in areas where human rights violations prevail (Bowring-Lossock, 2006; Edment, 2002; Ewers, 2002; Mohan, Slade, & Fahy, 2004; National Forensic Nurses' Research and Development Group, 2008; Timmons, 2010; Woods, 2002).

CASE STUDY

Marla is a 17-year-old transgendered male-to-female who is currently on hormone therapy, but has not undergone gender reassignment surgery. She was admitted to the inpatient forensic psychiatric unit after stabbing her female partner while intoxicated with methamphetamine. The court placed her in custody on charges of assault and ordered a psychiatric assessment. During the admission interview, Marla reports that she has been homeless intermittently since leaving home at age 13. As a teenager, she was the victim of gang rape by male classmates. She has been sexually assaulted on several other occasions, has been the victim of intimate partner violence in her last two relationships, and has struggled with substance abuse (alcohol, cocaine, methamphetamine, and ecstasy) since adolescence. She states that she was "high" at the time of the assault. Marla exhibits traits of borderline personality disorder; she is alternately remorseful, angry, and then seductive. She has extensive lateral scars on her forearms and multiple facial piercings.

Treatment Issues

Custody: Marla identifies as female, but anatomically is still male.

Safety: She has significant risk factors for self-harm.

Substance Abuse: She has a long history of significant drug use that has exacerbated poor impulse control.

Mental Health: Developing a therapeutic alliance with Marla is highly problematic. She demonstrates mood lability, poor impulse control, a scant history of trusting relationships, and a chaotic lifestyle. She also is highly suspicious of institutionalized care and interventions, as she has lived on the edges of society for a long period of time. There are likely strong symptoms of PTSD from sexual traumas and interpersonal violence.

Psychosocial support is lacking in her life: She has no contact with her family of origin, and has been living with her partner, so will be homeless when released. Many of her relationships fail due to her instability and lability, so her friendships are short-lived or superficial. She has few work skills as she is poorly educated and has no stable income.

Milieu: Marla will project much of her chaos onto the unit milieu and the treatment team. Expectations must be clearly delineated and limits strictly enforced to prevent breakdown of the milieu.

REFERENCES

Aiyegbusi, A. (2002). Nursing interventions and future directions with women in secure services. In A. W. Kettles, *Therapeutic interventions for forensic mental health nurses* (pp. 136–150). London, UK: Jessica Kingsley Publishers.

American Psychiatric Association. (2000). *The practice of electroconvulsice therapy: Recommendations for treatment, training, and privileging* (2nd ed.). Washington, DC: American Psychiatric Publishing.

American Psychiatric Association. (2013). *Diagnostic and statistical manual of mental disorders.* Washington, DC: American Psychiatric Publishing. Retrieved April 6, 2014, from psychiatryonline.org: dsmpsychiatrylonline.org/book. aspx?bookid = 556

BBC UK. (2014). *FGM: UK's first female genital mutilation prosecutions announced.* Retrieved November 14, 2014, from BBC News UK, www.bbc.com/news/uk-26681364

Bowring-Lossock, E. (2006). The forensic mental health nurse: A literature review. *Journal of Psychiatric and Mental Health Nursing, 13*(6), 780–785.

Buchman, D. Z., Skinner, W., & Illes, J. (2010). Negotiating the relationship between addiction, ethics, and brain science. *American Journal of Bioethics Neuroscience, 1*(1), 36–45. Retrieved April 1, 2014, from http://www.tandfonline.com/doi/abs/10.1080/21507740903508609#.VNhVCex0zDc

Burrows, S. (1995). Suicide: The crisis in the prison service. *British Journal of Nursing, 4*(4), 215–218.

Cabelus, N. (2011). Human trafficking. In V. A. Lynch & J. B. Duval, *Forensic nursing science* (2nd ed., pp. 531–535). St. Louis, MO: Elsevier/Mosby.

Chandley, M. (2002). Nursing interventions and future directions with severely assaultive patients. In A. W. Kettles, *Therapeutic interventions for forensic mental health nurses* (pp. 102–119). London, UK: Jessica Kingsley Publishers.

Chen, S. (2010). *Pressure for female genital cutting lingers in the US.* Retrieved March 27, 2014, from CNN Health, www.cnn.com/2010/HEALTH/05/21/america.female.genital.cutting/

Collins, M. (2000). The practitioner new to the role of forensic psychiatric nurse in the UK. In A. R. Kettles, *Forensic nursing and the multidisciplinary care of the mentally disordered offender* (pp. 27–34). London, UK: Jessica Kingsley Publishers.

Corvo, K., Dutton, D. G., & Chen, W. Y. (2008). Toward evidence-based practice with domestic violence perpetrators. *Journal of Aggression, Maltreatment and Trauma, 16*(2), 111–130.

Dale, T. (2014). *Egypt faces its first FGM trial.* Retrieved November 24, 2014, from Independent.com, www.independent.co.uk/news/world.africa/egypt-faces-first-fgm-trial-95554247.html

Das, K., Murray, K., Driscoll, R., & Nimmagadda, S. R. (2011). A comparative study of healthcare and placement needs among older forensic patients in a high secure versus medium/low secure hospital settings [Letter]. *International Psychogeriatrics, 23*(5), 847–848.

Economist, T. (2014). *The dark net is thriving.* Retrieved Jan 19, 2015, from www.businessinsider.com, www.businessinsider.com/illicit-e-commerce-the-amazons-of-the-dark-night-2014-10

Edment, H. (2002). Nursing intervention and future directions in community care for mentally disordered offenders. In A. W. Kettles, *Therapeutic interventions for forensic mental health nurses* (pp. 225–239). London, UK: Jessica Kinsley Publishers.

Equality Now. (n.d.). *Female genital mutilation in the US factsheet.* Retrieved March 27, 2014, from Equality Now, www.equalitynow.org/FGM_in_US_FAQ

Ewers, P. I. (2002). Nursing interventions and future directions with the severely mentally ill. In A. W. Kettles, *Therapeutic interventions for forensic mental health nurses* (pp. 92–101). London, UK: Jessica Kingsley Publishers.

Faria, M. A. (2013). Violence, mental illness and the brain: A brief history of psychosurgery; Part I-from trephination to lobotomy. *Surgical Neurology International, 4,* 49.

Finn, C. (2011). Relationship crimes. In V. A. Lynch & J. B. Duval, *Forensic nursing science* (2nd ed., pp. 370–379). St. Louis, MO: Elsevier/Mosby.

Green, C., Andre, G., Kendall, K., Looman, T., & Polvi, N. (1992). Study of 133 suicides among Canadian federal prisoners. *Forum on Corrections Research, 4*(3), 17–19.

Heck, N. C., Flentje, A., & Cochran, B. N. (2013). Offsetting risks; High school gay-straight alliances and lesbian, gay, bisexual, and transgender (LGBT) youth. *Psychology of Sexual Orientation and Gender Diversity, 1,* 81–90.

Huf, G., Coutinho, E. S., Adams, C. E., & TREC-SAVE Collaborative Group. (2012). Physical restraints versus seclusion room for management of people with acute aggression or agitation due to psychotic illness (TREC-SAVE): A randomized trial. *Psychological Medicine, 42*(11), 2265–2273.

Hughes, P., & Kerr, I. (2000). Transference and countertransference in communication between doctor and patient. *Advances in Psychiatric Treatment, 6,* 57–64.

Institutes of Medicine (US) Committee on Gay, Lesbian, Bisexual and Transgender Health Issues and Research Gaps and Opportunities. (2011). *The health of lesbian, gay, bisexual and transgender people: Building a foundation for better understanding.* Washington, DC: National Academies Press.

Justice Policy Institute. (2008). *Substance abuse treatment and public safety.* Retrieved November 22, 2014, from Justice Policy, www.justicepolicy.org/images/upload/08_01_re[_drugtx_ac-ps.pdf

Kaltman, E. (2013). *Carol Troberman criminal defense DUI lawyers blog.* Retrieved February 28th, 2014, from Orange County DUI Lawyers Blog, www.orangecountyduilawyersblog.com/2013/9/insanity-defense-cases/

Kaplan, H., Sadock, B., & Grebb, J. (1994). *Synopsis of psychiatry* (7th ed.). Baltimore, MD: Williams & Wilkins.

Kirby, S. C., & Cross, D. J. (2002). Socially constructed narrative interventions: A foundation for therapeutic alliances. In A. Kettles, *Therapeutic interventions for forensic mental health nurses* (pp. 187–205). London, UK: Jessica Kingsley Publishers.

Lauden, K. (2010). *AAP retracts controversial policy on female genital cutting.* Retrieved March 28, 2014, from Medscape Multispecialty, www.medscape.com/viewarticle/722840

Livingston, J. D., Nijdam-Jones, A., & Brink, J. (2012). A tale of two cultures: Examining patient-centered care in a forensic mental health hospital. *Journal of Forensic Psychiatry and Psychology, 23*(3), 345–360.

Marsh, I., Melville, G., Morgan, K., Norris, G., & Cochrane, J. (2011). *Crime and criminal justice.* Abingdon, Oxon, UK: Routledge.

Mason, T. (2011). Psychiatric forensic nursing. In V. A. Lynch & J. B. Duval, *Forensic nursing science* (2nd ed., pp. 441–450). St. Louis, MO: Elsevier/Mosby.

Mason, T., Lovell, A., & Coyle, D. (2008). Forensic psychiatric nursing skills and competencies: I role dimensions. *Journal of Psychiatric and Mental Health Nursing, 15*(2), 118–130.

McClelland, N. (2001). Assessment and clinical risk. In N. H. McClelland, *Forensic nursing and mental health disorders in clinical practice* (pp. 11–20). Oxford, UK: Reed Educational and Professional Publishing Ltd.

Mohan, R., Slade, M., & Fahy, T. A. (2004). Clinical characteristics of community forensic mental health services. *Psychiatric Services, 55*(11), 1294–1298.

Motiuk, L. L., & Porporino, F. J. (1991). *The prevalence, nature and severity of mental health problems among federal male inmates in Canadian penitentiaries.* Retrieved Feb 19, 2014, from http://WW.csc-scc.gc.ca/text/rsrch/reports/r24/r24e.sjtml

Mullen, P. E. (2000). Forensic mental health. *British Journal of Psychiatry, 176,* 307–311.

National Forensic Nurses' Research and Development Group. (2008). *Forensic mental health nursing capabilities, roles and responsibilities.* London, UK: Quay Books Division, MA Healthcare Ltd. Retrieved from http://www.quay-books.co.uk/content/site121/filessamples/670978185642362_000000003 19.pdf

Park, M., Cho, S. H., & Hong, H. J. (2015). Prevalence and perpetrators of workplace violence by nursing unit and the relationship between violence and the perceived work environment. *Journal of Nursing Scholarship, 47*(1), 87–95.

Peplau, H. (1952). *Interpersonal relations in psychiatric nursing.* New York, NY: Putnam & Sons.

Peternelj-Taylor, C. A. (2006). Forensic nursing. In W. Mohr, *Psychiatric-mental health nursing* (6th ed., pp. 381–382). Philadelphia, PA: Lippincott, Williams & Wilkins.

Petrila, J. (2004). Emerging issues in forensic mental health. *Psychiatric Quarterly, 75*(1), 3–19.

Petrila, J. (2006). Patterns of practice in mental health courts: A national survey. *Law & Human Behavior, 30*(3), 347–362.

Polvi, N. (1992). A study of 133 suicides among Canadian federal prisoners. *Forum on Correctional Research, 4*(3), 17–19.

Rasmussen, K. G., Rummans, T. A., & Richardson, J. W. (2002). Electroconvulsive therapy in the medically ill. *Psychiatric Clinics of North America, 25*(1), 177–193.

Redlich, A. S. http://www.ncbi.nlm.nih.gov/pubmed/?term = Steadman%20HJ%5BAuthor%5D&cauthor = true&cauthor_uid = 16775775

Sadock, B. J., & Sadock, V. A. (2007). *Kaplan and Sadock's Synopsis of Psychiatry* (10th ed.). Philadelphia, PA: Lippincott, Williams & Wilkins.

Schafer, P. (2002). Nursing interventions and future directions with patients who constantly break rules and test boundaries. In A. Kettles, P. Woods, & M. Collins (Eds.), *Therapeutic interventions for forensic mental health nurses* (pp. 56–71). London, UK: Jessica Kingsley Publishers.

Stojkovic, S. (2007). Elderly prisoners: A growing and forgotten group within correctional systems vulnerable to elder abuse. *Journal of Elder Abuse and Neglect, 19*(3/4), 97–117.

Stokowski, L. (2007). *Alternatives to restraint and seclusion in mental health settings.* Retrieved Jan 19, 2015, from www.medscape.com, www.medscape.com/viewarticle/555686

Substance Abuse Mental Health Services Administration. (2004). *The DASIS report: Substance abuse treatment admissions referred by the criminal justice system 2002.* Retrieved March 27, 2014, from SAMSHA.gov: www.samsha.gov/data/2k4/Cjreferrals/Cjreferrals.htm

Substance Abuse and Mental Health Services Administration. (2005). *National Survey on Drug Use and Health Report: Illicit drug use in persons arrested for serious crimes.* Washington, DC: Substance Abuse and Mental Health Services Administration. Retrieved March 27, 2014, from SAMHSA.gov/data/2k5/arrests/arrests.htm:www.samhsa

Tasman, K. U. (2013). *The cultural context of clinical assessment: In the psychiatric interview: Evaluation and diagnosis.* Retrieved January 19, 2015, from WileyOnlineLibrary: DOI: 10: 1002/9781118341001.ch3

The National Child Abuse Traumatic Stress Network. (2006). Trauma among lesbian, gay, bisexual, transgender, or questioning youth. *Culture and Trauma Brief, 1*(2). Retrieved May 1, 2014, from www.nctsnet.org/nctsn_assets/pdfs/culture_and_trauma_brief_LGBTQ_youth.pdf

TheGuardian.com. (2014). *Parents who allow female genital mutilation will be prosecuted.* Retrieved Nov 18, 2014, from theguardian.com, www.theguardian.com/society/2014/jul/22/parents-allow-female-genital-mutilation-prosecuted-cameron-law

Timmons, D. (2010). Forensic psychiatric nursing: A description of the role of the psychiatric nurse in a high secure psychiatric facility in Ireland. *Journal of Psychiatric and Mental Health Nursing, 17*(7), 636–646.

U.S. Department of State. (2013). *Trafficking in persons report 2013.* Washington, DC: U.S. Department of State. Retrieved April 6, 2014, from www.state.gov: www.state.gov/j/tip/tiprpt/2013/2105433.htm

United Nations Office on Drugs and Crimes. (2014). *World drug report 2014.* New York, NY: United Nations. Retrieved from http://www.unodc.org/documents/data-and-analysis/WDR2014/World_Drug_Report_2014_web.pdf

Walsh, P. K. (2001). Referral to admission. In N. H. McClelland, *Forensic nursing and mental health disorders in clinical practice* (pp. 1–10). Oxford, UK: Reed Educational and Professional Publishing Ltd.

Waltz, T. J., Campbell, D. G., Kirchner, J. E., Lombardero, A., Bolkan, C., Zivin, K., Lanto, A. B., Chaney, E. F., & Rubenstein, L. V. (2014). Veterans with depression in primary care: Provider preferences, matching, and care satisfaction. *Family Systems and Health, 32*(4), 366–377.

White, T. (2001). Assessing suicide risk: Taking it step by step is your best bet. *CorrectCare*, (Summer), 35–49.

Woods, P. C. (2002). Forensic nursing interventions and future directions for forensic mental health practice. In A. W. Kettles, *Therapeutic interventions for forensic mental health nurses* (pp. 240–245). London, UK: Jessica Kingsley Publishers.

World Health Organization. (2014). *World health organization*. Retrieved February 16, 2014, from http://www.who.int/mental_health/prevention/suicide/suicideprevent/en/

CHAPTER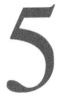

Forensic Correctional Nursing

Georgia L. Perdue
MaryAnne C. Murray
Wesley A. Rivera

OBJECTIVES

At the completion of this chapter, the learner will be able to:

- Synthesize the history and theory of correctional nursing.
- Explain the concept of "deliberate indifference" and what it means in the correctional setting.
- Identify the key concepts and issues of correctional nursing.
- Describe the impact of special populations in the correctional environment.
- Identify future issues in corrections and their impact on the practice of correctional nursing.

KEY TERMS

Inmate: A person who is confined to an institution, such as a jail, prison, or hospital.

Kite or sick call slip: A document that is used to communicate medical needs to medical staff or to request medical attention.

Chronic care clinic: A clinic held to address chronic medical illnesses, such as diabetes, hypertension, seizures, or infectious diseases.

Custody staff: An individual who is responsible for the custody, care, and security of individuals who are in jail, prison, or incarcerated.

Booking: An area in which an inmate who is brought to the facility conveys personal information; the staff obtains records information about the crime; and the individual is fingerprinted, photographed, and searched; receives a medical examination and obtains clearance; and is relieved of his or her personal property.

Housing unit: Location where an inmate is assigned to sleep or live while incarcerated. Jails are locally operated, short-term facilities that hold inmates awaiting trial or sentencing or both, and inmates sentenced to a term of less than 1 year, typically misdemeanants.

Jail: A "locally-operated, short term facility[y] that hold[s] inmates awaiting trial or sentencing or both, and inmates sentenced to a term of less than 1 year, typically misdemeanants" (Bureau of Justice Statistics, n.d.).

Prison: A "long term facility[y] run by the state or the federal government and [that] typically hold[s] felons and inmates with sentences of more than 1 year. Definitions may vary by state" (Bureau of Justice Statistics, n.d.).

HISTORY AND THEORY

Correctional nursing has a long and varied history. Incarceration of a person who violated laws and rules set forth by society dates to the formation of states as social organizations. Correctional history can be summed up by the four "R"s (King, 2008):

- Retribution (First societal form of punishment)
- Restraint (1700s)
- Rehabilitation (Late 1800s)
- Reintegration or Re-entry (Twentieth century)

The following timeline presents a perspective on how laws have evolved through the centuries. The United States (US) laws effecting correctional history will be discussed in depth, while laws that did not provide significant changes affecting behavior will be mentioned only briefly.

Prehistoric: Urukagina (reigned ca. twenty-fourth century BC?) First written text on clay tablets outlining behavior and consequences for unacceptable behavior

2100–2050 BC: Code of UR-Nammu, which established extant legal test arranged in casuistic form

1792–1750 BC: Code of Hammurabi, King of Babylon

529 AD: Justinian Code—Ancestor of laws used today from the Byzantine Empire

604: 17th Article Constitution of Japan developed by royalty regarding the moral and philosophical aspects of law

640: Roman law

653: T'ang Code: Developed a standard forum of procedures in law

1100: First law school opened in Italy; specialized in teaching the laws of antiquity

1200: Magna Carta put into law by the King of England and today's laws in England evolved from this

1689: English Bill of Rights

1692: Salem Witch Trials; used gossip, unbacked accusations, hearsay, stories to convict people

1740: South Carolina Slave Code stripped all black slaves of legal protection

1776: Declaration of Independence severed US ties with Great Britain

1782: David Tyree accused of treason; public opinion turned against execution

1864: The Geneva Convention agreed on the neutrality of ambulances and military hospitals during war

1945: Nuremburg War Crimes Trials; tried crimes against humanity during World War II (Stahl, 2014)

By the late 1700s, BC, written language was developed with codes or guidelines by which society could conduct its behavior. The Code of Hammurabi was the first written set of laws by Hammurabi, King of Babylon, 1792–1750 BC (Gadd, 1965). The Code consisted of 282 rules based on punitive behavior and penalties for violation of the laws King Hammurabi deemed appropriate (Koeller, 2003). This concept, known as *lex talionis*, the law of retaliation or "an eye for an eye," was based on the premise that people were punished for their behavior as a form of vengeance. Numerous ancient civilizations, such as Sumerian, Egyptian, and Mosaic, also used vengeance as punishment, often meted out by the victims themselves for behavior that violated the rules set forth (O'Conner, 2012; Welch, 2003).

Ancient Greek philosophers, such as Plato, started to develop the theory of basing punishment on correcting or reforming behavior to comply with the laws, rather than using only punitive punishment. This theory was based on the belief that lawbreakers could learn from having to pay a monetary fine rather than being imprisoned. Consequently, the poorest of society were usually imprisoned, because they were unable to pay the fine. Romans were the first to use confinement in the form of prison as punishment. Creativity in incarceration was evident. Romans imprisoned lawbreakers in cages, quarries, and existing buildings. Rome's wealthy were often placed under house arrest until trial, provided they behaved themselves. Rome's poor did not fare as well. Ancus Marcius, the fourth king of Rome (640–616 BC), constructed a dungeon for detention in the existing sewers below Rome. Prisoners who were awaiting trial or execution were held in a dark, damp area 6½-feet high and 30-feet wide, still present today, and named Mamertine Prison after the Roman god Mars. Human waste was present, creating not only miserable living conditions but spreading diseases due to the unsanitary conditions. Prisoners who were condemned to die were thrown in this underground room, giving rise to the term *"to be cast into prison"* (Heaton, 2014). If the prisoner died prior to trial or execution, the iron door which opened into the main sewer of Rome, called the *Cloaca Maxima*, was opened and the body cast into the Tiber River for disposal (Heaton, 2014).

Middle Ages: In the Middle Ages, officials and the monarchy held the rights to imprison persons. The possession of the right to imprison citizens confirmed the official's authority over others. Physical forms of punishment continued to flourish. Public shaming, such as shunning, stocks, whipping, mutilation, and loss of life, were commonly used (Spierenburg, 1998). During the rule of King Edward I (1239–1307), misdemeanors were still being punished by whipping, mutilation, branding, or by removal of a hand or foot; felonies were punished by decapitation (Spierenburg, 1998).

Eighteenth Century: In the eighteenth century, public opinion turned against executions and torture, and persons perpetuating such acts were considered violent and sadistic. In 1782, David Tyrie, accused of treason, was the last man in British history who was sentenced to be drawn, hanged, castrated, disemboweled, burnt, beheaded, and quartered. After his sentence was carried out, he was placed in a coffin and buried by the sea. Later, his body was dug up by sailors who took the body and cut it into thousands of pieces with each sailor carrying away a piece of his body to show their shipmates (ExecutedToday.com, 2011). Because of this history, the drafters of the Eighth Amendment to the US Constitution as part of the Bill of Rights concluded: "Excessive bail shall not be required, nor excessive fines imposed, nor cruel and unusual punishments inflicted" (U.S. Constitution amendment VIII, 2002). This was interpreted to forbid torture or wanton infliction of pain and suffering, including any punishment that could be considered inhuman or that violated a person's dignity (Findlaw.com, 2013). Mass incarceration as a deterrent gave way to prison reform. The concept of rehabilitation was again visited (Foucault, 1995). By 1786, the United States began to notice English reform policies concerning the incarcerated. The Pennsylvania Quaker community urged the Commonwealth to adopt laws reflecting more humane treatment of criminals that promoted prevention of future harm to society. To achieve this, Pennsylvania passed legislation that all inmates not sentenced to death were required to perform public projects, such as building roads or forts, via penal servitude (McClennan, 2008). These individuals would provide a free source of labor to the Commonwealth while providing a deterrent to unlawful behavior. However, this public penal servitude was a dismal failure. The prison workers frequently engaged in disorderly conduct at the worksite, resulting in physical mistreatment of the prisoners that drew criticism from the citizenry witnessing the mistreatment (McClennan, 2008). Next came the idea of placing criminals in a house of repentance, where the imprisoned would be subjected to bodily pain, labor, watchfulness, solitude, and silence, joined with cleanliness and a simple diet (Kann, 2005). This served to keep the incarcerated out of the public eye.

During the time of prison reform, health care was delivered; nurses provided the first recorded care in 1797, coinciding with the opening of the Newgate Prison in New York City. The warden, Thomas Eddy, believed that criminals could be rehabilitated, so he provided the first prison hospital, pharmacy, and school (ANA, 2007). The profession of nursing was organized into the Nursing Society of Philadelphia in 1836, with an instructional school for nurses opening in 1850 (ANA, 2007).

Nineteenth Century: In the nineteenth century, prison conditions deteriorated in the United States, forcing the federal government to become involved. Because inmates were crowded together in dormitories, violence was commonplace. One of the earliest cases filed concerned the right of an inmate to health care in the state of North Carolina in 1926. A prisoner was injured during arrest and required surgery. Because of the lack of a qualified surgeon in the county in which the prisoner was arrested, he was taken to a hospital out of the county for care. The surgeon, Dr. Spicer, performed surgery at the behest of the county sheriff. The surgery was successful and the surgeon presented the bill for his services to the sheriff. The sheriff in turn presented the bill to the County Board of Commissioners for payment. The Board refused payment, reasoning that they had not authorized the sheriff to take the prisoner out of the county for treatment. The case wound its way to the Supreme Court of the State of North Carolina, which held, "It is but just that the public be required to care for the prisoner, who cannot, by reason of the deprivation of his liberty, care for himself" (*Spicer v. Williamson*, 1926; p. 293; Moore, 2005).

Twentieth Century: By the twentieth century, prisons had become places of security out of the public eye, surrounded by fencing, razor or electric wire, rocks, and other barriers to deter or prevent escape. Motion sensors, lighting, armed patrol guards, and dogs were all used to ensure security (Sheridan, 1996). In 1953, European countries adopted the *European Convention on Human Rights*, specifically, Article 3, which states "No one shall be subjected to torture or to inhuman or degrading treatment or punishment" (European Court of Human Rights, 1953; p. 6).

In the 1960s, the US courts began to examine more closely the medical treatment of inmates. One of the first federal cases involved the condition of prisons in the State of Alabama. Evidence revealed shortages of staff, equipment, and supplies (*Newman v. Alabama*, 1972). Inmates were used to provide medical care to fellow inmates. The court found that the practices resulted in "a degree of neglect of basic medical needs of prisoners that could justly be called 'barbarous' and 'shocking to the conscience'" (*Newman v. Alabama*, 1972; p. 281).

By the 1970s, violence and prisoner uprisings occurred frequently. Civil rights organizations filed lawsuits to improve conditions, citing violations of the Eighth Amendment against using cruel and unusual punishment. Courts forced prisons to improve living conditions by providing prisoners adequate living space, a bed, three meals a day, medical care, and opportunities for educational and rehabilitative programs. In addition to medical care, housing came under scrutiny. Housing an offender can range from placement in an individual cell with a central day room, to a confined room where the prisoner eats, sleeps, and maintains hygiene, to open pods that house multiple prisoners in a barracks-style living arrangement. Prisoners can also be separated by type of offense, race, ethnicity, and sexual orientation to prevent inmate-on-inmate violence.

Two primary models exist for housing. The first, remote supervision, allows for the officer to observe the prison population from a remote position. This can include secure desk positions or towers. Remote-controlled doors, cameras, restraints, and alarms are all employed to control movement of prisoners (Latessa & Smith, 2011). The second is direct supervision, where the officer monitors the prisoners from within the population, creating a more visible presence (Carlson & Garrett, 2008).

Incarcerated persons are more likely than the general public to have health issues (i.e., substance abuse, drugs, and alcohol; communicable disease; mental illness; and generally poor health (Moore, 2005)). Homelessness and incarceration may exacerbate these problems.

Inmates frequently come from disadvantaged social and cultural groups that either do not seek out medical care on a routine basis or have a negative response to the healthcare system. They are also less likely to seek out preventative care and are more susceptible to exposure to harmful environmental factors (Glaser & Greifinger, 1993). Mental illness is also disproportionately higher with the incarcerated population than the community (NPR, 2011).

While incarcerated, factors negatively effecting the incarcerated include crowding, lack of privacy, and isolation from family and friends. Women in particular are at risk when incarcerated. An estimated 25% of all women in prison suffer from mental illness. This includes depression, bipolar disorder, schizophrenia, posttraumatic stress disorder (PTSD), and addictions (NCCHC, 2011). Diabetes, human immunodeficiency virus (HIV), and sexually transmitted diseases are higher in incarcerated females than the male population (ANA, 2013). Providing primary and preventive services, such as breast cancer screening and yearly PAP smears, are essential (NCCHC, 2011). These interventions have an enormous impact on public health. Lack of care impacts both the family and community when the inmate is released. Untreated issues lead to increased utilization of public resources and higher recidivism rates once the female inmate is released (Women's Health Encyclopedia, 2011). Pregnant females need both physical and mental needs to be addressed while in custody. Provisions for the birth and care of the infant are part of this planning (NCCHC, 2011). Children of women who are incarcerated are at greater risk of being displaced and ending up in foster care, which adds to the stress of incarceration (PBS, n.d.).

Local governments are legally obligated to provide health care to the incarcerated population. The legal framework came in the 1976 landmark Supreme Court case of *Estelle v. Gamble* (1976). In this case, the state prisoner, J. W. Gamble, a prisoner working for the State of Texas, injured his back when a bale of cotton fell on him while he was unloading a truck. He filed his lawsuit *pro se* by submitting a handwritten document after his numerous attempts to obtain help for his severe back pain. A medical assistant treated him on numerous occasions, as did a prison physician and an outside physician. During this time, inmate Gamble also complained of chest pain with accompanying symptoms. Medical treatment was delayed for 4 days by the correctional staff. The Court found for the defendant as it viewed Gamble's failure to receive proper medical care as inadvertent. However, this case established the principle that the deliberate failure of prison authorities to address the medical needs of an inmate constitutes the unnecessary and wanton infliction of pain described in the Eighth Amendment. The Supreme Court ruled that prisoners have the right to be free of "deliberate indifference to [their] serious medical needs" (*Estelle v. Gamble*, 1976; p. 106). Every claim by a prisoner that he or she has not received adequate medical treatment is not a violation of the Eighth Amendment. The Court clarified that "a complaint that a physician has been negligent in diagnosing or treating a medical condition does not state a valid claim of medical mistreatment under the Eight Amendment" (*Estelle v. Gamble*, 1976; p. 106). To be successful, the prisoner must assert a claim that the acts or omissions are "sufficiently harmful to evidence deliberate indifference to [his or her] serious medical needs. It is only such indifference that can offend 'evolving standards of decency,' in violation of the Eighth Amendment" (*Estelle v. Gamble*, 1976; p. 106).

> The Court stated: The elementary principles establish the government's obligation to provide medical care for those whom it is punishing by incarceration. An inmate must rely on prison authorities to treat his medical needs; if the authorities fail to do so, those needs will not be met. In the worst cases, such a failure may actually produce physical "torture or a lingering death," . . . the evils of most immediate concern to the drafters of the Amendment. In less serious cases, denial of medical care may result in pain and suffering which no one suggests would serve any penological purpose . . . The infliction of unnecessary suffering is inconsistent with contemporary standards of decency as manifested in modern legislation codifying the common view that "[i]t is but just the public be required to care for the prisoner, who cannot, by reason of the deprivation of his liberty, care for himself (*Estelle v. Gamble*, 1976; p. 103–104).

From litigation based on *Estelle v. Gamble* (1976), three basic guarantees emerged. First is the right to access to medical care. This means that when an inmate seeks medical care, a medical triage mechanism must exist for the guards to alert the medical staff of a need. This sick call or medical triage usually consists of the inmate providing the medical staff with a written request, commonly called a kite. The second right is access to professional medical judgment. Whatever the medical staff deems is necessary and prudent should be undertaken without delay. Courts will not determine which of two treatments should be undertaken, but rather, seek to ensure that medical personnel make decisions concerning the nature and timing of medical care. The facility must also use equipment designed for medical use, in locations conducive to medical functions, and for reasons that are purely medical (Rold, 1998). Lastly is the right to the care that the medical professional orders. This care should not be impeded or delayed; the custody staff should facilitate medical care and ensure that the inmate receives the care ordered in a timely fashion (Rold, 1998). The constitutional standard does not require an express intent to inflict pain or suffering, rather, it depends on the defendant's state of mind. Further, the defendant must be aware and disregard a substantial risk of harm. The defendant (facility) does not need to be aware or understand that a lack of action can cause danger; however, this can be surmised if the presenting facts indicate that a clear risk of injury or death is incumbent given a failure to act (Rold, 1998).

The US Constitution requires that prisons and jails provide care only for "serious medical needs" (*Estelle v. Gamble*, 1976; p. 106). The cases of *Duran v. Anaya* (1986) and *Ramos v. Lamm* (1983) define a medical need as "serious" if a physician has diagnosed the condition as mandating treatment or if the condition is so obvious that even a layperson would easily recognize the necessity for a physician's attention. Any condition that causes pain, discomfort, or threat to good health is considered serious (*Dean v. Coughlin*, 1989). To fall within the bounds of the Eighth Amendment, serious conditions need not be life-threatening. In *Lugo v. Senkowski* (2000), prisoner Lugo had a stent surgically placed in his kidney to treat a kidney stone. Lugo was released from prison shortly after this surgery with no discharge information regarding expectations or followup treatment for the removal of the stent. He suffered severe pain. The U.S. District Court for the Northern District of New York found that his Eighth Amendment rights were violated because "[t]he State has a duty to provide medical services for an outgoing prisoner who is receiving continuing treatment at the time of his release for the period of time reasonably necessary for him to obtain treatment 'on his own behalf'" (*Lugo v. Senkowski*, 2000; p. 115). As a result of the *Lugo* case, it was further determined that since treatment began while prisoner Lugo was in custody, the State was obligated to complete the treatment course. Because of this decision, prisons must now provide discharge planning to a prisoner when released (NCCHC, 2014b).

The concept of providing health care to incarcerated persons is best summed up by stating: Prisoners are being punished for their crime, "[b]ut the punishment is loss of liberty – not loss of a limb, of eyesight, or of bowel function" (Puleo & Chedekel, 2011). When people were initially incarcerated, the goal was to restrict liberty of movement, not deprive them of a hand, foot, or bodily function. The primary purpose of prisons and jails is not to provide health care; it is to confine lawbreakers and protect society from these criminals for determined amounts of time. Together with confinement comes the obligation to provide shelter, food, and medical care. It is well known that delaying necessary medical treatment can exacerbate a problem with associated increases in costs when the treatment is finally undertaken. Failure of correctional officers to facilitate obtaining prescribed treatment or hindering medical staff has resulted in lengthy, protracted litigation. The combined awards of attorney's fees, damages, and injunctions regarding delivery of medical services have led to costly legal monetary judgments assessed against the institution (Rold, 1998).

Because health care to the incarcerated individual is secondary to the primary purpose of confinement, no governing bodies (aside from the judicial system) provide a mechanism for disciplinary or fining violations. Some organizations that recommend standards for jails and prisons are the National Commission on Correctional Health Care (NCCHC, 2014a; 2014b), the American Correctional Association (ACA, 2004), and the Bureau of Prisons. The United Nations' Standard Minimum Rules for the Treatment of Prisoners articulates acceptable confinement standards for the incarcerated, but it is largely ignored (U.S. Department of State, 2012). Although these organizations provide frameworks for humanely incarcerating people, they provide no monetary incentives or sanctions for lack of compliance. Membership in or accreditation by one of these organizations is strictly voluntary. Therefore, none of these entities can be construed as representing the whole of correctional health care (Faiver, 1998). However, by implementing the standards, the organization establishes a clear framework of acceptable standards to follow.

According to its most recent statistics, the International Centre for Prison Studies' World Prison Population List states that "[m]ore than 10.2 million people are held in penal institutions throughout the world" (Walmsley, 2013; p. 1). This does not include those incarcerated in military detention centers. Also lacking in the count are individuals incarcerated in China and North Korea, which are estimated to total another 800,000 persons (Walmsley, 2013). This translates into an enormous public health challenge. Inmates are usually from economically disadvantaged sections of society. Whether through lack of access to health care, inadequate education, or addictions, offenders' health care can be erratic, unorganized, or nonexistent (Dole, 2006). Frequent health problems noted upon admission to jails and prisons are hypertension, diabetes, and addictions to alcohol, tobacco, and/or other drugs. Large numbers of offenders suffer from mental health issues, which can be challenging to address in custody. Each prisoner has to contend with his or her criminal behavior, as well as his or her physical and mental health while incarcerated. Frequently, the inmate is so profoundly mentally ill as to be unable to assist in a defense until completing the process of acute withdrawal and medical stabilization. Unfortunately, this takes time (NPR, 2011).

Globally, discussion of health care for the incarcerated is largely silent and one can only guess the reasons why. Amnesty International found conditions in Chad "so deplorable that they amount to cruel, inhuman and degrading treatment or punishment" (Amnesty International, 2012; p. 68). In Venezuela, in 2012, 45,000 persons were imprisoned in an area designed for 14,500 (Zamorano, 2012). The list of examples goes on. Added to the problem of overcrowding are the compounding issues of lack of sanitation and food, and contact with violent persons frequently resulting in injury, illness, and even death (Walmsley, 2012).

Because of financial concerns and an increase in the incarcerated population, providing medical care will become more of a challenge in this economic climate.

INTERSECTING SYSTEMS AND SERVICES

- The correctional nurse is instrumental in providing medical care to the incarcerated population. According to the American Nurses Association (ANA), the essence of correctional nursing is caring for and respecting the human dignity of the incarcerated (ANA, 2013). Further, correctional nurses work through correctional and legal systems to provide this care. These systems consist of the domains of research, education, and critical thinking while conferring with fellow medical professionals to provide quality care to the incarcerated (ANA, 2013). As described by Ann Moak in her article, *Defining a Correctional Nurse*, correctional nurses are one part security; one part emergency department nurse; one part primary care nurse; and if working in an infirmary, one part critical care nurse (Moak, 2010).
- Globally, nurses are providing the bulk of health care to the incarcerated. Nurses are not in corrections to assist with punishment; they are there as medical professionals to provide competent health care. They do this through education, advocacy, and delivery of care that is based on community standards (ANA, 2013). In Canada and the United Kingdom (UK), nurses working in the correctional arena are becoming more proactive and implementing standards to guide their care. Canada has established a legal mandate to provide every incarcerated person with essential healthcare and reasonable access to nonessential medical care (Miller, 2013). In the United Kingdom, the Royal College of Nursing (RCN) established principles of nursing practice that apply to all settings, including criminal justice (Dale & Woods, 2002). By becoming more proactive, the RCN nurses in 2012 decided on eight principles and plan to expand on these to guide them in the correctional setting (Knox, 2013).
- When the correctional nurse interacts with inmates in the clinic, booking area, and housing units, he or she must possess excellent critical thinking skills. These include services and skills comparable to working in public health, disease management, emergency nursing, mental health, outpatient services, and chronic and acute care. A corrections nurse must be well versed in all aspects of medical and nursing care, and keep current on nursing trends. The correctional nurse must also be skilled in assessment and negotiation skills (ANA, 2007).
- Forensic nurses partner with others in health care and the legal and social systems to assist in determining a cause when psychological or physical injury has occurred. Forensic nurses are able to articulate the scientific reasons and the resulting consequences by integrating knowledge of forensic and nursing sciences in their assessments (IAFN & ANA, 2009). Forensic nurses use the realms of education, scientific research, nursing practice, and consultation with others to provide care to their patients (IAFN & ANA, 2009).

Although correctional nurses provided the first known health care to offenders in 1797, the ANA has recognized correctional nursing as a specialty only since 1985. The Task Force on Standards of Nursing Practice in Correctional Facilities under the direction of the Executive Committee of the Council of Community Health Nurses published *Standards of Nursing Practice in Correctional Facilities* (Schoenly & Knox, 2013). Although having standards of nursing practice in correctional facilities is largely unique to the United States, globalization of the need to obtain higher education for nurses will bring about quality, consistency, and common standards of practice. Common educational standards are necessary to regulate the nursing profession in which lives depend on specific competencies (Baumann & Blythe, 2008). Correctional nursing is "the practice of nursing and delivery of patient care within the unique and distinctive environment of the criminal justice system" (ANA, 2007; p. 1). Jails, prisons, juvenile detention centers, and facilities that provide community corrections and inpatient and outpatient drug-abuse treatment have a nurse employee on staff (Schoenly & Knox, 2013). Nurses overwhelmingly are the largest group of caregivers in the correctional system in the United States as compared to other medical professionals (i.e., physicians) (ANA, 2013). Having nurses in a confined setting allows arrestees – many of whom are homeless and have co-occurring mental health and substance abuse issues and are known to frequently cycle through the criminal justice system – to access needed medical care (Puleo & Chedekel, 2011). Unfortunately, often, a lack of appropriate, affordable medical/mental health care or/and housing and money exist to support treatment programs in the offenders' community, once a person is released. While in custody, these prisoners are able to address their medical/social needs (ANA, 2013).

- Many systems and services intersect on a daily basis to provide the incarcerated person with assistance while in custody. Health staff can consist of a physician, administrator, nurses, physician assistants, nurse practitioners, dentist, and mental health and substance abuse professionals (NCCHC, 2003). If the correctional facility is located in a rural setting and is unable to provide inhouse services/staff, a memorandum of understanding (MOU) or a contract needs to exist between the facility and the needed medical identity for the correctional facility to provide the needed service. Frequently, mental health and dental services are contracted out into the community to provide these services to the inmates and meet standards of practice appropriate to the correctional facility, whether it is prison or jail (ANA, 2013).

- Another rapidly growing segment of correctional care is outsourcing of inmate housing and medical care to private companies. Private companies contract for the complete management and operation of correctional facilities. These private, for-profit companies are able to provide the facility with increased cost-savings due to eliminating the duplication of components necessary for efficient operation (policies, practices, bulk purchasing, and experience) by virtue of numerous systems (corrections.com, 2000). The negative aspect of this option is the loss of control for the facility especially in a rural setting in terms of staffing, full-time equivalent (FTE) positions for healthcare staff, and hours of healthcare services available. Recent literature reveals that private companies are unable to provide services more cost-effectively than the correctional facility can (corrections.com, 2000).

- Telehealth is also becoming a viable alternative for delivering health care to inmates because of the cost-savings associated with its use and the ability to reach persons anywhere. Use of computer functions for provision of specific medical care via computer can save time and permit more patient coverage. One healthcare provider with particular expertise can serve numerous facilities that lack a specialty skill component on their staff (Heller, Oros, Durney-Crowley, 2013).

- The nurse must maintain professional boundaries while advocating for the best interest of the inmate. Although it is rare, nurses have been known to cross the professional boundary and develop inappropriate relationships with the incarcerated; their actions jeopardize the safety and security of their peers, correctional staff, and the prisoner (ANA, 2007). The nurse must maintain professional boundaries during interactions with the prisoner and articulate and appropriately document in the medical chart the findings and the care rendered. These can become blurred when a personal relationship develops. Confidentiality must be maintained even in the presence of correctional staff that is often tasked with monitoring the prisoner during medical care (ANA, 2007). Further, because physical contact between the nurse and the prisoner is discouraged or prohibited, the nurse must develop excellent interpersonal communication skills to convey expressions of caring (ANA, 2013).

In 1985, the ANA established standards for the practice of nursing in correctional settings, which were the first such national nursing standards to be developed. Canada and the United Kingdom have since expounded on their standards of practice to include correctional nursing (Knox, 2013). The definition of nursing practice in the correctional setting is:

> [T]he provision of primary care services for the population from the time of entry into the system, through transfers to other institutions, to final release from custody. Primary health services in this field include the use of all aspects of the nursing process in carrying out screening activities, providing direct healthcare services, analyzing individual health behaviors, teaching, counseling, and assisting individuals in assuming responsibility for their own health to the best of their ability, knowledge, and circumstances (Northrup, 1987; p. 253).

Further, the provider of care should not be limited by personal attitudes or beliefs, and should provide unbiased care to all inmates. Each inmate should be cared for in a professional, nonjudgmental way.

- Correctional nursing is essentially involved in every domain that impacts the daily life of the inmate; it is considered a partner in the correctional staff system (ANA, 2013). The correctional nurse must have excellent critical thinking skills, attention to detail, ability for clinical decision-making, and a working knowledge of the standards of professional practice, particularly when he or she is employed at a small or rural correctional facility where no physician is physically on duty. The correctional nurse must be able to quickly recognize an emergency and provide the correct treatment to prevent untoward outcomes (ANA, 2013).

Over centuries, the debate has raged whether incarceration is for punitive or rehabilitative purposes. One author proposed that in addition to rehabilitating the person, incarceration serves three distinct functions: retribution, deterrence, and isolation or removal from society (Alschuler, 2003). Limiting the incarcerated person's freedom – while maintaining public safety and security and providing for the health and well-being of the inmate population – is the recurring goal of incarceration (ANA, 2007). Frequently, persons not associated with incarceration (e.g., the community) view correctional facilities as isolated institutions where supposed horrors, such as rape, harsh treatment, and beatings, stay within the confines of the institution (ANA, 2013). This lack of understanding can reduce correctional nurses' satisfaction with their jobs and lead to burnout and frustration (ANA, 2013).

Correctional nurses are faced with continuingly changing scenarios for providing health care to inmates who may cycle through the system even before healthcare changes can be instituted. This cycling can result in incomplete treatments, missed diagnoses, and missed opportunities to educate inmates on health issues. This cycling may also alter the correctional nurse's attitude toward inmates in that the nurse may feel it is futile to treat inmates as they are not in custody long enough to complete treatment. In a study conducted in 2013, nurses' attitudes were measured using the Attitudes Toward Prisoners Scale (ATPS), which was administered to 146 nurses practicing at 19 correctional facilities in 5 states. Demographic data collected included age, education, gender, and length of time working in corrections. Results showed two factors were associated with attitude: age and whether the nurse worked in a jail or prison setting. Overall attitude scores for correctional nurses were lower (more negative) than the scores of previously measured groups, which included correctional officers, police officers, community members, and others involved with corrections (Shields & de Moya, 1997).

- The delivery of health care is a collaborative effort between the security staff, mental health staff, medical staff, and substance abuse treatment staff. Unreasonable barriers to care must be avoided. Examples of barriers include punishing inmates for seeking treatment, uncooperative behavior, and holding sick call at hours that are not conducive for the inmate to attend or that conflict with another activity the inmate is attending (e.g., court, religious services, and classes). Permitting unreasonable delays before an outside healthcare provider sees an inmate is also an example of hindering or impeding the access to care (NCCHC, 2003). A highly effective systematic plan of care can be achieved through the cooperative effort of a collaborative team approach. Custody staff is a vital link in carrying out the prescribed health treatments and needs of the inmates. If this cooperation between custody staff and the clinical staff is lacking, the healthcare staff, the mental health staff, and the drug abuse treatment staff will be hindered in their ability to perform their professional duties (NCCHC, 2003). The team must work together to ensure cooperation rather than competition. The overarching goal is to have a positive patient healthcare outcome (Lee, Palmbach, & Miller, 2006).

- Cost of care should not be a consideration or a valid defense for failing to provide adequate medical care. Inmates in correctional facilities are entitled to essential elements of hygiene; adequate sanitary living conditions; adequate drinking water; competent medical, psychological, and dental care; medically prescribed drugs and diets; drug/alcohol detoxification; use of exercise and recreational areas; and visitor and telephone calls (*Finney v. Arkansas Board of Corrections*, 1974; *O'Conner v. Donaldson*, 1975). Only Nordic prisons (Denmark, Sweden, Finland, and Norway) fare better in treatment of the incarcerated. Nordic prisons focus on inmate rights, which are of paramount concern. The ultimate goal is to teach offenders that their choices have consequences, both good and bad, which result in more favorable outcomes for the education and rehabilitation of offenders. Nordic prisons are also limited in size. One hundred inmates per institution is normal and the system strives to keep the incarcerated person in close proximity to his or her families. Regardless of the crime, sentences are imparted, so the incarcerated person will be released while still living (Ward et al., 2013).

PRACTICE AND PREVENTION

Correctional nursing is a diverse nurse-driven system that is based on professional practice, critical thinking skills, ongoing education, situational awareness, and the importance of sound assessment skills. The practice of correctional nursing begins at intake or when a patient arrives at the facility and moves on through the sick call, wellness checks, immunizations, and chronic care process, to discharge or release.

- The assessment: The nurse's ability to perform a head-to-toe nursing assessment, interview for history of present illness, and gather historical and healthcare data helps provide the same level of care the inmate would receive in the community. The correctional nurse must determine if an inmate has special needs, help prevent illness from spreading throughout the facility, or by his or her assessment, prevent an inmate from dying from an illness, injury, or substance withdrawal. The correctional nurse must know when a higher level of care is indicated and be able to refer a patient to the hospital setting to prevent morbidity or mortality. A nurse's role is critical to the health of the inmate and each encounter builds upon a professional therapeutic relationship between the patient and the caregiver with collaboration among other health professionals and a focus on evidence-based care.

- The intake screening: According to the National Commission on Correctional Health Care (NCCHC) standards, the receiving (intake) screening is performed on all inmates upon their arrival at the facility so that emergent and urgent health needs of the new inmates are met in a timely manner (NCCHC, 2014b). A receiving (intake) screening is a process of focused questions and observations designed to prevent newly arrived inmates from being admitted to the facility's general population with a potential threat to their own health and safety or that of another inmate. The goal is to identify current and past illnesses or health conditions; assess for emergency situations among new arrivals; assess for communicable and infectious diseases; identify patients who have a history of mental illness or are at risk for suicide; obtain information on dental problems, pregnancy, allergies, substance use, and so forth; and identify patients with known illnesses and those who are currently on medications so they may receive further assessment, referral, and continued treatment. This intake screening process requires expert clinical assessment skills and appropriate healthcare training on history-taking to obtain adequate data to evaluate necessary placement of the inmate. Along with identifying an inmate's special needs or risk status, the screening findings lead to referrals or affect housing assignments. Occasionally, a screening for health clearance will be performed in an emergency department of a local hospital prior to the patient being transferred to the detention facility. This is often performed when the arresting officers is aware that the offender has a medical condition or recent injury.

Although booking officers are required to conduct a medical questionnaire as part of the booking process (receiving an inmate into the facility), it is imperative that appropriately trained healthcare staff conducts an intake screening and review of the inmate's health and mental health conditions. Inmates are not always forthcoming with officers regarding information about medical issues. They may fear retaliation or lack of confidentiality. The correctional nurse's role in the intake screening process is to gather valuable information on the inmate's medical and mental health so that proper care is initiated from the beginning of incarceration, and to protect the safety and welfare of other inmates, as well as the correctional and support staff. The intake screening is also a time when an inmate is provided with information on access to care and how to contact the medical services department.

Nursing staff performing the intake screening can have a positive effect in helping inmates perceive that medical personnel are concerned about the inmates health issues and that they will be taken care of while incarcerated. Early screening, referral to a provider when indicated, and rapid initiation of nursing treatment protocols for treatment of common disorders that are site-specific help prevent morbidity, mortality, and liability suits.

According to the NCCHC, the four purposes of the intake screening are:

- To identify and meet any urgent health needs of those being admitted;
- To identify and meet any known or easily identifiable health needs that require medical intervention prior to the health assessment (see the initial health assessment or physical);
- To identify and isolate inmates who appear potentially contagious; and
- To appropriately obtain a medical clearance when necessary (NCCHC, 2014b).

Other health screenings occur in the correctional setting to assess inmates prior to assignments for work duties, prior to admission to some treatment programs, and when they are placed in segregation (NCCHC, 2014a). The intake screening can be abbreviated for returning inmates, such as transfers or those who serve weekend sentences in a jail setting. These screens are designed to capture any changes in condition or newly prescribed medications. Frequently, additional data are gathered on drug or alcohol use, communicable diseases, mental illness symptoms, pregnancies, and recent hospitalizations (Schoenly & Knox, 2013).

A focused screening is performed on inmates involved in altercations within the facility. This screening focuses on injury and trauma at the time of the incident and frequently requires additional documentation so that security personnel can complete an investigation. The documentation includes a written description of injuries, appropriate referrals to mental health for followup care, and a clear statement of any comments made by the patient regarding the incident. The correctional nurse does not perform a forensic examination for the purpose of gathering evidence, but refers the patient to an appropriate emergency facility if indicated (NCCHC, 2014a).

- The initial physical: According to NCCHC requirements and recommendations, the physical examination is to be completed by the fourteenth day of incarceration. It involves an objective hands-on evaluation of the individual, including inspection, palpation, auscultation, and percussion (NCCHC, 2014b). This examination is a full head-to-toe physical, and is performed by a specially trained registered nurse, an advanced practice registered nurse (APRN), a physician, or a certified physician assistant (PA-C). The physical examination functions as a more detailed tool to obtain information on family and patient history, physical or mental illnesses, medications, and surgical history or hospitalizations. It includes a dental screening and education on dental care while incarcerated, laboratory testing as indicated, and placement or referral into a chronic care system to treat asthma, diabetes, hypertension, HIV infection, and other chronic diseases. During this examination, staff also has an opportunity to provide the inmate with valuable health education information on health care and disease topics.

- Chronic care clinics: The nurse's role as part of a multidisciplinary team is essential for chronic disease management in the correctional environment. Chronic diseases now affect more than one third of inmates in federal prisons, state prisons, and local jails (Schoenly & Knox, 2013; Wilper et al., 2009). Many factors affecting a high proportion of the incarcerated population influence the rates of chronic diseases. Some of these include ethnic minorities, hypertension, obesity, cigarette smoking and substance abuse, poor diets, and longer sentences (Sabol, Minton, & Harrison, 2007). The inmate population is also aging, and have an accelerated physiological aging of approximately 10 years as compared to those who have never been incarcerated (Smyer & Burbank, 2009). Other differences between the incarcerated population and general population include a wide variety of literacy skills and, in many cases, absence of family involvement.

    National medical consensus groups have developed guidelines for chronic disease management to reduce morbidity and mortality from hypertension, dyslipidemia, diabetes, HIV, and asthma. NCCHC and the American Correctional Association (ACA) have both adopted and endorsed these guidelines for chronic care disease management. In late 2002, NCCHC published the first set of guidelines designed for correctional settings, which adapted guidelines from the JNC 6&7, the American Diabetes Association's diabetic guidelines, and the National Asthma Education Program. The NCCHC continues to review and incorporate community standard guidelines into its recommendations on correctional clinical practice (NCCHC, 2014a; 2014b).

    Individualized treatment plans are vital to the ongoing management of these patients. Teaching patients about their disease processes and treatment goals is crucial. This patient education is also one of the tenets of the American Nurses Association's *Correctional Nursing: Scope and Standards of Practice* (ANA, 2013). Nurses can impact the patients' understandings of medications, side effects, and disease processes and assist them in making informed choices regarding their health care.

    In many facilities, professional nursing staff use standardized forms for followup care of chronic conditions in between the patients' provider visits. At these visits, nursing staff members review medications with patients, and obtain and review diagnostic studies and monitoring, such as blood pressures or blood glucose levels (NCCHC, 2014b). Again, this offers a valuable opportunity for education and patient teaching.

- Nurse sick call: In 1976, the Supreme Court decision in *Estelle v Gamble* resulted in guaranteed, mandated requirements for inmate medical care. Access to care is a fundamental right. As a result, inmates must have access to medical staff and a way to communicate the need for care. From this requirement, a sick call system was developed in correctional settings to provide access to care in a timely manner. Upon intake, the inmates are educated about how to access care and the facility's procedures for sick call. Medical staff reviews the requests and all patients have the opportunity to request services daily (NCCHC, 2014b). Some systems post a list on which the inmates sign up and then report to the clinic to be seen by a health professional; some require completion of a sick call request form; and others offer sick call daily as part of nursing rounds. Nursing and medical staff should initiate sick call and manage all sick call requests once the patients fill them out. Some facilities have locked boxes and nursing staff maintain the keys; other facilities have the patients directly hand their request slips to nursing staff during medication passes or rounds each day. This provides the patients with confidentiality and ensures that no limitations are placed on to access to care.

    The sick call system utilizes the entire nursing process. At most facilities, a nursing staff member reviews each sick call slip to determine acuity and need for referral, and to assist with prioritizing scheduling due to limited resources. In many instances, sick call clinics are scheduled daily to address the nonemergency healthcare requests and needs.

During sick call, the nursing staff often uses nursing protocols to provide interventions to patients. Nursing assessment protocols are written guidelines for nurses to undertake to evaluate a patient's complaint and to provide the interventions (NCCHC, 2014b). Nursing administration develops the nursing protocols and the responsible physician then reviews them every year (NCCHC, 2014b). Each nursing professional using the protocols must have documentation of training and competency. Protocols specify use of over-the-counter medications unless an emergency or life-threatening situation is being assessed. Each site must have written policy and procedures addressing the use of nursing procedures (NCCHC, 2014b). States differ on scope of practice; all nursing protocols must comply with the state's Nurse Practice Act. All treatments with prescription medication must have the written or verbal order of a licensed practitioner. Some states require signatures within a certain timeframe so that the patient will be evaluated.

- Infirmary care: Many jail and prison settings have large housing areas, which are set up to treat inmate patients with special needs or increased medical acuity. Some are referred to as special housing units and others as medical observation, infirmary, or mental health special housing. If the site is accredited and medical services contracts specifically address the staffing needs of its special units, each area is staffed according to state requirements and standards. Nursing staff often provides additional care services such as maintaining intravenous lines and administering tube feedings, performing complicated wound care and dressing changes, providing acute mental health care, or offering services found in long-term care settings. The care provided in the special housing areas can be short- or long-term but consists of services that cannot be given in the general population housing. These special units are typically located near the medical nursing station or main medical area so that staff may evaluate the inmates during each shift and have ease of access.

  Like other medical encounters, care provided in the special housing units is documented in the medical record, including education or specific instructions given to the inmate. Logs of admission and discharge are kept as well.

  An infirmary houses patients who have conditions that require skilled nursing care 24 hours a day and a daily provider visit. A provider must admit the inmate to the infirmary and discharge him or her when appropriate. Security personnel do not have authority to place an inmate in the infirmary. For infirmary admission, a physician or nonphysician provider (APRN or PA-C) must evaluate the inmate and write an admission order. Within 24 hours, the clinician must complete a physical examination and the nursing staff must create the nursing care plan. Release from an infirmary setting also requires an order by the provider. A discharge summary outlining the care received and ongoing treatment plans is required (NCCHC, 2014b).

- Infection control: In most jails and prisons, inmates live in close quarters and have limited access to soap and water. Many of these prospective patients have poor hygiene, poor self-care skills, and mental illness. Because of variations in information-sharing between and among correctional jurisdictions, the possibility of infection and transmission of diseases is higher in these environments (Bick, 2007).

  Nursing in these environments can be challenging in requiring diligence regarding infectious diseases and parasites. Nurses must screen the inmates on intake for infectious diseases such as tuberculosis (TB), parasites, and airborne or other illnesses. Correctional employees and medical staff are often at risk for exposure to blood-borne pathogens during daily work duties. The NCCHC requires each accredited facility to have an exposure control plan and policy and procedures in effect to address infection control (NCCHC, 2014b).

  The infection control program is site-specific and focuses on accurate, consistent surveillance of ongoing episodes of infection. This process is used to monitor and evaluate the care of the inmates and to monitor for infections that pose a high risk of morbidity and mortality. Monitoring includes communicable diseases, healthcare-associated infections, unusual infections, unusual organisms or parasites, post-hospital discharge infections, or other trends noted within the facility. Common diseases seen in the correctional environment include hepatitis, ectoparasites, HIV, influenza, Staph infections such as methicillin-resistant *Staphylococcus aureus* (MRSA), norovirus, TB, sexually transmitted infections, and varicella (Schoenly & Knox, 2013; CDC, 2012a; CDC, 2012b).

Each facility usually has an infection control committee. Infection control data and reports should be shared at least quarterly in the medical meetings with custodial administration. State and local public health officials rely on healthcare providers, laboratories, and other public health personnel to report to state and local health departments regarding the occurrence of noticeable diseases. Without such data, trends cannot be accurately monitored, unusual occurrences of diseases might not be detected, and the effectiveness of intervention activities cannot be easily evaluated.

Requirements for reporting noticeable diseases are mandated by state laws or regulations; the list of reportable diseases differs in each state. The Centers for Disease Control and Prevention (CDC) and the Council of State and Territorial Epidemiologists have established a policy that requires state health departments to report cases of selected diseases to the CDC's National Noticeable Diseases Surveillance System (NNDSS).

Sites use standard precautions as defined by the CDC and the WHO. These standards combine the features of univeral precautions and body substance isolation to reduce transmission risks of blood-borne pathogens and those of moist body substances.

Aspects of standard precautions include disinfection and sterilization of instruments and equipment; monitoring of sterilization; the appropriate labeling and safe handling of laboratory specimens; and the use of retractable needles, single-use equipment, blood-spill cleanup kits, personal protective equipment (such as gloves, masks, and gowns to protect both the healthcare worker and patients), and other special equipment as needed to maintain a safe environment for staff. Limitations for infection control in the correctional setting include issues such as access to running water, location and availability of supplies, safety issues with violent offenders, and limitations of security.

- Medication management and documentation: Medication management within the correctional setting carries its own set of challenges and restrictions. Inmates usually receive their medications on a scheduled pill pass where inmates present to a window or staff members go to the housing units to provide medications directly to the patients. Most facilities use patient-specific medication. Nursing staff is expected to follow the regulations and laws of each state with regard to who can pass the medication and how it is accomplished. Controlled medications are kept on count with multiple signatures for documentation, verification, and disposal. These drugs are monitored during each shift by nursing staff and documentation is imperative. Inmates in segregation areas require different security measures, which can increase the amount of time needed to provide medications and care. Medications can be in blister packs, bottles, or other packaging options. For security reasons, most facilities prohibit glass, except for items such as insulin and nitroglycerin. Some facilities permit inmates to keep their chronic medications or over-the-counter medications on their person; others require each dose to be delivered by nursing staff (NCCHC, 2014b).

In the correctional setting, communication is vital, not only to the patient/inmate population but also among health professionals. Part of this process includes the necessary and appropriate documentation. Documentation supports the nurse by detailing the care provided to the patient, demonstrating quality of care, and providing evidence if needed in a court process. The legal process for use in courts and obeying the US federal mandates of the Health Insurance Portability and Accountability Act (HIPAA) require patients to provide consent for release of medical records. The medical chart is considered a legal document and all medical care staff maintains confidentiality of personal health information. Clarity of documentation benefits the patient and other caregivers in the provision or continuity of care. In correctional settings, one may see both paper and electronic medical records (EMR). Either of these records must be complete. Medical staff members are responsible for scanning documents and records to ensure that dates and signatures are attached. The records are organized on a site-specific basis but include sections for progress notes, orders, diagnostic results, and medications.

The format for noting in progress notes in the correctional environment follows that of the community. Most systems support the subjective, objective, assessment, and plan (SOAP) protocol for noting. Important details are to avoid abbreviations and opinions in noting (NCCHC, 2014b). A standard practice in all settings, including corrections, is the assumption that if something is not documented, it has not been done. Nursing staff must take ownership of this vital process in the care continuum.

POPULATIONS AT RISK

Incarcerated persons are more likely than the general public to have health issues (i.e., substance abuse, drugs and alcohol, communicable disease, mental illness, and generally poor health) (Moore, 2005; WHO 2007b; WHO, 2014). Homelessness and incarceration may exacerbate these problems.

- Mental illness and substance abuse: An estimated 72% of the incarcerated population has comorbidity of serious mental illness coupled with substance abuse (ANA, 2013). In a meta-analysis of global literature on mental health and prisoners, Fazel and Seewald (2012) found that 10% of incarcerated men and 14% of incarcerated women had diagnoses of major depression. Prevalence of psychosis was 3.6% for incarcerated male prisoners and 3% in female prisoners (Fazel & Seewald, 2012). In Greece, mental health problems, followed by hepatitis, are the health issues most negatively impacting quality of life among incarcerated men (Togas, Raikou, & Niakas, 2014). Offenders are disposed to antisocial behavior in the form of criminal mindsets, problems with impulse control, and poor coping skills. These can lead to difficult behavior, which can be projected toward the caregiver (Ross & Drake, 1992).

  Since the 1980s, when the United States began to systematically defund the public mental healthcare system, increasing numbers of individuals with mental illness have been incarcerated for behaviors that may be symptomatic of their mental disorders (Torrey et al., 2014). Worldwide, more than half of all offenders suffer from mental illness (WHO, 2012). In state prisons, offenders with mental illness were twice as likely as others to have been homeless in the year prior to their arrests (Torrey et al., 2014). In women's prisons, nearly three out of four offenders have a mental illness (Harner & Burgess, 2011). Offenders with mental illness are more vulnerable in many ways. For example, these ill offenders are twice as likely as mentally healthy offenders to be injured in fights during their incarcerations.

- Depression: An offender who suffers from a major depressive disorder (MDD) experiences symptoms that may include some or all of the following: diminished interest in previously pleasurable activities, sadness and hopelessness, insomnia, fatigue, alteration in food intake, feelings of failure, difficulty concentrating, attention deficits, psychomotor retardation or agitation, and active or passive thoughts of suicide. Treatment of MDD usually involves prescription of antidepressant medications, such as selective serotonin reuptake inhibitors (SSRIs) and selective norepinephrine reuptake inhibitors (SNRIs). Examples of SSRIs include fluoxetine (Prozac), paroxetine (Paxil), citalopram (Celexa), and sertraline (Zoloft). Venlafaxine (Effexor) and duloxetine (Cymbalta) are well-known SNRIs. Some common side effects of SSRIs and SNRIs include nausea during initial dosing, impaired libido or blunted sexual response, increased energy, heavy sweating, and an increased tendency toward bruising and bleeding. Older tricyclic antidepressants (TCAs) are usually not used in correctional facilities because of their side effects, narrow therapeutic windows, and the ease with which they can be hoarded and used for suicide attempts. The exception to this TCA undesirability is trazodone (Oleptro), which may be used to induce sleep. Even with low doses, patients may feel residual morning sedation. At high doses of trazodone, male patients may suffer from priapism, which can require emergent intervention. Occasionally, other TCAs, particularly amitriptyline (Elavil) or nortriptyline (Pamelor) may be used to treat chronic pain issues. Monoamine oxidase inhibitors (MAOIs) are seldom used in correctional facilities because of their interactions with common foods and other medications (Burns, 2005).

Fiscal considerations dictate use of narrow formularies that emphasize lower-cost generic pharmaceutical agents. Thus, an inexpensive SSRI, such as citalopram (Celexa), is likely to be included in a formulary, while its half-sibling, escitalopram (Lexapro), is likely excluded; brand medications may cost more than ten times greater than their generic versions. Similarly, immediate release formulations are favored over sustained release (SR) and extended release (XR) preparations, because of costs rather than efficacy. Psychiatric medications often comprise a disproportionately large share of an institution's pharmaceutical expenses.

- Anxiety disorders: An offender who suffers from an anxiety disorder is a candidate for SSRI medication such as fluoxetine (Prozac), paroxetine (Paxil), or citalopram (Celexa), because these medications have anxiolytic properties and can significantly decrease symptoms of anxiety as well as depression. Although benzodiazepines (BZDs) are famous for reducing anxiety, they have a high potential for abuse and interactions with other medications, so they are rarely used to treat chronic anxiety in persons who are incarcerated. Diazepam (Valium), lorazepam (Ativan), and alprazolam (Xanax) are among the most popular BZD anxiolytics. Serotonin stabilizer buspirone (BuSpar), antihistamine hydroxyzine (Vistaril), and sympatholytic beta-blocker propranolol (Inderal) are popular nonaddicting options for treating anxiety.
- Posttraumatic stress disorder: Posttraumatic stress disorder (PTSD) is a mental disorder in which a person who has survived what he or she believes to be a life-threatening event suffers from nightmares, flashbacks, and/or intrusive thoughts of re-experiencing that traumatic event (Harner & Burgess, 2011). Common symptoms of this disorder include hyperarousal, anxiety, fear, and ineffective coping skills. Many offenders acquire PTSD during their incarceration experiences. Paroxetine (Paxil) and sertraline (Zoloft) are popular SSRIs approved for treatment of PTSD. Prazosin (Minipress), an antihypertensive agent that may be dosed at bedtime or twice per day, is also commonly prescribed to reduce hyperarousal and decrease nightmare activity (Keller, 2012).
- Psychosis: Psychosis is a mental state in which a person loses contact with reality. Psychosis may be a symptom of a thought disorder, such as schizophrenia, or of a severe mood disorder, such as bipolar affective disorder. Behavioral issues, including stimulant abuse and/or lack of sleep, may induce psychosis. Treatment with antipsychotic medications targets the positive symptoms (delusions, hallucinations, disorganized speech, and disorganized behavior) and negative symptoms (narrowing range of emotional expression, interactions with others, and self-motivation). First-generation antipsychotic agents (FGAs), like chlorpromazine (Thorazine) and haloperidol (Haldol), and second-generation or atypical antipsychotic agents (SGAs or AAPs) may be prescribed to help stabilize moods and reduce symptoms of psychosis. Popular SGAs, including olanzapine (Zyprexa) and quetiapine (Seroquel), carry risks of weight gain and hyperglycemia, so patients on these medications must be monitored for these side effects. Body mass index (BMI), waist circumference, weight, and fasting blood glucose are typically monitored in persons taking antipsychotic medications. Antipsychotic medications may be augmented with other agents, such as anticonvulsants and/or mood stabilizers. Electrocardiograms (ECGs) are required upon initiation of certain antipsychotics or mood-stabilizing agents.

Correctional nurses may work in forensic psychiatric units wherein suspects and offenders are evaluated for competency to understand the charges against them and to participate in their own defenses. Newly sentenced offenders with mental health issues may begin their terms of confinement in specialty prison units where their needs are assessed to determine their optimal feasible placement so that they can most successfully integrate into institutional culture.

With the deinstitutionalization of persons with mental illnesses since the 1960s, jails and prisons have become the placement for people whom detoxification centers and hospitals are unable to treat due to violent behavioral issues (ANA, 2013). Because persons with mental illness may find it difficult to distinguish right from wrong, they often find themselves entangled with the legal system. When a prisoner is booked into custody, if the prisoner's behavior is noncompliant, under the influence, or violent, the correctional nurse must first determine the cause of this behavior. The correctional nurse must begin his or her assessment at the initial contact. Speaking with the prisoner is telling. The nurse may determine if the inmate is under the influence or is exhibiting a mental illness. Laboratories have developed rapid, multiple panel urine tests that give a presumptive result for the drug tested. Equipment is available that can screen for various drugs of abuse. "Breathalyzer" machines are available to measure alcohol levels. These, along with written protocols, all aid the nurse with his or her decision-making. Critical thinking skills are essential to this process (NCCHC, 2003).

Upon admittance to the facility, a mental health screening and evaluation should be performed to determine the prisoner's mental status. This evaluation must include any current or past history of psychiatric hospitalization; suicidal ideation or attempts; violent behavior; any cerebral trauma or seizures; whether any sex offenses were committed; and whether the prisoner may be gravely disabled, or pose a danger to self and others (NCCHC, 2003).

When an inmate screens positive for a history of mental health issues, he or she needs to be referred to a qualified mental health professional. If the inmate is suicidal or in an acute mental health crisis, appropriate precautions must be taken or the inmate should be transferred to the appropriate mental health facility (NCCHC, 2003). According to the Bureau of Justice Statistics, suicide is the number one cause of death in jails, but not in prisons (NCCHC, 2011). In this setting, the interaction between the medical staff, mental health staff, and security staff is essential and can make the difference between a successful suicide attempt or a failed one (NCCHC, 2011).

An offender's use of substances may impact his or her care throughout the incarceration—from arrival at jail through release upon completion of the sentence. Correctional nurses must be able to recognize symptoms of intoxication and withdrawal from alcohol as well as from a variety of street and prescription drugs. Nurses must know and follow their institutions' policies and procedures regarding detoxification and withdrawal. Although it can be difficult for offenders to obtain alcohol and drugs within their correctional institution, substances can be obtained or manufactured onsite through the underground prison economy. *Pruno*, also called *julep*, is a fruit-based alcoholic beverage brewed by offenders. Offenders who consume pruno or alcohol-based hand sanitizers may require detoxification and other medical attention (Weinstein, Kim, Mack, Malavade, & Saraiya, 2005). Symptoms of alcohol and benzodiazepine withdrawal include nausea/vomiting, tremulousness, and anxiety; in severe cases, hallucinations, seizures, and death may result. Symptom severity may be monitored using the Revised Clinical Institute Withdrawal Assessment for Alcohol (CIWA-Ar) scale (Sullivan, Sykora, Schneiderman, Naranjo, & Sellers, 1989). Chlordiazepoxide (Librium), carbamazepine (Tegretol), haloperidol (Haldol), clonidine (Catapres), and gabapentin (Neurontin) are among the medications that may be selected to treat withdrawal symptoms (Bayard, McIntyre, Hill, & Woodside, 2004).

For persons who are addicted to opioids, incarceration often precipitates an acute withdrawal period lasting from several days to 2 weeks, depending on the substance. Opioid withdrawal is characterized by mydriasis, photophobia, rhinorrhea, diaphoresis, nausea/vomiting, muscle cramping (hence the slang term *kicking*), diarrhea, blood pressure elevation, irritability, and an overall feeling of malaise. Symptom severity may be measured and monitored using the Clinical Opiate Withdrawal Symptoms Scale (COWS) (Wesson & Ling, 2003). Symptoms of opioid withdrawal may be mitigated with the use of medications such as a *kick kit*, including clonidine (Catapres) to reduce blood pressure, methocarbamol (Robaxin) for muscle cramping, and dicyclomine (Bentyl) to reduce gastric motility and diarrhea. Although opioid withdrawal may be intensely uncomfortable, it usually does not carry the severe health risks of alcohol or benzodiazepine withdrawal. However, in pregnant offenders, opioid withdrawal may precipitate miscarriage or fetal demise and daily methadone (Dolophine), which is not teratogenic, is the preferred treatment until after delivery (Wong, Ordean, & Kahan, 2011). Some jurisdictions recognize the value of methadone maintenance treatment (MMT) for offenders, especially those already participating in MMT programs at the time of their arrest, in order to promote long-term sobriety. Research continues on offenders who receive MMT to determine its impact on reducing healthcare expenses and recidivism (O'Donnell & Trick, 2006).

A higher proportion of injection drug use (IVDU) occurs among female prisoners than male. Both are likely to continue using while incarcerated, primarily to relax, whereas before incarceration, they used for recreation and to forget their problems. Worldwide, it is estimated that up to 25% of injection drug users begin injecting in prisons where access to clean needles is rare and needle-sharing is common. Opioid replacement therapy can be a powerful intervention to reduce risky behaviors, particularly those that increase exposure to HIV, and to support therapeutic interventions in drug-dependent prisoners (Jurgens, 2007). Research indicates that IVDU is particularly common when prisoners regain their freedom; one study reported IVDU relapse on the day of release for 82% of the former inmates who returned to IVDU (Jurgens, 2007). The World Health Organization recommends that incarcerated persons have access to clinical trials for HIV therapies, equivalent to that of nonprison populations, and without pressure to participate in research studies (Jurgens, 2007).

Although substance abuse treatment (SAT) for incarcerated individuals has demonstrated efficacy in reduced recidivism and decreased healthcare costs, correctional facilities may offer fewer psychosocial treatment services now than in previous years due to cost-cutting measures. The US Supreme Court has ruled that offenders have no constitutional right to chemical dependency treatment (Weinstein et al., 2005). Jails that offer SAT may make it available throughout a person's incarceration (Center for Substance Abuse Treatment, 2005). In prisons, SAT may be delayed until an offender's release date nears, because the introspection and interpersonal treatment activities may soften an offender's demeanor to the point where he or she may become more vulnerable within the prison population.

- Ethnic minorities: Ethnic minority persons in the United States are incarcerated at rates much higher than those of Caucasian Americans. In 2010, African-American males were almost seven times more likely than Caucasian-American males to be incarcerated. Hispanic-American males were more than twice as likely as Caucasian-American males to be incarcerated. At the same time, African-American women were three times as likely, and Hispanic women nearly twice as likely as Caucasian-American women to be imprisoned. A number of sociocultural issues contribute to these disproportionate incarceration rates, including poverty, substance abuse, work in the sex trade, and untreated mental illness (CDC, 2014).

- Religious minorities: A 2004 study by the Christian Research Institute (Holding, 2004) found that about 65% of offenders in US jails and prisons reported having Christian beliefs. A low of 4% of Florida inmates and high of about 14% of New York inmates identified with Islamic beliefs. The predominant Islamic group was the Nation of Islam. Smaller religious groups, such as Jehovah Witnesses, Latter Day Saints (Mormons), Santeria, and Native American religions were cited as representing fewer than 1% of the prison populations studied. Holding (2004) found that custodial staff frequently expressed anti-Islamic sentiments which seemed often to be related to the popularity of Islam among African-American offenders who rejected Christianity, ostensibly as a "white man's religion," and converted during their incarcerations. Similarly, Jews represent about 1% of prison populations (Bloomfield, 2013), a smaller portion of offenders than their statistical share of the American population. Arenberg (2009) found rampant anti-Semitism and strongly held stereotypes among his fellow offenders in a New York state prison. He details the complex relationships between the dominant white groups (the *skinheads*, the Aryan Brotherhood, Nazis), as well as ethnic minority groups and gangs, which he had to negotiate during his lengthy incarceration. According to Arenberg, many of his fellow offenders had lived their lives in very circumscribed geographic areas and had never met a Jew prior to encountering him. He opines this is why negative stereotypes of Jews were so pervasive: that the offenders had not had experiences with Jews to counter cultural caricatures.

The American Civil Liberties Union (ACLU) cites activities to protect the rights of religious minorities to practice their religions in correctional institutions. Examples of these rights include Sikhs' rights to maintain untrimmed beards (ACLU, 2011), Sabbath work exemptions for Seventh Day Adventist inmates, kosher meals for Jewish offenders, and halal meals for

Islamic offenders (ACLU, 2013). The freedom to practice their religion is important for offenders to help them maintain hope and plan for re-entry into society. Religious groups such as Prison Congregations of America (promoting Christian worship), the Aleph Institute's Spark of Light Program (serving Jewish offenders), Chuck Colson's Prison Fellowship (serving Evangelical Christians), Paulist Prison Ministry (serving Roman Catholics), and Muslim Prison Ministry exist to help offenders. These organizations promote spirituality among the offenders, creating a supportive community within the institutions and linking them with congregations in the free world that are ready to welcome and support the offenders when they re-enter society.

Many religious groups exist to meet the spiritual needs of offenders. Prison Congregations of America develops church communities in prisons, which partner with sponsoring congregations in their respective local communities to promote Christian worship, fellowship, service, and support for re-entry (Prison Congregations of America, n.d.). Muslim prison chaplaincy programs support offenders' total spiritual transformation by helping them obtain halal foods, religious literature, and fellowship, while also seeking to quell non-Muslims' fears that offenders gathering for prayer may be radicalizing and planning sedition (Dooghan, 2006; Pluralism Project, Harvard University, n.d.).

Nurses can support offenders' participation in activities that help satisfy their spiritual needs by becoming educated about the religious requirements and dietary rules for participants in the various religious groups. Nurses can advocate for clinic scheduling that will not interfere with religious services and holidays (e.g., scheduling Muslim patients for visits on days other than Fridays, and supporting their need to eat before and after daylight hours during Ramadan), as well as ensuring nonporcine insulin for Muslim and Jewish diabetics. Other groups work to support spirituality and reduce despair and violence within penal institutions, including those who have created spirituality-focused communities within prisons. Among these are the David Lynch Foundation (2015), which promotes transcendental meditation, and the North American Vipassana Prison Project (2013), whose work teaching meditation in an Alabama prison was detailed in the film *The Dhamma Brothers* (2007). These programs offer benefits to offenders and correctional staff in terms of decreased violence in the institutions, and to society in terms of reduced recidivism rates among participants.

- Veterans: Veterans of the US armed forces represent about 9% of the population in US jails and prisons, which is lower than the percentage of all veterans comprising the US population (US Census Bureau, 2012a; US Census Bureau, 2012b). Only about 20% of the armed forces veterans actually serve in combat duty, and thus, not all veterans are at an elevated risk of PTSD. When compared with their peers who have not served in the military, veterans who are remanded to prison are less likely to have previous criminal offenses and more likely to have committed violent crimes for which they are given longer sentences (Noonan & Mumola, 2007).

As the numbers of women serving in combat areas increase, the numbers of female veterans increase. As of September 2013, women represented 10.3% of the US armed forces veteran population in the United States. That percentage is anticipated to increase to 50% by 2030 (HHS, 2013). Female veterans are more likely than male veterans to be unemployed or underemployed, and homeless. Also, female veterans are 20 times more likely than their male counterparts to suffer from military sexual trauma (MST). Estimates range from 30% to 84% of female veterans suffering MST and sexual harassment while in uniform. These traumatic experiences combined with the dangers of war yield a greater prevalence of PTSD among female veterans, resulting in increased rates of substance abuse and lifestyle dysfunction, including criminal activity. Although the Veterans Health Administration works to create programs to serve the needs of female veterans, many do not access the services for which they are eligible, including programs that could provide sentencing alternatives. Currently, about 1,400 female veterans are incarcerated in US jails and prisons (National Resource Center on Justice Involved Women, 2013). Incarceration rates of women veterans in the United Kingdom are also on the rise with a large number returning from the wars in Iraq and Afghanistan with psychological problems (Doward, 2010).

- Sexual minorities: Incarcerated lesbian, gay, bisexual, transgender, queer/questioning and inter-sexed (LGBTQI) individuals are particularly vulnerable to victimization by other offenders and facility staff. Of these, transgender persons are at greatest risk of sexual abuse (Smith, Loomis, Yarussi, & Marksamer, 2013).

A transgender individual is a person whose anatomical gender does not match the person's self-perceived gender. He or she may identify with what the world may consider the opposite sex. Transgender experience may range from cross-dressing occasionally, to full time dressing in the garb of the desired gender and "passing" as that gender. Transgender persons may or may not obtain medical care for completing the transition. Such medical care may include hormone injections, mastectomy or breast implants, and gender reassignment surgery involving removal or remodeling of the vagina or penis to match the desired gender. For males who choose the surgical transition to live as females, additional procedures, such as surgical revision of large Adam's apples, pinning of protruding ear pinna, and electrolysis to remove facial hair, are often undertaken (Bradford, Reisner, Honnold, & Xavier, 2013).

A transgender person should be addressed and described in terms of his or her gender identity. Thus, a male-to-female person should be described as "she" and vice versa. The sexual identity of a transgender person may be heterosexual, homosexual, or bisexual. A male-to-female transgender person may identify as lesbian and be sexually attracted to both naturally born and transgender women (Smith et al., 2013).

Transgender persons experience multiple discriminations in our society. Although gay and lesbian individuals are often regarded as sinners and outcasts in religious families, transgender persons may be perceived as abominations in that their trans-sexuality is considered a declaration that God has erred in giving them the wrong bodies (Whitehead, 2006). Although homosexuality itself is no longer considered a mental illness, gender dysphoria and trans-sexuality can contribute to major depressive disorder and ineffective coping skills (Bradford et al., 2013).

Incarcerated transgender persons should be assessed for housing in the facilities appropriate to their targeted gender or to their special needs, and they should have access to private toilets where their genitals are not displayed to others. Each transgender offender's status should be reviewed every 6 months to determine any change in gender status and whether the care plan must be revised. Any physical searches should be performed by persons of the target gender, or by females, as transgender individuals are often regarded as more feminine. Searches or examinations should not be performed solely to determine the person's genital status; rather, each offender's statement of gender identity should be accepted and his or her right to privacy regarding gender status should be protected (Smith et al., 2013).

In addition to routine care appropriate to all incarcerated individuals, nursing care for transgender offenders must ensure that medical screenings appropriate for the genetic and target gender are performed (e.g., prostate examinations for older transgender women, and women's health examinations for transgender men), as gender specific internal organs are not ordinarily removed in gender reassignment surgeries. Nurses may also administer hormone injections, using appropriate techniques to minimize the discomfort and leakage associated with these steroids (Coleman et al., 2011).

The LGBTQI community includes women who are sexually attracted to other women, men who are sexually attracted to other men, and individuals who are sexually attracted to men and women. Not all men who have sex with men identify as homosexual or gay (men who have sex with men, but who do not consider themselves as gay or bisexual are sometimes described as "being on the down low"). Some persons self-identify as pansexual or omnisexual, meaning they are sexually attracted to all gender variations. Intersex individuals may have anatomical features of both genders, and may self-describe as genderqueer (Coleman et al., 2011).

LGBTQI offenders are at risk of victimization from other offenders and staff members who resent their refusal to comply with societal norms for expression of gender and sexuality. Transgender and intersex persons are especially vulnerable to offensive behavior by others who are pruriently interested in their sexual experiences. Sometimes, in order to protect LGBTQI offenders from populations that might prey upon them, the LGBTQI offenders are housed in special pods for sexual minorities. This isolation may reduce certain types of victimization, but it may have the unintended consequence of excluding the LGBTQI offenders from desirable programs of education and employment, library access, or other special services (Coleman et al., 2011).

- Aging offenders: As the numbers of offenders increase in the United States, the numbers of incarcerated individuals over age markers of 50 and 65 also increase (Aday & Krabill, 2012). Many states consider offenders *elderly* at age 50 because incarcerated persons tend to have increased signs of physical aging when compared to their not-incarcerated age cohort, due to factors including drug and alcohol abuse and lack of access to preventive and primary care services (Mitka, 2004). The deprivations and stressful nature of prison life further accelerate the aging process (Arkin, 2013). The graying of our incarcerated population poses special challenges in the management of offenders. A study of elderly male prisoners in England and Wales found that more than 80% had documented chronic medical diseases, of which the highest prevalence was psychiatric, cardiovascular, musculoskeletal, and pulmonary issues, in descending order (Fazel, Hope, O'Donnell, Piper, & Jacoby, 2001).

Offenders already serving long sentences and chronic recidivists are wiser to prison culture and may have lesser acculturation needs than those who are first incarcerated at middle age and beyond. When they are healthy, prison-wise individuals age in place in institutions that generally are designed to accommodate the needs of younger individuals. Typical mobility assistance fixtures such as handrails, grab bars in bathrooms, and wide doorways to accommodate wheelchairs, are lacking and not easily or inexpensively retrofitted. Assistive devices like walkers and wheelchairs are more cumbersome in these institutions, and supports such as special shoes and prosthetic devices may not be readily available (Snyder, van Wormer, Chadha, & Jaggers, 2009).

Older persons serving for first convictions generally have committed serious crimes, such as murder and sexual offenses, or perhaps, significant white-collar crimes (Aday & Krabill, 2012). For example, New York businessman Bernard Madoff of Investment Securities, LLC, was arrested in December 2008 for bilking investors out of $50 billion in a 16-year-long Ponzi scheme. In 2009, the 71-year-old Madoff pleaded guilty and was sentenced to 150 years in prison (Frank & Efrati, 2009). In some cases, the newly incarcerated offenders may have a diminished capacity to understand the implications of their crimes and display minimal resilience for developing coping skills (Aday & Krabill, 2012). In the United Kingdom, factors contributing toward the increased numbers of elderly prisoners include trends toward delayed reporting and prosecution of child sex abuse, the pursuit of decades-old cold case crimes, and lengthier sentences (O'Brien, Tewaniti, Hawley, & Fleming, 2006). The needs of aging female prisoners are rarely addressed in literature or policy planning.

Older persons incarcerated for the first time, if they have previously lived in poverty, may have a paradoxical improvement in their quality of life. Access to medical, dental, and psychiatric care may create a new sense of physical well-being at the same time the offender may be struggling to adapt to a loss of freedom, loss of family and friend relationships, learning a new culture and language, and developing new self-preservation skills. Often, offenders who come from poverty have had less preventive care, have lower overall health status, and require more care for chronic conditions than do their peers who are not incarcerated (Snyder et al., 2009). In addition, older offenders are at increased risk of aggression from younger and stronger offenders (Aday & Krabill, 2012).

Initial health screenings for older offenders should pay special attention to functional impairments and their needs for assistive devices, such as spectacles, modified lighting to reduce glare, hearing aids, and mobility issues.

For those offenders who arrive with medication regimens already established, institutional formularies may not include the specific medications or dosing methods to which the individuals are accustomed. Thus, these offenders' adjustments to incarceration may be compounded by physical dysregulation due to forced medication changes.

- Physical disabilities: Offenders with physical disabilities may need to be moved to special living units that can accommodate their altered capabilities. Some larger jails and prisons have onsite skilled nursing facilities for those offenders whose needs include skilled assistance with their activities of daily living. In some American states, varying security nursing homes are established to provide health-oriented residential care for infirm older adult offenders and younger offenders with disabilities. Recent new prison construction in Australia includes consideration of the special needs of the elderly and persons with disabilities (O'Brien et al., 2006).

  Hospice care may be available for offenders in standard facilities and those in dedicated nursing facilities for offenders. New York State has established a hospice prison facility where health professionals provide state-of-the-art care for offenders whose deaths are imminent. Costs of care for offenders in this institution are more than double the costs for the general prison population in New York. California offers a less costly alternative in training offenders to provide hospice care for other offenders. The California programs provide training in dementia care to "Gold Coat" offenders (so named for their distinctive garb) who earn about $50 per month for providing compassionate supervision to other offenders who suffer from Alzheimer's and other dementias. The Gold Coat caregivers assist with feeding, activities of daily living, and protecting the most vulnerable older adult offenders from others who would do them harm. In addition, the Gold Coat caregivers advise the facility staff members about their charges' aberrant behaviors and help discriminate between dementia-related excitability and volitional acting out (Belluck, 2012). In Queensland, Australia, some inmates are given the opportunity to earn caregiving certification so that they can help provide for the needs of older adult prisoners and those with disabilities (O'Brien et al., 2006).

- Compassionate release: The Federal Bureau of Prisons has established a compassionate release program, whereby an offender can petition for early release from prison due to a compelling personal or community need. Compassionate release is not a pardon or a parole, but rather, recognition that some cases merit release of an offender due to his or her terminal illness or the needs of a dependent child that cannot be met in any other reasonable way (DOJ, 2013; Savage, 2013). The correctional nurse may be called upon to assist in providing documentation to support a petition for compassionate release. In 2002, France instituted a system of medical parole, allowing judges to grant early release of elderly prisoners at any time in their prison sentences when their conditions are terminal or incompatible with prison life and management (O'Brien et al., 2006).

- Women in prison: Female offenders comprise 6.6% of federal and state prison systems in the United States and 4.6% in England (Ministry of Justice, 2015). Female inmates are the fastest growing segment of America's incarcerated populations. The number of female offenders in the United States has more than doubled from 2001 to 2010 and has increased 825% since 1973 (Zust, 2009). Hispanic women are twice as likely, and African-American women are four times as likely as Caucasian women to be imprisoned in the United States. The vast majority of the women in prison have been convicted of nonviolent crimes and especially drug-related crimes. Many are already victims of trauma, and they further suffer abuse while they are incarcerated (Harner & Burgess, 2011; Zust, 2009). In some jurisdictions with fetal protection policies, pregnant drug abusers are incarcerated for violation of drug trafficking laws (e.g., for delivering drugs to their fetuses) (Fentiman, 2009).

  When single mothers of young children are incarcerated, their families are more likely to disintegrate than the families of male offenders (Brown & Motiuk, 2005; Waldman, 2013; Zust, 2009). Because there are fewer female offenders, there are fewer institutions to house them, and due to the paucity of female correctional facilities, female offenders tend to experience greater geographical distance from their families.

  Correctional institutions and their medical budgets tend to be tailored toward the needs of the male majority. Incarcerated women have a greater need for medical care targeting reproductive health and chronic illnesses, such as diabetes, cardiovascular disease, hypertension, malnutrition, and sexually transmitted infections including HIV/AIDS (WHO, 2007a). Women also have greater tendencies toward mood disorders and need greater access to psychiatric/mental health care to cope with the stresses inherent in prison life (Zust, 2009). One study found that 73% to 75% of female offenders suffer from mental health problems (James & Glaze, 2006; Van Voorhis, 2013).

The needs of pregnant offenders may be the most challenging of all incarcerated subpopulations. Six percent of female offenders in the United States are pregnant at the time they are admitted to prison, and one in four women have been pregnant in the year prior to their incarceration (Lewis, 2005). Pregnant offenders who have drug addictions need careful assessment of their recent substance abuse so that appropriate detoxification can be provided. For example, an opioid addict may require maintenance doses of methadone to prevent premature labor or fetal demise (ACOG, 2014). Although pregnant offenders may have adequate prenatal care within their institutions, they are unlikely to have birth attendants with whom they have already formed trusting relationships. In some penal systems, these women are handcuffed to gurneys or beds during labor and delivery. This practice prolongs labor and damages a woman's dignity at a time when she is tremendously vulnerable physically and psychologically. In many correctional systems, a newly delivered offender has little or no chance to interact with her newborn. The missed opportunity for that parental bond has lasting negative implications for both in the mother–infant dyad (Cardaci, 2013).

Although a few women's prisons have established special programs for pregnant and parenting offenders, even the most progressive of these programs have time limitations, and separation looms with the child's first birthday or other anticipated event. Nurses serving pregnant and parenting female offenders may provide extensive health education in prenatal care, birth planning, labor coaching, infant care, and psychosocial support around the issues of loss and longing for the offenders' growing children, as well as working to educate offenders about their rights, inform the public and lawmakers about the need for humane laws, and ensure the protection of offenders' dignity throughout their care (Cardaci, 2013).

- Families of offenders: The arrest, trial, conviction, sentencing, and incarceration of a person are extremely stressful events for the individual and his or her family. Through the judicial process, the individual may experience shame, anxiety, anger at the system, and worry about family members. The family and friends may be concerned about the individual's welfare, the drain on the family's financial resources due to legal defense costs, the individual's lost wages, the family's standing in the community in the aftermath of the crime, the care of the individual's children and/or spouse, and the logistics of including the person in the family's life despite the forced separation (Bernstein, 2005; Savage, 2013).

Penal institutions have their own policies about visitation and correspondence. Visiting hours may be subject to change, depending upon the individual's location within the institution, the level of security, and any special conditions of the facility at a given time. Transfers are made to accommodate the offender's special conditions and/or the needs or convenience of the system. An offender may be moved within an institution, or between institutions, and families may not be notified until transfers have occurred. Thus, a family may journey a significant distance to visit an incarcerated family member, only to learn that he or she is no longer at that location (Bernstein, 2005).

When an offender begins to serve a lengthy sentence, he or she may be sent to an evaluation or assessment center initially, and then transferred to a facility with whatever special programs may match the offender's needs, wants, and security level. As the time served passes and the release date approaches, he or she may be offered lower security options with work opportunities and, eventually, halfway-house status.

Prisons tend to be situated at some distance from urban centers, where public transportation may be difficult to impossible. Visiting family members must move through a variety of steps to visit, including getting onto the individual's approved visitor list, arranging for travel (which usually requires having a car and gas money or the ability to persuade someone to provide transportation), arranging for lodging if the travel distance is great, procuring needed or wanted items requested by the offender, and managing the emotional impact of the visitation (Harner & Burgess, 2011).

Some states lack adequate facilities to house their incarcerated populations and contract with other states or private prison corporations to host their offenders for a fee. This can pose tremendous hardships for the offenders and their families who may find themselves forcibly separated by thousands of miles (Pelaez, 2014). One Washington State offender was housed in a southern state for several years. Although his extended family had made elaborate arrangements to bring his school-aged children across the state for periodic visits, when he was moved out of state, the distance became too great and he completely missed several years of his children's lives. For families with limited financial means, even within-state travel can be daunting. For family members with disabilities, distance travel and discomforts can be prohibitive. Few organizations exist to help offenders' families defray the costs of visitation (Bernstein, 2005).

When a state has few female offenders, or limited housing capability, there may be no options to support visitation. One northwestern state has one female prison and three juvenile prisons, all of which are in the western half of the state divided by mountains and travel challenges that are difficult in good weather and insurmountable in winter.

Even telephone communications can be costly and vexing. Offenders may be required to make outgoing calls via collect only, which can double or triple the reasonable costs of telephone calls. If the offender's calls have highly emotional content, the family members may become resentful and refuse to accept the calls. Also, the family members may simply be unable to afford the padded costs of the telephone calls (Bernstein, 2005).

Offenders often cannot receive mail or phone calls from other prisons. A family with multiple offenders may lose touch completely for months or years. One juvenile offender's parents were in separate prisons and could not make direct communication, so the child who longed for parental love depended upon the kindness of aunts and uncles to deliver the messages of familial care (Bernstein, 2005).

- Sex offenders: A great body of mythology surrounds the prosecution, incarceration, and outcomes of persons convicted of sex crimes. Despite popular opinion, most sex offenders do not have histories of being sexually victimized in childhood. However, about 30% of juvenile and adult offenders have histories of childhood physical and sexual abuse. Some who offend against children are pedophiles who have sexual preferences for children, but most who offend against children have thinking problems that result in their sexual acting out against available victims who may be of any age. Adult sex offenders who remain in their communities and obtain treatment are less likely to reoffend than those who are incarcerated and do not receive treatment (Center for Sex Offender Management, 2000). The stiff penalties and long prison sentences demanded by outraged citizens tend not to deter sexual offenders from recidivism. Juvenile sex offenders are predominantly males who commonly choose child victims. In some cases, juveniles have been convicted and remanded to prison for unwittingly having consensual sex with partners found to be more than 2 years younger than themselves.

  Sex offenders, especially those who sexually abuse children, are reputed to be particularly despised in jail and prison populations. For this reason, state and federal prisons offer special programs for sex offenders who are amenable to treatment. The Federal Bureau of Prisons (n.d.) offers voluntary sex offender treatment programs at nine sites in the northeast, south, and central US. The State of Washington offers sex offender treatment at one site for males and one site for females. Fewer than 7% of those who complete treatment are eventually returned to prison. Violent sex offenders who are determined to be likely to re-offend may undergo an evaluation process by which they may be civilly committed to secure housing in a special facility. For civil commitment offenders (those confined to a mental health hospital setting), annual reviews determine whether they may be safely released to their communities or whether continued detainment can be supported (Washington State Department of Corrections, 2014). In the United Kingdom, the number of sex offenders in England and Wales has risen by more than a third over the last 5 years. There are more than 40,000 registered sex offenders living in these areas and being monitored by probation services. The sentences are increasing and high numbers of offenders in prison are committing violent and sexual offenses (Swinford & Amin, 2014).

- Juvenile offenders: In the United States, offenders under age 18 may be housed in community-based housing, such as group homes with highly structured environments, juvenile-only correctional facilities, or adult prisons, depending on the nature of their crimes and resulting sentences. Although the number of juveniles in correctional facilities rose from 1985 to 1997, the percentage of incarcerated juveniles remained at about 0.5% of the prison population throughout this period. For violent offenders, some states hold juveniles in segregated incarceration (e.g., special facilities for ages 14 to 18 vs. special facilities for ages 19 to 24), while others use straight adult incarceration where juvenile offenders sentenced as adults are not differentiated in adult prisons. Another option is graduated incarceration, whereby juvenile offenders may remain in juvenile facilities until age 18 at which time they are transferred to adult facilities to serve the remainders of their sentences (Strom, 2000). Other nations' practices may vary. In Greece, for example, youthful offenders are incarcerated in juvenile facilities until age 21 (Togas et al., 2014).

In juvenile institutions, offenders may lack connections with parents or other family members to celebrate their accomplishments. The juvenile prison may offer educational opportunities for the youths to complete high school in a public school on the campus of the prison, attend coaching toward earning a General Equivalency Diploma (GED), or participate in vocational programs such as welding, auto body repair, mechanics, and woodworking. When a juvenile offender accomplishes a milestone, such as high school graduation, the correctional nurses may attend the graduation ceremony acting *in loco parentis* to support the offender and offer further encouragement.

- Immigration and Customs Enforcement (ICE) prisons: The ICE describes itself as "the largest investigative arm of the Department of Homeland Security. ICE is a 21st century law enforcement agency with broad responsibilities for a number of key homeland security priorities" (ICE, n.d., p. 2). The Enforcement and Removal Directorate in 2012 housed 34,260 undocumented aliens for average stays of 27 days each in more than 240 facilities around the United States (ICE, n.d.). The activities of the ICE are controversial in that the numbers of detainees and the costs of their incarceration have doubled in the years between 2005 and 2010. Three large corporations, which operate private-for-profit detention facilities in Texas, Georgia, and Arizona, manage more than one-third of the ICE detainees and have actively lobbied for public policies promoting their industry. Many of the ICE detainees are confined in private-for-profit facilities. Detainees complain of inadequate health care, lack of access to legal representation, and an inability to communicate with their families and friends. Of the 126 ICE detainees who died in custody from October 2003 through October 2011, a total of 17 had asphyxia listed as the cause of death. These deceased detainees ranged in age from 21 to 51, with a median age of 27 years. Of these deaths, only four were in facilities staffed with the ICE Health Service Corps (American Friends Service Committee, n.d.; Detention Watch Network, 2011). Correctional nurses often act as a liaison with security staff and assist this population in accessing health care and social services.

- Political prisoners: Political prisoners around the world seek opportunities for relief of their suffering. When Pope Francis I made a visit to the Philippines in 2015, a group of 32 activists representing 491 political prisoners fasted 24 hours to draw the Pope's attention to their plight. Similar efforts were made during visits made by Pope John Paul II in 1981 and 1995 (Gamil, 2015). Journalists are at particularly high risk of incarceration due to their professional reporting, which oppressive regimes seek to stifle. The Committee to Protect Journalists (2014) notes that 221 journalists were incarcerated worldwide, the second highest number since statistics were first gathered in 2000. China has the highest number at 44, followed by Eritrea at 23, and Ethiopia at 17. Russia is listed as having one and the United States is not listed as having journalist political prisoners (Committee to Protect Journalists, 2014).

CONCEPTS AND ISSUES

- Context for care: Inmate patients within the correctional setting often present dilemmas to nursing staff with regard to security or custody versus care. Nursing staff must work within the aspects of security to provide medical care while maintaining constant awareness of their surroundings and remembering that they are working within a correctional setting. Boundary setting is a necessary aspect of correctional nursing, which differs significantly from community care. Incarcerated patients can be especially manipulative and dangerous, and they may be highly skilled at abusing the system.

  Questions often arise regarding the cost-effectiveness of providing treatment programs in corrections versus an attitude of warehousing inmates. Many inmates are under the influence of drugs and alcohol when arrested, and statistics show that the costs of treatment programs per inmate versus incarceration are significant at a ratio of about 10 to 1. It actually is cheaper to provide programs for treatment and followup care, which also reduces recidivism in this population (Miranda, 2009). An English study of the effectiveness of treatment in the prison services found that the benefits of treatment and the impact on reducing offending behaviors along with the improvement of health outweighed the cost of the programs (Harrison, Cappello, Alaszewski, Appleton, & Cooke, 2003).

- Deinstitutionalization: In order to address deinstitutionalization, one must first discuss the factors contributing to why the inmate would need to be deinstitutionalized. When first admitted into custody, the penal institution requires inmates to relinquish control of their autonomy and freedom to make choices over their daily lives. Choices range from clothing, food, when to sleep and what hours to be awake, showering communally with strangers when told to, and having no say on who will share their living quarters with them. This can be a difficult process and some never adjust. Conversely, others adjust so successfully that they gradually lose the capability of contributing any control or decision-making to their lives. Although it is rare, some institutionalized persons become so incapable of making decisions regarding themselves that, given the opportunity, they are unable to do so and they flounder (Haney, 2002).

  This loss of control over person, space, and decisions in custody also extends to behavior. If the inmate acts out in an unacceptable manner, the consequences are swift. The institution may so fully control the inmate's actions that any internal controls the inmate once possessed regarding his- or herself may decay or fail. The inmate may no longer be able to make decisions regarding him/herself and thus be positioned for failure when released from custody (Haney, 2002). Feelings of decreased self-worth flourish with this lack of control.

  This type of institutionalization is particularly problematic when the person is released and attempts to re-enter free society. The person who has been institutionalized for a lengthy time may no longer have the skills or ability to confront complicated problems or conflicts, especially when these are unexpected. If the person is lacking any relationships with family, friends, or counselors who would provide a safety net, the person's chances of success drop dramatically as his or her ability to cope is stunted. It is not uncommon for the incarcerated person to suffer ending of relationships (via divorce, death, or shunning), which also increases the psychological despair and turmoil that is associated with institutionalization (Haney, 2002).

  Self-survival is so important that the incarcerated individual must adhere to whatever is necessary for survival. The cultural behaviors are driven by gangs and are well established within the prison walls. Once a person gains admission to a gang, the inmate may find that even if he or she is released from custody, that person may not be able to leave the gang life behind and reintegrate into society (Haney, 2002).

  Deinstitutionalization or releasing the inmate from prison after a long sentence does not come without a price. According to Haney, after an offender serves time, reintegration into society can be problematic (Haney, 2002). When released, the cost of long-term care, including housing and medical programs, is lower, and affords the person the chance to function in society. However, with increased independence and freedom from the structured environment of prison, problems may arise with the inability of the inmate to make rational choices about his or her life. This creates the negative risk to deinstitutionalization. A parent re-entering into a child's life cannot be expected to resume full parental responsibilities while his or her own life is compromised. This holds true for spouses and other familial/social relationships as well (Wall & Andersen, 2013).

According to the global organization, Human Rights Watch, in 2009, 56% of state offenders and 45% of federal offenders had symptoms or a recent or chronic history of mental health problems. Correctional facilities were never meant to house and care for persons with mental illness but with the closing of psychiatric hospitals starting in the 1960s, incarceration has become the holding centers for this population. Mental illnesses, including schizophrenia, bipolar disorder, major depression, and so forth, are two to four times more prevalent among the incarcerated than the general public (Human Rights Watch, 2009). Releasing persons who have mental illness is fraught with unforeseen problems.

Individuals who could not be institutionalized against their will have the chance of becoming homeless or returning to jail/prison, as they often do not possess the coping skills to function without supervision. Many of these soon-to-be deinstitutionalized persons have a mental illness, which only augments the likelihood of failure when they are released from jails and prisons into the general population. Once released, because of the lack of oversight and laws regarding human rights, these persons are not forced to accept treatment. This has the spiraling effect of intensifying their symptoms. In conjunction with their deteriorating behavior, relationships are impacted. Where family, friends, or neighbors once provided a safety net, the behavior of the person with mental illness fragments these relationships, resulting in further isolation, exacerbating the problem and increasing the chance for re-arrest (Human Rights Watch, 2009).

President Kennedy's 1963 establishment of Community Mental Health Centers accelerated the trend toward deinstitutionalization of this population. With the introduction of Medicare and Medicaid in the 1960s, the federal government began to assume responsibility for the cost of mental health care. In 1974, the Supplemental Security Income promoted deinstitutionalization especially for the elderly by promoting the need for comprehensive community mental health care. This was an ambitious goal, which was never fully realized due to financial issues and scattered approaches. Consequently, to this day, many persons with mental illness are left adrift, turning to illegal drugs and alcohol for self-treatment of their symptoms. The World Health Organization (WHO) examined the need to shift mental health intervention for common mental health disorders in India (WHO, 2012). With so many, it is only a matter of time before they become entangled in the legal system (Human Rights Watch, 2009).

To be deinstitutionalized successfully is to relearn how to live and function in the free world. If coping skills are poor or absent and the inmate has no safety net, chances are good that he or she will reoffend and return to incarceration, thus continuing the arrest–release cycle. Society needs to focus on this relearning program to find ways to aid in the successful transition of the institutionalized inmate to a successfully deinstitutionalized person in society.

- Institutional rape: The Prison Rape Elimination Act (PREA) was enacted in 2003 to require that all correctional facilities in the United States collect and report to the Bureau of Justice data on sexual assaults in prisons, jails, and detention facilities, and to take steps to protect incarcerated individuals from sexual victimization (Prison Rape Elimination Act, 2003). Correctional facilities must ensure that their staff be trained in methods of protecting offenders from victimization by other offenders, and that those who have been victimized can report that victimization without fear of reprisal. Facilities must also demonstrate their zero tolerance for staff perpetration of sexual assaults (National Center for TransGender Equality, 2012). This law offers additional protections to members of at-risk populations.

- Services: Jails and prisons are not only for confining lawbreakers; they now serve to provide the incarcerated with services (i.e., mental health, educational, vocational, religious, and rehabilitation classes as well as other services that intersect daily with the inmate's life). These intersecting systems and services are provided with the expectation that the inmate's life will be improved and the revolving-door effect will diminish. Many offenders obtain their General Education Diplomas (GED), and higher education while incarcerated. Others learn a vocational trade that will provide them an opportunity for gainful employment when released. Further, businesses in the community may contract with jails, community corrections, and prisons to provide employment to the confined (as in community corrections) or the recently released. This service is important because the reality is that numerous entities and businesses will not employ a person who has served time in a penal institution or has a criminal record (Mohr, 2013).

Alternatives to incarceration are conditional sentences that are served outside the prison or jail walls. These have gained in popularity in the last decade mainly due to financial reasons with overall goals of reducing recidivism, crime in the community, and the prison and jail population. Requirements for acceptance into one of these programs are based on conditions that must be met by the offender. Another form of incarceration alternative is Community Corrections, which is part of the justice system. This system includes both adult and juvenile offenders. The Community Corrections provides services while imposing sanctions that are court-ordered. Community Corrections seeks to keep offenders within the community while providing for public safely. Participants are carefully screened for appropriateness to participate in the programs and held accountable to the program goals set for them. These may be making restitution to their victims, obtaining education, or being gainfully employed while maintaining ties to the community (Evans, 1996).

Candidates for these programs are carefully screened for eligibility and success. Candidates for these programs are low-risk and or first-time offenders. They also must be gainfully employed or have a medical reason for not having a job or attending school (Mohr, 2013). The advantage is twofold: (1) the offender can continue to function in the outside world and still be productive to society and (2) the prison and jail community is not burdened with housing the person. Those offenders granted alternative sentences are still expected to follow the terms and conditions of their sentence. The advent of Global Positioning Satellite (GPS) technology has allowed law enforcement to monitor the exact location of the offender by use of satellites at any time. Because of the increased effectiveness of GPS tracking, when an offender violates the terms of his parole, he can be rearrested without delay. The cost is also advantageous; the approximate cost of $3,500 per year offers a significant cost-savings to the state over the expense of housing each prisoner in a facility (Sipes, 2009).

In conclusion, inmates frequently come from disadvantaged social and cultural groups that either do not seek out medical care on a routine basis, or have a negative response to the healthcare system. They are also less likely to seek out preventative care and are more susceptible to exposure to harmful environmental factors (Glaser & Greifinger, 1993). Mental illness is also disproportionately higher with the incarcerated population than the community (NPR, 2011).

While incarcerated, factors negatively affecting these persons include crowding, lack of privacy, and isolation from family and friends. Women, in particular, are at risk when incarcerated. An estimated 25% of all women in prison suffer from mental illness. These include depression, bipolar disease, schizophrenia, PTSD, and addictions (NCCHC, 2011). Diabetes, HIV, and sexually transmitted diseases are higher in incarcerated females than the male population (ANA, 2013). Providing primary and preventive services such as breast cancer screening and yearly PAP smears are essential (NCCHC, 2011). These interventions have an enormous impact on public health. Lack of care impacts both the family and community when the inmate is released. Untreated issues lead to greater use of public resources and increased recidivism rates once the female inmate is released (Women's Health Encyclopedia, 2011).

Pregnant females have both physical and mental needs to be addressed while in custody. Provisions for the birth and care of the infant are part of this planning (NCCHC, 2011). Children of incarcerated women are at greater risk of being displaced and ending up in foster care, which adds to the overall stress of incarceration (PBS, n.d.).

Finally, no jail, prison, juvenile facility, or community corrections can function without medical care. Rena Murtha, a pioneer in correctional nursing care in the 1970s describes entering the correctional facility where the nurse was seen as a "tool of the warden, a slave of the physician and an unknown to the patient" (ANA, 2013; p. 2). Today, this no longer holds true. Now the nurse is considered an integral member of the correctional staff. Further, the nurse works in concert with the correctional security staff to provide a safe, clean, humane environment for the incarcerated population (ANA, 2013).

- Patient population characteristics impacting care
  - Seclusion and restraint impact of isolation on behaviors: Healthcare staff members monitor patients while they are in seclusion or restraints. The NCCHC standards require minimum numbers of contacts by healthcare staff, depending on the level of isolation in which an inmate is housed. Special assessments and followup evaluations are provided for vulnerable populations, and records of inmates are reviewed to assess the increased risk of adverse impact on mental illness or medical conditions (NCCHC, 2014b). Each site must have site-specific policies that address the care and monitoring of inmates in seclusion or restraints.
  - Ethics and human rights: Another area of debate is that of caring for inmates and their rights to care while they are on death row or pending execution. Capital punishment brings about its own dilemmas, but for nurses, care of inmates on death row falls within the expected right for medical treatment. Staff working with these patients often must separate themselves from the capital punishment question and focus on nursing care (NCCHC, 2014b). The questions that arise with this population include whether they have the right to the same level of care as that of inmates in a general population: Do they have a right to receive or provide organs for transplant? At what point do nurses separate themselves from these individuals? The NCCHC standards specify that medical staff members do not participate in executions, but nurses are called upon to keep patients healthy enough to participate in their executions (NCCHC, 2014b).
  - Self-harm and suicide: Offenders in jails and prisons are at greater risk of self-harm and suicide than persons who are not incarcerated. Cutting and scratching one's body may be an ineffective means of coping with stress, a cry for attention, or a practice in desensitization to pain and lowering one's inhibitions toward further self-injury. An individual who cuts his or her body may commit suicide accidentally by causing a more serious injury than was intended, or gradually and deliberately escalating the series of injuries in preparation for completing a suicide (Joiner, 2007).

    All personnel working with offenders in correctional institutions bear responsibility for the safety of the offenders. Staff should receive focused training in suicide prevention, and this should be updated and reviewed during annual training. Jail staff should be aware that intoxicated male offenders in jails are at greatest risk for impulsive behaviors such as suicide. Hanging is the most commonly implemented method of suicide among offenders (Hayes, 2005). Suicide rates among incarcerated individuals have decreased dramatically in recent decades, perhaps due to the positive impact of suicide prevention programs. As of 2002, the rates of suicide were 47 per 100,000 offenders in local jails and 14 per 100,000 offenders in state prisons. In both settings, suicide rates among violent offenders were more than twice the rates for nonviolent offenders (Mumola, 2005).

    Correctional nurses must be alert to offenders' presentations at medication dispensing times, in the healthcare center, and for behavior that deviates from baseline. Sadness, receipt of bad news, family crises, and despondency observed or reported by other staff should lead to suicide risk assessment and intervention according to the institution's protocols.
  - Gang affiliations: Offenders who band together to protect themselves from other groups of offenders form prison gangs. Membership is often based upon national origin or ethnicity. Although some gangs claim to promote understanding of religion (e.g., Aryan Brotherhood) or ethnic culture (e.g., Neta), their purposes are more focused on exerting power and control within correctional institutions. Gang activities include violence against rival gangs and correctional personnel plus purveyance of drugs and other contraband within correctional institutions. Many prison gangs have corollary organizations in the free world. Deliberate

and unwitting transgressions against gang members are punishable by violence and death (DuFresne, 2010; Knox, 2012).

Gang members may be recruited from within the community or within correctional institutions. Initiation rituals often include displays of loyalty by committing acts of violence against rivals and withstanding violence against oneself. Gang members are said to be "beaten in and beaten out," but the reality is that disaffiliation from some gangs may result in death. In correctional institutions, gangs may strongly influence their members to avoid health care in general and mental health care in particular (Chaiken, Thompson, & Shoemaker, 2005).

Gang members may be identified by their tattoos, graffiti, symbolic language, and gestures. Tattoos may have insignia with religious (e.g., the rosary and Our Lady of Guadalupe are popular among Hispanic men) or historical themes (e.g., lightning bolts and swastikas feature prominently in the tattoos of the Aryan Brotherhood), and memorials to living or deceased family or gang members. Some writers understand facial tattoos to be statements that the individuals do not ever expect to participate in the broader dominant culture. In some jurisdictions, support is available to absorb the cost of tattoo removal for persons renouncing gang affiliations (Chaiken, Thompson, & Shoemaker, 2005).

Forensic nurses in the correctional setting must become aware of gangs and their influence in the particular institution, as gang issues must be considered when scheduling and transporting offenders to health services. Members of rival gangs must not be scheduled in proximity to each other as violence may result. In addition, within institutions, victims of violence avoid divulging the truth about attacks upon themselves, requiring that nurses understand the various mechanisms of injuries. Skin infections from amateur tattoos and scarification are common health conditions that nurses must recognize and treat.

FUTURE ISSUES

- Education: A person can enter the field of correctional nursing with a licensed practical nurse/licensed vocational nurse (LPN/LVN) licensure. The LPN/LVN can pass medications, assist with patient care, and work as part of the healthcare team. Duties depend on scope of practice in the state where one works. Some facilities use medication technicians and other supportive personnel under the supervision of a registered nurse (RN). The unique challenges of the correctional environment permit the RN to work autonomously and exercise extensive assessment and critical thinking skills. Once a nurse begins a career in corrections, additional learning opportunities are available from the American Correctional Association (ACA) and the NCCHC. Both organizations offer basic and advanced certification in correctional health care. In the United Kingdom, to work as a prison nurse, one needs to be a qualified RN, preferably in the areas of adult, mental health, or learning disabilities. The nurse may be directly employed by the National Health Service (NHS) or the facility (NHS, 2006). Graduate programs in forensic nursing are currently available at colleges and universities, such as Duquesne University and Fitchburg State University. Boston College offers a post-Masters certificate while other online certificate options are available from institutions such as University of California, Riverside. In 2006, the ACA established a certification program, offering nurses certification in two specialty categories: certified correction nurse manager (CCN/M) and certified corrections nurse (CCN) (ANA, 2007).

    Advanced practice nurses (APRN) are also employed extensively in corrections. The APRN functions as the primary care provider for the inmate patient and performs diagnosis and treatment for acute, chronic, and psychiatric illness. This provider assesses the patient, orders and interprets diagnostic studies, and orders medications according to the practice act of the state in which the facility is located.

- Career opportunities and growth: Correctional nursing provides unique growth opportunities and career options. Many of the private companies that now provide contracted medical services to the inmate patient population offer increasing growth opportunities in management up to and including executive nurse leadership positions, such as vice president of nursing or chief nursing officer. These companies have multiple facilities and both clinical and operational management positions are available. As a correctional nurse, one can start out as a night shift RN and progress to charge nurse, director of nursing, health services administrator, and then to a regional or national-level management position.

- Research and evidenced-based practice: Nurses will be called upon to play a greater role in the medical care of the incarcerated patient. To provide this care, nurses must implement a holistic approach, which is sensitive to the culture, age, and gender of a growing and diverse population (ACA, 2004). According to the ANA's *Correctional Nursing: Scope and Standards of Practice* (2013), "[T]he correctional registered nurse attains knowledge and competence that reflect current nursing practice" (p. 52). In addition, a need exists to use research findings and evidence-based practice to expand the nurse's skills and professional knowledge.

Previous research studies in correctional nursing have been practice-focused, including the exploration of the unique correctional environment and its impact on the correctional nurse (Schoenly & Knox, 2013). Almost and her colleagues (2013) reviewed and researched education and work environments in the correctional nursing setting. The Nursing Department of the University of Connecticut in conjunction with Connecticut Division of Corrections conducted research on development of a competency-based training and orientation program for correctional nurses that used mobile training centers and simulation (Shelton, Weiskopf, & Nicholson, 2010). Studies have examined the impact of the custody environment on correctional nursing (Maroney, 2005); boundary studies relate to correctional nursing and the care of inmates (Weiskopf, 2005).

Clinical research in correctional facilities requires informed consent and must follow the statutory regulations for vulnerable populations. This greatly decreases clinical research trials involving offenders in the United States (IOM, 2007). Correctional research is "dominated by epidemiological studies (e.g., surveys; 39%) and correlational designs (27%). Other studies are described as examining behavioral issues (14%), medical outcomes (5%), case studies (6%), nonmedical experiments (1%), or 'other' (8%). An alternative classification of study content reveals that health status questions (43%) and personality characteristics (19%) are the focus of most research. Other studies deal with aspects of being confined (10%) or reentry into the community (11%) or bear no clear relationship to prisoner status (9%)" (IOM, 2007; p. 62–63). An example of clinical studies in the correctional environment is that of Moser (n.d.), who researched a cardiovascular risk reduction intervention as a clinical trial in the Kentucky prison system. Today, both NCCHC (2014b) and the ACA (2004) have specific limits on human subjects research in jails and prisons; the US federal government has established regulations as well (HHS, 2009; DOJ, 1999).

Barriers to participation in evidence-based practice in the correctional setting include environment, resources, time constraints, and limitations imposed by security rules. Options for nursing input include quality improvement studies, workflow management, infection control studies, and outcome studies used as part of NCCHC accreditation (2014b).

As a result of these obstacles, correctional nurses are challenged to use research principles to move forward and drive their practice by participating in and developing studies to evaluate the concepts of caring in a patient relationship in the correctional setting, measuring boundaries, and developing professional practice and clinical issues specific to this practice setting, such as application of community standards in the correctional setting for pain management, patient education, substance abuse, and palliative care (Schoenly & Knox, 2013).

Correctional healthcare nursing is a rapidly expanding specialty that will continue to evolve in conjunction with the increasing incarcerated population. The challenges of the environment and the requirements of correctional nurses to maintain consistent practice make this a complicated role with multiple opportunities for growth.

CASE STUDIES

CASE STUDY #1

Steve is an African-American male who was arrested tonight for public intoxication. He reports that he has diabetes, had a heart attack last month, has high blood pressure, and drinks nightly. During the intake assessment, he states he has been homeless for about 6 months and does not eat regularly. He denies having money for medications and mentions that he was diagnosed with bipolar disorder a few years ago.

Intake Issues:
    Medical—alcohol history and abuse
    – diabetes, no medication
    – hypertension, no medication
    – cardiac history
    – bipolar disorder

Social—homeless
    – poor diet
    – no social supports

- What are the greatest risks for this patient?
- What issues should be addressed immediately?
- What would be the care plan for this individual?

CASE STUDY #2

A 22-year-old female patient was arrested when she and her boyfriend were driving through a drug-ridden part of the city and an acquaintance of her boyfriend approached on foot as the car was stopped at a stoplight. The acquaintance went to the driver's side of the car and shook hands with the boyfriend. Soon the police swarmed in as part of an emphasis patrol. Although the patient denied having anything to do with that exchange, she was in the vehicle at the time the alleged drug buy occurred. She was convicted of possession of methamphetamine with intent to sell.

When she arrives at the women's prison, she is a thin and frightened-looking young woman. The forensic nurse performing the initial screening notes a number of pockmark scars on the patient's right antecubital fossa and notes that she signs her name with her left hand. When the nurse asks about drug use, the patient denies it. The nurse continues the examination and asks whether the patient has been tested for hepatitis, and she responds, "You just assume I'm a druggie, but I'm not!" The nurse proceeds with the examination and learns that the patient's last menstrual period began about 4 months ago. The patient exclaims that she cannot be pregnant because she has been having some light bleeding every month. She has attributed the altered menses to the stress of incarceration and going to trial.

- What are the greatest risks for this patient?
- What issues should be addressed immediately?
- What would be the care plan for this individual?

REVIEW QUESTIONS

1. According to the Eighth Amendment to the United States Constitution, what class of Americans is constitutionally guaranteed health care?

2. What constitutes *deliberate indifference* on the part of a correctional institution?

3. How has deinstitutionalization of persons with mental illness affected jails and prisons in the ensuing years?

4. How important is mental health screening in a correctional facility?

REFERENCES

Aday, R. H., & Krabill, J. J. (2012). Aging offenders in the criminal justice system. *Marquette Elder's Advisor, 7*(2), Article 4. Retrieved February 22, 2015, at http://scholarship.law.marquette.edu/elders/vol7/iss2/4

Alschuler, A. W. (2003). The changing purposes of criminal punishment: A retrospective on the past century and some thoughts about the next. *University of Chicago Law Review, 70*(1), 1–22.

American Civil Liberties Union (ACLU). (2011). *ACLU files lawsuit on behalf of California inmate subjected to baseless religious discrimination.* Retrieved March 31, 2014, from https://www.aclu.org/prisoners-rights-religion-belief/aclu-files-lawsuit-behalf-california-inmate-subjected-baseless-rel

American Civil Liberties Union (ACLU). (2013). *ACLU, Michigan corrections settles religious freedom lawsuit.* Retrieved March 31, 2014, from http://www.aclumich.org/issues/halal/2013–11/1894

American College of Obstetricians and Gynecologists (ACOG), Committee on Health Care for Underserved Women and the American Society of Addiction Medicine. (2014). Opioid abuse, dependence, and addiction in pregnancy. *Committee Opinion, 524.* Retrieved February 22, 2014 from http://www.acog.org/-/media/Committee-Opinions/Committee-on-Health-Care-for-Underserved-Women/co524.pdf?dmc=1&ts=20150223T1549415167

American Correctional Association (ACA). (2004). *Performance-based standards for adult local detention facilities* (4th ed.). Alexandria, VA: ACA.

American Friends Service Committee. (n.d.). *List of detainee deaths October 2003-October 31, 2011.* Retrieved March 31, 2014, from https://afsc.org/document/ice-detainee-deaths-2003–2011

American Nurses Association (ANA). (2007). *Correctional nursing: Scope and standards of practice,* Silver Spring, MD: Nursesbooks.org.

American Nurses Association (ANA). (2013). *Correctional nursing: Scope and standards of practice* (2nd ed.). Silver Spring, MD: Nursesbooks.org.

Amnesty International. (2012). *Chad: "We are all dying here" – Human rights violations in prisons.* London, England: Amnesty International. Retrieved February 19, 2015, from http://www.amnestyusa.org/research/reports/chad-we-are-all-dying-here-human-rights-violations-in-prisons

Arenberg, D. (2009). David Arenberg reflects on being Jewish in State prison: A reflection on anti-Semitism on the yard. *Southern Poverty Law Center Intelligence Report, 136.* Retrieved February 18, 2015, from http://www.splcenter.org/get-informed/intelligence-report/browse-all-issues/2009/winter/a-jew-in-prison

Arkin, D. (2013). Exploding number of elderly prisoners strains system, taxpayers. *NBCNews.com.* Retrieved February 23, 2015, from http://usnews.nbcnews.com/_news/2013/06/29/19192029-exploding-number-of-elderly-prisoners-strains-system-taxpayers

Baumann, A., & Blythe, J. (2008). Globalization of higher education in nursing. *Online Journal of Issues in Nursing, 13*(2), manuscript 4. doi: 10.3912/OJIN.Vol13No02Man04

Bayard, M., McIntyre, J., Hill, K. R., & Woodside, J., Jr. (2004). Alcohol withdrawal syndrome. *American Family Physician, 69*(6), 1443–1450.

Belluck, P. (2012). Life with dementia. *New York Times.* Retrieved February 22, 2015, from http://www.nytimes.com/2012/02/26/health/dealing-with-dementia-among-aging-criminals.html?pagewanted = all

Bernstein, N. (2005). *All alone in the world: Children of incarcerated parents,* New York, NY: New Press.

Bick, J. A. (2007). Infection control in jails and prisons. *Healthcare Epidemiology, 45*(15), 1047–1055.

Bloomfield, D. (2013). Jews in prison stick with faith to cope with flood of anti-Semitism. *Jewish Daily Forward.* Retrieved March 31, 2014, from http://forward.com/articles/186868/jews-in-prison-stick-with-faith-to-cope-with-flood/?p=all

Bradford, J., Reisner, S. L., Honnold, J. A., & Xavier, J. (2013). Experiences of transgender-related discrimination and implications for health: Results from the Virginia Transgender Health Initiative Study. *American Journal of Public Health, 103*(10), 1820–1829.

Brown, S. L., &. Motiuk, L. L. (2005). *The dynamic factor identification and analysis (DFIA) component of the offender intake assessment (OIA) process: A meta-analytic, psychometric, and consultative review* (Research Report R-164). Ontario, Canada: Correctional Service Canada.

Bureau of Justice Statistics. (n.d.). *FAQ detail: What is the difference between jails and prisons?* Retrieved February 22, 2015, from http://www.bjs.gov/index.cfm?ty=qa&iid=322

Burns, K. (2005). Psychopharmacology in correctional settings. In C. Scott & J. Gerbasi (Eds.), *Handbook of correctional mental health* (pp. 89–108). Washington, DC: American Psychiatric Publishing.

Cardaci, R. (2013). Care of pregnant women in the criminal justice system. *American Journal of Nursing, 113*(9), 40–48.

Carlson, P. M., & Garrett, J. S. (2008). *Prison and jail administration: Practice and theory,* Sudbury, MA: Jones & Bartlett Learning.

Center for Sex Offender Management, U.S. Department of Justice. (2000). *Myths and facts about sex offenders.* Retrieved February 20, 2015, from http://www.csom.org/pubs/mythsfacts.html

Center for Substance Abuse Treatment, Substance Abuse and Mental Health Services Administration. (2005). *Substance abuse treatment for adults in the criminal justice system* (Treatment Improvement Protocol [TIP] Series 44). Rockville, MD: U.S. Department of Health and Human Services. Retrieved March 23, 2014, from http://www.ncbi.nlm.nih.gov/books/NBK64123/

Centers for Disease Control and Prevention (CDC). (2012a). *TB in correctional facilities in the United States.* Retrieved March 31, 2014, from http://www.cdc.gov/TB/topic/populations/correctional/default.htm

Centers for Disease Control and Prevention (CDC). (2012b). *Hepatitis C & incarceration.* Retrieved March 31, 2014, from http://www.cdc.gov/hepatitis/Settings/corrections.htm

Centers for Disease Control and Prevention (CDC). (2014). *HIV in correctional settings.* Retrieved March 31, 2014, from http://www.cdc.gov/hiv/risk/other/correctional.html

Chaiken, S., Thompson, C., & Shoemaker, W. (2005). Mental health interventions in correctional settings. In Scott, C., & Gerbasi, J. (Eds.), *Handbook of correctional mental health* (pp. 109–131). Washington, DC: American Psychiatric Publishing.

Coleman, E., Bockting, W., Botzer, M., Cohen-Kettenis, P., DeCuypere, G., Feldman, J...Zucker, K. (2011). Standards of care for the health of transsexual, transgender, and gender-nonconforming people, version 7. *International Journal of Transgenderism, 13,* 165–232. Retrieved February 18, 2015, from http://www.wpath.org/uploaded_files/140/files/IJT%20SOC,%20V7.pdf

Committee to Protect Journalists. (2014). *2014 prison census: 221 journalists jailed worldwide.* Retrieved January 25, 2015, from https://www.cpj.org/imprisoned/2014.php

Dale, C., & Woods, P. (2002). *Caring for prisoners: RCN prison nurses forum roles and boundaries project.* London, England: Royal College of Nursing.

David Lynch Foundation. (2015). *Transcendental meditation in prison: Freedom behind bars.* Retrieved March 31, 2014, from http://www.davidlynchfoundation.org/prisons.html

Dean v. Coughlin, No. 84 Civ. 1528, 1989 WL 82421 (S.D.N.Y. July 12, 1989).

Detention Watch Network. (2011). *The influence of the private prison industry in the immigration detention business.* Retrieved March 31, 2014, from https://afsc.org/resource/az-private-prison-report/ICE-resources

Dole, P. J. (2006). *Caring for offenders: Correctional nursing.* St. Louis, MO: Elsevier/Mosby.

Dooghan, J. K., & U.S. Army Command and General Staff College. (2006). *Muslim prison ministry: Hindering the spread of the radical, militant, violent and irreconcilable wing of Islam.* Fort Leavenworth, KS: School of Advanced Military Studies.

Doward, J. (2010). Number of armed forces' veterans in jail "on the rise." *TheGuardian.com.* Retrieved February 22, 2015, from http://www.theguardian.com/society/2010/jan/10/armed-forces-veterans-prison-population

DuFresne, D. (2010). Top 10 US prison gangs. *ListVerse.* Retrieved February 18, 2015, from http://listverse.com/2010/12/11/top-10-us-prison-gangs/

Duran v. Anaya, 642 F. Supp. 510 (D.N.M. 1986).

Estelle v. Gamble, 429 U.S. 97, 97 S. Ct. 285, 50 L. Ed. 2d 251 (1976).

European Court of Human Rights, Council of Europe. (1953). *European convention on human rights.* Strasbourg, France: European Court of Human Rights. Retrieved February 19, 2015, from http://www.echr.coe.int/Documents/Convention_ENG.pdf

Evans, D. G. (1996). Defining community corrections. *Corrections Today.* Retrieved from http://www.thefreelibrary.com/Defining+community+corrections.a018826973

ExecutedToday.com. (2011). *1782: David Tyrie, The last hanged, drawn, and quartered.* Retrieved February 18, 2015, from http://www.executedtoday.com/tag/david-tyree/

Faiver, K. L. (1998). *Health care management issues in corrections.* Baltimore, MD: United Book Press, Inc.

Fazel, S., & Seewald, K. (2012). Severe mental illness in 33,588 prisoners worldwide: Systematic review and meta-regression analysis. *British Journal of Psychiatry, 200,* 364–373.

Fazel, S., Hope, T., O'Donnell, I., Piper, M., & Jacoby, R. (2001). Health of elderly male prisoners: Worse than the general population, worse than younger prisoners. *Age and Ageing, 30*(5), 403–407.

Federal Bureau of Prisons. (n.d.). *Custody and care: Sex offenders.* Retrieved March 21, 2014, from http://www.bop.gov/inmates/custody_and_care/sex_offenders.jsp

Fentiman, L. C. (2009). In the name of fetal protection: Why American prosecutors pursue pregnant drug users (and other countries don't). *Pace Law Faculty Publications.* New York, NY: Pace University School of Law. Retrieved March 23, 014, from http://digitalcommons.pace.edu/do/search/?q=fentiman&start=0&context=153428

FindLaw.com. (2013). *Rights of inmates.* Retrieved February 18, 2015, from http://files.findlaw.com/pdf/civilrights/civilrights.findlaw.com_other-constitutional-rights_rights-of-inmates.pdf

Finney v. Arkansas Board of Corrections, 505 F.2d 194 (8th Cir. 1974).

Foucault, M. (1995). *Discipline and punishment: The birth of the prison.* New York, NY: Random House.

Frank, R., & Efrati, A. (2009). "Evil" Madoff Gets 150 Years in Epic Fraud. *Wall Street Journal.* Retrieved February 20, 2015, from http://www.wsj.com/articles/SB124604151653862301

Gadd, C. J. (1965). Hammurabi and the end of his dynasty. In *Cambridge ancient history* (rev. ed.) (Vol. 2) (Ch. 5).

Gamil, J. T. (2015). Political prisoners fast to grab Francis' attention. *Philippine Daily Enquirer.* Retrieved January 25, 2015, from http://globalnation.inquirer.net/117033/political-prisoners-fast-to-grab-francis-attention/

Glaser, J. B., & Greifinger, R. B. (1993). Correctional health care: A public health opportunity. *Annals of Internal Medicine, 118*(2), 139–145.

Haney, C. (2002). *The psychological impact of incarceration: Implications for post-prison adjustment.* Washington, DC: Urban Institute.

Harner, H., & Burgess, A. W. (2011). Using a trauma-informed framework to care for incarcerated women. *Journal of Obstetric, Gynecologic, and Neonatal Nursing, 40*(4), 469–475.

Harrison, L., Cappello, R., Alaszewski, A., Appleton, S., & Cooke, G. (2003). *The effectiveness of treatment for substance dependence within the prison system in England: A review.* Canterbury, England: Centre for Health Services Studies. Retrieved February 21, 2015, from http://www.kent.ac.uk/chss/docs/etdd.PDF

Hayes, L. M. (2005). Suicide prevention in correctional facilities. In C. Scott & J. Gerbasi (Eds.), *Handbook of correctional mental health* (pp. 69–88). Washington, DC: American Psychiatric Publishing.

Health Insurance Portability and Accountability Act (HIPAA). Public Law No. 104–191, 110 Stat. 1936, (enacted August 21, 1996).

Heaton, C. (2014). *Roman prisons.* Retrieved from www.unrv.com/government/roman-prisons.phys

Heller, B. R., Oros, M. T., & Durney-Crowley, J. (2013). *The future of nursing education: Ten trends to watch.* Washington, DC: National League for Nursing. Retrieved from http://www.nln.org/nlnjournal/infotrends.htm

Holding, J. (2004). Faith behind the fence: Religious trends in US prisons. *Christian Research Institute, 27*(6). Retrieved March 31, 2014, from http://www.equip.org/articles/faith-behind-the-fence-religious-trends-in-us-prisons/

Human Rights Watch. (2009). *Mental illness, human rights, and US prisons: Human Rights Watch statement for the record to the Senate Judiciary Committee Subcommittee on Human Rights and the Law.* Retrieved from http://www.hrw.org/news/2009/09/22/mental-illness-human-rights-and-us-prisons

Institute of Medicine (IOM) (US) Committee on Ethical Considerations for Revisions to DHHS Regulations for Protection of Prisoners Involved in Research. (2007). Today's prisoners: Changing demographics, health issues, and the current research environment. In L. O. Gostin, C. Vanchieri, & A. Pope (Eds.), *Ethical considerations for research involving prisoners* (pp. 29–72). Washington, DC: National Academies Press. Retrieved June 17, 2015, from http://www.ncbi.nlm.nih.gov/books/NBK19877/

International Association of Forensic Nurses (IAFN) & American Nurses Association (ANA). (2009). Forensic Nursing: Scope and Standards of Practice. Silver Spring, MD: Nursesbooks.org

James, D., & Glaze, L. (2006). *Mental health problems of prison and jail inmates.* Washington, DC: Bureau of Justice Statistics.

Joiner, T. (2007). *Why people die by suicide.* Cambridge, MA: Harvard University Press.

Jurgens, R. (2007). *Effectiveness of interventions to address HIV in prisons.* Geneva, Switzerland: World Health Organization. Retrieved January 25, 2015, from http://whqlibdoc.who.int/publications/2007/9789241596190_eng.pdf

Kann, M. E. (2005). Concealing punishment. In *Punishment, prisons, and patriarchy: Liberty and power in the early American republic.* New York, NY: New York University Press.

Keller, D. M. (2012). Prazosin relieves nightmares and sleep disturbance in PTSD. *Medscape.com.* Retrieved February 21, 2015, from http://www.medscape.com/viewarticle/760070

King, L. N. (2008). *Mission matters: Professional identity and correctional medicine.* Quincy, MA: 2nd Annual Academic and Health Policy Conference on Correctional Health Care.

Knox, C. (2013). International perspectives on nursing practice within the criminal justice setting. *Essentials of Correctional Nursing.* Retrieved from http://www.essentialsofcorrectionalnursing.com/2013/10/22/international

Knox, G. (2012). *The problem of gangs and security threat groups (STGs) in American prisons and jails today: Recent findings from the 2012 NGCRC national gang/STG survey.* Peotone, IL: National Gang Crime Research Center. Retrieved March 31, 2014, http://www.ngcrc.com/corr2012.html

Koeller, D. (2003). Hammurabi, king of Babylon 1792 -1750 BC. *WebChron: The Web Chronology Project.* Retrieved from http://www.the nagain.info/;WebChron/MiddleEast/Hammurabi.html

Latessa, E. J., & Smith, P. (2011). *Corrections in the community* (5th ed.). New York, NY: Taylor and Francis.

Lee, H., Palmbach, T., & Miller, M. (2006). *Henry Lee's crime scene handbook.* London, England: Elsevier Ltd.

Lewis, C. (2005). Female offenders in correctional settings. In C. Scott & J. Gerbasi, (Eds.), *Handbook of correctional mental health* (pp. 155–185). Washington, DC: American Psychiatric Publishing.

Lugo v. Senkowski, 114 F. Supp. 2d 111 (N.D.N.Y. 2000).

Maroney, M. K. (2005). Caring and custody: Two faces of the same reality. *Journal of Correctional Health Care, 11,* 157–169.

McClennan, R. M. (2008). *The crisis of imprisonment: Protest, politics, and the making of the American penal state. 1776–1941.* New York, NY: Cambridge University Press.

Miller, A. (2013). Providing principled health care in prison. *Canadian Medical Association Journal, 184*(4), E-183-E-184.

Ministry of Justice, National Offender Management Service & HM Prison Service. (2015). *Prison population statistics and Prisons and probation statistics.* Retrieved February 18, 2015, from https://www.gov.uk/government/collections/prisons-and-probation-statistics

Miranda, L. (2009). Jail vs. treatment for drug offenders. *Treatment Solutions.* Retrieved June 16, 2015, from http://www.treatmentsolutions.com/301//

Mitka, M. (2004). Aging prisoners stressing health care system. *Journal of the American Medical Association, 292*(4), 423–424.

Moak, A. (2010). *Defining a correctional nurse.* Retrieved from http://www.corrections.com/news/article/24280-defining-a-correctional-nurse

Mohr, G. (2013). Integrated criminal justice systems: Working collaboratively to reduce recidivism. *Corrections Today, 75*(4), 28–31.

Moore, J. (2005, Fall). Public health behind bars: Health care for jail inmates. *Popular Government,* 16–23. Retrieved February 17, 2015, from http://sogpubs.unc.edu/electronicversions/pg/pgfal05/article2.pdf

Moser, D. K. (n.d.). *Testing a cardiovascular risk reduction intervention in the Kentucky state prison system* [PowerPoint presentation]. Retrieved from http://www.correctionalhealthconference.com/sites/correctionalhealthconference.com/files/Testing%20a%20Cardiovascular%20Risk%20Reduction%20Intervention%20in%20the%20_0.pdf

Mumola, C. J. (2005). *Suicide and homicide in state prisons and local jails.* Washington, DC: Bureau of Justice Statistics.

National Center for Transgender Equality. (2012). *LGBT people and the Prison Rape Elimination Act.* Retrieved March 1, 2014, from www.Transequality.org

National Commission on Correctional Health Care (NCCHC). (2003). *Correctional mental health care: Standards and guidelines for deliveries of service.* Chicago, IL: NCCHC.

National Commission on Correctional Health Care (NCCHC). (2011). *Guidelines for the management of an adequate delivery system.* Chicago, IL: NCCHC.

National Commission on Correctional Health Care (NCCHC). (2014a). *Standards for health services in jails.* Chicago, IL: NCCHC.

National Commission on Correctional Health Care (NCCHC). (2014b). *Standards for health services in prisons.* Chicago, IL: NCCHC.

National Health Service (NHS). (2006). *Prison nursing.* Retrieved February 22, 2015, from http://www.nhscareers.nhs.uk/explore-by-career/nursing/careers-in-nursing/prison-nursing/

National Public Radio (NPR) Staff. (2011). *Nation's jails struggle with mentally ill prisoners.* Retrieved from http://www.npr.org/2011/09/04/140167676/nations-jails-struggle-with-mentally-ill-prisoners

National Resource Center on Justice Involved Women. (2013). *Responding to the needs of women veterans involved in the criminal justice system.* Retrieved March 31, 2014, from http://cjinvolvedwomen.org/sites/all/documents/WomenVeterans.pdf

Newman v. Alabama, 349 F. Supp. 278 (M.D. Ala. 1972).

Noonan, M. E., & Mumola, C. J, (2007). *Veterans in state and federal prison, 2004.* Washington, DC: Bureau of Justice Statistics. Retrieved February 21, 2015, from http://www.bjs.gov/content/pub/pdf/vsfp04.pdf

North American Vipassana Prison Project. (2013). *Vipassana meditation as taught by S. N. Goenka in the tradition of Sayagyi U Ba Khin.* Retrieved February 18, 2015, from http://www.prison.dhamma.org/en/na

Northrup, C. E. (1987). Nursing practice in correctional facilities. In C. E. Northrup & M. E. Kelly, *Legal issues in nursing.* St. Louis, MO: Mosby.

O'Brien, M., Tewaniti, T., Hawley, J., & Fleming, D. (2006). Managing elderly offenders. *Australian Correctional Leadership Program.* Retrieved January 25, 2015, from www.csa.intersearch.com.au.2006344.MAN.pdf

O'Conner v. Donaldson, 422 U.S. 563, 95 S. Ct. 2486, 45 L. Ed. 2d 396 (1975).

O'Conner, T. (2012). Early history of corrections. *Megalinks in Criminal Justice.* Retrieved from http://www.drtomoconnor.com/1050/1050lect01.htm

O'Donnell, C., & Trick, M. (2006). *Methadone maintenance treatment and the criminal justice system.* Washington, DC: National Association of State Alcohol and Drug Abuse Directors, Inc. Retrieved February 21, 2015, from http://www.nasadad.org/resource.php?base_id = 650

Pelaez, V. (2014). The prison industry in the United States: Big business or a new form of slavery? *GlobalResearch. com.* Retrieved February 22, 2015, from http://www.globalresearch.ca/the-prison-industry-in-the-united-states-big-business-or-a-new-form-of-slavery/8289

Pluralism Project, Harvard University. (n.d.). Muslim chaplaincy in the U.S. Plurism.org. Retrieved February 22, 2015, from http://www.pluralism.org/religion/islam/issues/prison-ministry

Prison Congregations of America. (n.d.). A congregation in a prison - Really? *Prisoncongregations.org.* Retrieved February 21, 2015, from http://www.prisoncongregations.org/

Prison Rape Elimination Act (PREA). Public Law No. 108–79, 117 Stat. 972 (enacted September 4, 2003). Retrieved February 23, 2015, from http://www.gpo.gov/fdsys/pkg/PLAW-108publ79/pdf/PLAW-108publ79.pdf

Public Broadcasting Service (PBS). (n.d.). *Now with Bill Moyers: Women, prison, and children.* Retrieved from http://www.pbs.org/now/society/womenprisoners.html

Puleo, T., & Chedekel, L. (2011). Inmate health-care costs rise: Complaints about inadequate care expose taxpayers to even steeper longterm costs. *The Republican Newsroom.* Retrieved February 19, 2015, from http://www.masslive.com/news/index.ssf/2011/04/inmate_healt-care_costs_rise_c.html

Ramos v. Lamm, 713 F.2d 546 (10th Cir. 1983).

Rold, W. J. (1998). Legal considerations in the delivery of health care services in prisons and jails. In M. M. Puisis (Ed.), *Clinical practice in correctional medicine* (pp. 345–350). St. Louis, MO: Mosby.

Ross, M. W., & Drake, S. (1992). Mad, bad and dangerous to know: Dimensions and measurements of attitudes toward injecting drug users. *Drug and Alcohol Dependence, 30,* 71–74.

Sabol, W. J., Minton, T. D., & Harrison, P. M. (2007). *Prison and jail inmates at midyear 2006.* Washington, DC: U.S. Department of Justice, Office of Justice Programs. Retrieved February 25, 2014, from https://www.ojp.usdoj.gov/bjs/abstract/pjim06.htm

Savage, C. (2013). Justice dept. seeks to curtail stiff drug sentences. *New York Times.* Retrieved February 22, 2015, from http://www.nytimes.com/2013/08/12/us/justice-dept-seeks-to-curtail-stiff-drug-sentences.html?pagewanted=all

Schoenly, L., & Knox, C. (2013). *Essentials of correctional nursing.* New York, NY: Springer Publishing Co.

Shelton, D., Weiskopf, C., & Nicholson, M. (2010). Correctional nursing competency development in the correctional managed health care program. *Journal of Correctional Health, 16,* 299.

Sheridan, F. (1996). Security and control: Perimeter security. In M. D. McShane & F. P. Williams (Eds.), *Encyclopedia of American prisons* (pp. 681–684). New York, NY: Taylor & Francis.

Shields, K. E., & de Moya, D. (1997). Correctional health care nurses' attitudes toward inmates. *Journal of Correctional Health Care, 4*(1), 37–59. Retrieved from jcx.sagepub.com/content/4/1/37/abstract

Sipes, L. A., Jr. (2009). GPS tracking of criminal offenders. Corrections.com: Where criminal justice never sleeps. Retrieved from http://www.corrections.com/news/article/22961

Smith, B., Loomis, M., Yarussi, J., & Marksamer, J. (2013). *Policy review and development guide: Lesbian, gay, bisexual, transgender, and intersex persons in custodial settings.* Washington, DC: National Institute of Corrections, U.S. Department of Justice. Retrieved February 17, 2015, from www.wcl.american.edu/endsilence/documents/Module4_PREAGuidedPolicieshandouts.pdf

Smyer, T., & Burbank, P. M. (2009). The U.S. correctional system and the older prisoner. *Journal of Gerontological Nursing, 35*(12), 32–37.

Snyder, C., van Wormer, K., Chadha, J., & Jaggers, J. W. (2009). Older adult inmates: The challenge for social work. *Social Work, 54*(2), 117–1124.

Spicer v. Williamson, 191 N.C. 487, 132 S.E. 291 (N.C. 1926).

Spierenburg, P. (1998). *The body and the State: Early modern Europe.* Retrieved from http://books.google.com/books?id=bwvH5ce94elC&pg=PA44

Stahl, M. (2014). Development of law. *Timetoast.com.* Retrieved from http://www.timetoast.com/timelines/development-of-law-14

Strom, K. (2000). *Profile of state prisoners under age 18, 1985–97.* Washington, DC: Bureau of Justice Statistics.

Sullivan, J. T., Sykora, K., Schneiderman, J., Naranjo, C. A., & Sellers, E. M. (1989). Assessment of alcohol withdrawal: The revised clinical institute withdrawal assessment for alcohol scale (CIWA-Ar). *British Journal of Addiction, 84*(11), 1353–1357.

Swinford, S., & Amin, A. (2014). *Number of sex offenders in England and Wales rises by more than a third in five years.* Retrieved January 28, 2015, from http://www.telegraph.co.uk/news/uknews/law-and-order/10627796/Number-of-sex-offenders-in-England-and-Wales-rises-by-more-than-third-in-five-years.html

Togas, C., Raikou, M., & Niakas, D. (2014). An assessment of health related quality of life in a male prison population in Greece associations with health related characteristics and characteristics of detention. *BioMed Research International,* 2014, article ID 274804, doi:10.1155/2014/274804

Torrey, E. F., Zdanowicz, M. T., Kennard, A. D., Lamb, H. R., Eslinger, D. F., Biasotti, M. C., & Fuller, D. A. (2014). *The treatment of persons with mental illness in prisons and jails: A state survey.* Arlington, VA: Treatment Advocacy Center. Retrieved February 20, 2015, from http://tacreports.org/storage/documents/treatment-behind-bars/treatment-behind-bars.pdf

U.S. Census Bureau. (2012a). *Table 52: Veterans by selected period of service and state: 2010.* Washington, DC: US Census Bureau.

U.S. Census Bureau. (2012b, December 31). *U.S. and world population clock.* Washington, DC: US Census Bureau.

U.S. Constitution amendment VIII. Superintendent of Documents, U.S. Government Printing Office. (2002). Retrieved February 22, 2015, from http://www.gpo.gov/fdsys/pkg/GPO-CONAN-2002/pdf/GPO-CONAN-2002-9-9.pdf

U.S. Department of Health and Human Services (HHS). (2009). *Protection of human subjects: Additional protections pertaining to biomedical and behavioral research involving prisoners as subjects,* 45 C.F.R. §§46.301-46.306.

U.S. Department of Health and Human Services (HHS), Health Resources and Services Administration, Maternal and Child Health Bureau. (2013). *Women's health USA 2013.* Rockville, Maryland: HHS.

U.S. Department of Justice (DOJ). (2013). *The Federal Bureau of Prisons' compassionate release program.* Washington, DC: DOJ.

U.S. Department of Justice (DOJ), Federal Bureau of Prisons. (1999, May 12). *Program statement number 1070.07.* Washington, DC: DOJ. Retrieved February 22, 2015, from http://www.justice.gov/oig/reports/2013/e1306.pdf

U.S. Immigration and Customs Enforcement (ICE). (n.d.). *A day in the life of ICE enforcement and removal operations.* Retrieved March 31, 2014, from https://www.ice.gov//about/offices/enforcement-removal-operations/

U.S. Department of State. (2012). *Report on international prison conditions.* Washington, DC: U.S. Department of State. Retrieved February 20, 2015, from http://www.state.gov/documents/organization/210160.pdf

Van Voorhis, P. (2013). *Women's risk factors and new treatments/interventions for addressing them: Evidence-based interventions in the United States and Canada.* Tokyo, Japan: United Nations Asia and Far East Institute for the Prevention of Crime and the Treatment of Offenders (UNAFEI). Retrieved February 17, 2015, from http://www.unafei.or.jp/english/pdf/RS_No90/No90_09VE_Van%20Voorhis.pdf

Waldman, A. (2013). Women are fastest-growing group of incarcerated persons in U.S. *Humane Exposures Blog.* Retrieved March 9, 2014, from http://humaneexposures.com/blog/women-are-fastest-growing-group-of-incarcerated-persons-in-u-s.html

Wall, J., & Andersen, S. M. (2013). Effective community supervision: Implementing a risk and needs assessment for offenders transitioning into the community. *Corrections Today, 75*(4), 36.

Walmsley, R. (2013). *World prison population list* (10th ed.). London, England: International Centre for Prison Studies. Retrieved February 18, 2015, from http://www.prisonstudies.org/sites/prisonstudies.org/files/resources/downloads/wppl_10.pdf

Ward, K., Longaker, A., Williams, J., Naylor, A., Rose, C. A., & Simpson, C. G. (2013). Incarceration within American and Nordic prisons: Comparison of national and international policies. *Engage: An International Journal for Research in Practice of Student-School Engagement, 1*(1), 36–47.

Washington State Department of Corrections. (2014). *Civil commitment of sexually violent offenders.* Retrieved March 31, 2014, from http://www.doc.wa.gov/community/sexoffenders/civilcommitment.asp

Weinstein, H., Kim, D., Mack, A., Malavade, K., & Saraiya, A. (2005). Prevalence and assessment of mental disorders in correctional settings. In C. Scott & J. Gerbasi (Eds.), *Handbook of correctional mental health* (pp. 43–68). Washington, DC: American Psychiatric Publishing.

Weiskopf, C. S. (2005). Nurses experience of caring for inmate-patients. *Journal of Advanced Nursing, 49,* 336–343.

Welch, M. (2003). A social history of punishment and prisons. In *Corrections: A critical approach* (2nd ed.) (pp. 16–39). New York, NY: McGraw-Hill.

Wesson, D., & Ling, W. (2003). The clinical opiate withdrawal scale (COWS). *Journal of Psychoactive Drugs, 35*(2), 253–259.

Whitehead, D. (2006). The Health Promoting Prison (HPP) and its imperative for nursing. *International Journal of Nursing Studies, 43*(1), 123–131.

Wilper, A. P., Woolhandler, S., Boyd, J., Lasser, K. E., McCormick, D., Bor, D. H., & Himmelstein, D. U. (2009). The health and health care of US prisoners: Results of a nationwide survey. *American Journal of Public Health, 99*(4), 666–672.

Women's Health Encyclopedia. (2011). *Prison health.* Retrieved from http://womenshealthency.com/p/prison-health/

Wong, S., Ordean, A., & Kahan, M. (2011). Substance use in pregnancy (Practice Guideline #256). *Journal of Obstetrics and Gynaecology of Canada, 33*(4), 367–384. Retrieved February 17, 2015, from http://sogc.org/wp-content/uploads/2013/01/gui256CPG1104E.pdf

World Health Organization (WHO). (2007a). *Effectiveness of interventions to address HIV in prisons.* Geneva, Switzerland: WHO. Retrieved January 25, 2015, from http://whqlibdoc.who.int/publications/2007/9789241596190_eng.pdf

World Health Organization (WHO). (2007b). *Health in prisons: A WHO guide to the essentials in prison health.* Copenhagen, Denmark: WHO. Retrieved February 17, 2015, from http://www.google.com/url?sa=t&rct=j&q=&esrc=s&source=web&cd=4&ved=0CDAQFjAD&url=http%3A%2F%2Fwww.euro.who.int%2F__data%2Fassets%2Fpdf_file%2F0009%2F99018%2FE90174.pdf&ei=fTjEVMfOD4OaNu-ngbAJ&usg=AFQjCNGs59e-I1jSHo6bhmX-S7yCt4YM_fw&bvm=bv.84349003,d.eXY

World Health Organization (WHO). (2012). Economic evaluation of a task-shifting intervention for common mental disorders in India. *Bulletin of the World Health Organization, 90,* 813–821. Retrieved January 1, 2015, from http://www.who.int/bulletin/volumes/90/11/12-104133/en/

World Health Organization (WHO). (2014). *Prisons and health.* Retrieved from http://www.euro.who.int/en/health-topics/health-determinants/prisons-and-health/publications/2014/prisons-and-health

Zamorano, A. (2012). Venezuela's prisons see security breakdown. *BBC News.* Retrieved from http://www.bbc.co.uk/news/world-latin-america-19003776

Zust, B. L. (2009). Partner violence, depression, and recidivism: The case of incarcerated women and why we need programs designed for them. *Issues in Mental Health Nursing, 30,* 246–251.

SUGGESTED RESOURCES

http://correctionalnurse.net
http://www.aca.org
http://www.achsa.org
http://www.americanjail.org
http://www.awec.us
http://www.ncchc.org
http://www.iafn.org/displaycommon.cfm?an=1&subarticlenbr=762
http://nursesincorrectionalfacilities.weebly.com/resources.html

CHAPTER 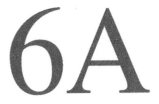 6A

Emerging Issues: Military Forensic Nursing

Michelle Ortiz

"Sexual harassment and sexual assault in the military are a profound betrayal – a profound betrayal – of sacred oaths and sacred trusts." Secretary of Defense Chuck Hagel to West Point Cadets (May 25, 2013).

OBJECTIVES

At the completion of this chapter, the learner will be able to:

- Provide an overview of the military forensic nursing program.
- Identify key pioneers in military forensic nursing.
- Distinguish between "restricted" and "unrestricted" reporting.
- Describe the sexual assault care training process for military personnel.

KEY TERMS

DoD: Department of Defense

DoJ: Department of Justice

FOB: Forward Operating Bases

JTF-SAPR: Joint Task Force – Sexual Assault Prevention and Response

NDAA: National Defense Authorization Act

SAPRO: Sexual Assault Prevention and Response Office

SARC: Sexual Assault Response Coordinator

SART: Sexual Assault Response Team

SecDef: Secretary of Defense

HISTORY AND THEORY

The United States military has long grappled with the issue of sexual assault within the organization. The American public was first introduced to the issue when news reports were saturated with the 1991 Tailhook scandal, which occurred at the Las Vegas Hilton. Ninety victims, both male and female, were subjected to varying levels of assault by Navy and Marine Corps aviators. In 1996, the Army moved to the forefront of media attention. The Aberdeen Proving Ground sex scandal investigated 12 male officers who allegedly sexually assaulted female trainee subordinates in the officers' charge. In 2003, the US Air Force Academy reported that 12% of female graduates had either been raped or were the victim of an attempted rape during their academic stay. Later that year, the Department of Defense (DoD) received 94 reports of sexual assault from soldiers in the areas of Iraq, Kuwait, and Afghanistan (DoD, 2004). In the year prior, these regions received only 24 reports of sexual assault (DoD, 2004). Globally, 901 reports were made in 2001, and 1,012 in 2003.

Further fueled by the shocking November 2003 article series, "Betrayal in the Ranks," authored by *Denver Post* reporter Miles Moffet, the DoD was forced to acknowledge the problem of sexual assault in the military and began taking a closer look at how to effectively address the problem. In 2004, then Secretary of Defense (SecDef) Donald Rumsfeld commissioned the "Care for Victims Task Force," which later became the Joint Task Force – Sexual Assault Prevention and Response (JTF-SAPR). This panel would serve as the single point of accountability and the center of gravity for sexual assault prevention and response policy across the services (DoD, 2004).

One of the hallmarks that resulted from this panel's work was the need for improved and standardized care delivery processes by the military healthcare system across the enterprise (DoD, 2004). The report specifically identified the need for the military to integrate specially trained sexual assault nurse examiners (SANEs) into its medical programs (Ferguson, 2008). Although "SANE care" was the specific recommendation and verbiage used by the task force, the unique care environments and military missions in which US soldiers, sailors, airmen, and marines serve necessitate forensic examination training for multilevel providers. Some of these mission environments present logistical challenges to the provision of care. Included in such environments are forward operating bases (FOBs) in combatant zones, submarines on surveillance missions that are unable to surface for extended periods of time, and remote locations, such as Diego Garcia, Antarctica, and small isolated African villages; other environments have reduced capabilities due to supply availability and manpower. "Timely access to quality forensic care can be a logistical challenge. However, this patient population is no less likely to be victimized than any other, and is deserving of the same caliber and effective standards of care afforded to civilian populations in the United States" (Ortiz, 2008; p. 44). By mandate, providers must be prepared to respond as directed by the governing instruction to the needs of the forensic patient.

Several pioneers in the area of military forensic nursing have filled unique roles and made enormous contributions to the acceptance of the discipline throughout the DoD. With their tenacity and perseverance, the care for military victims of violence and trauma has steadily improved. Some of these pioneers have retired from active service, but continue to serve the DoD in a civilian capacity; some are still on active duty serving their nation.

The pioneers who have helped to forge the path for forensic nursing in the military and Department of Veterans Affairs include, but are not limited to:

- Colonel Teresa Parsons, Colonel Heidi Warrington, and Nancy Emma of the US Army Nurse Corps

- Captain Susan Rist, Commander Lovette Robinson, Commander Cynthia T. Ferguson, Lieutenant Commander Alana Huber, and Lieutenant Commander Michelle Ortiz of the US Navy Nurse Corps
- Colonel Janet Barber Duval and Colonel Susan Hanshaw, US Air Force Nurse Corps
- Mary K. Sullivan, Department of Veterans Affairs

Although SANE practice is well represented among these trailblazers, it is not the only representation of forensic nursing in the DoD. Expertise in "other specialty areas, including human abuse and neglect, death investigation, intimate partner violence, and healthcare risk management" is also found among the ranks of military forensic nurses (Lynch & Duval, 2011; p. 623). "Military nurses ... have been tenacious in their determination to provide the highest quality of forensic services for those affected by violence, both victims and offenders" (Lynch & Duval, 2011; p. 624). Indeed, as the interest and popularity of forensic nursing continues to grow, the numbers of military nurses seeking advanced degrees and certifications in this discipline inevitably will also increase. This will have a positive impact on the availability and adaptability of the nurses providing care to military patients on multiple platforms and will be key in the effective prevention and response initiatives in the coming years.

INTERSECTING SYSTEMS AND SERVICES

In 2006, the now permanent DoD SAPR office released its most recent governing instruction, the DoDI 6495.02. Contained within were several key mandates: (1) Sexual assault responders must be provided training, (2) the additional option of "restricted" or confidential reporting must be available, and (3) a pathway must be provided for victims of sexual assault to access all support personnel and lines of service regardless of whether they choose to initiate an investigation.

This new instruction effectively created an "organizational chart" of intersecting systems that closely followed the sexual assault response team (SART) model in the military forensic care environment. With the SART model, various entities from legal, medical, and victim support intersect to assist the patient, based on his or her needs and wishes, the scenario presented, and the services for which the patient qualifies. If the patient opts for an unrestricted report, he or she will be afforded access to medical-forensic care. This includes followup appointments for laboratory specimens and medications, legal assistance, law enforcement involvement, a personal victim's advocate, a sexual assault response coordinator (SARC), religious supportive services, relocation assistance if desired, and mental health support, including survivor group access. In contrast, if a patient opts for a "restricted" report, he or she qualifies for the same services as those who choose the "unrestricted" report, with the following exception: no investigatory inquiry will be conducted and no prosecutorial legal assistance will be offered. To qualify for a restricted report, the victim must adhere to a strict policy of disclosure. Disclosure of the assault can only be made to the SARC, a victim's advocate, and medical personnel. Members of the chaplain corps were granted absolute confidentiality through SecNav Instruction 1730.9, which states, "Confidential communication includes acts of religion, matters of conscience, and any other information conveyed to a Navy chaplain in the chaplain's role as a spiritual advisor that is not intended to be disclosed to third persons...."

PRACTICES AND PROCESSES

Training and Education

One of the greatest challenges for the military healthcare system has been the development, execution, standardization, and tracking of SANE education for its care providers. DoD Instruction (DoDI) 6495.02 governs the training requirements for military sexual assault forensic examiners (SAFEs). This instruction refers directly to the 2013 edition of the Department of Justice's (DoJ)

National Protocol for Sexual Assault Medical Forensic Examinations, Adults/Adolescents, which outlines the following recommendations for "building the capacity" of forensic examiners:

- Encourage the development of specific knowledge, skills, and victim-centered approaches in examiners;
- Encourage advanced education and supervised clinical practice of examiners, as well as certification for all examiners; and
- Provide access to experts on anti-sexual assault initiatives who can participate in sexual assault examiner training, mentoring, proctoring, case review, photograph review, and quality assurance (DoJ, 2013).

The instruction further recommends that examinations be performed by examiners with "advanced education and clinical experience, if possible." This recommendation is difficult to execute and invest in; budgetary limitations and the delivery across multiple platforms of care pose challenges. Translation of the DoJ's 2013 training and education recommendations have been applied to various delivery modes across the services: one service expanded training to include a 3-week course with clinical skills assessment; another branch adopted computer-based technology as primary training, with a service-specific compact disc (CD) and competency requirements for registered nurses only; a third branch adheres to a 40-hour didactic training with hands-on skills assessment to demonstrate competency. A further difficulty is that the DoD does not officially recognize the specialty of forensic nursing.

CONCEPTS AND ISSUES

Recent, high-visibility media cases have exerted new pressures. The 2010 release of "The Invisible War" documentary, chronicling the problem and highlighting several victims of sexual assault, resulted in renewed attention. Other highly publicized media cases include:

- Naval Academy Midshipmen case, 2013; acquittal of all charges
- Army Brigadier General Jeffrey Sinclair, 2014; acquittal of the most serious sex charges, guilty of lesser charges, fined $20,000
- Head of US Air Force DoD SAPRO, 2013; guilty of reduced charges

These cases have helped to further fuel the anger of Congress and the American public to demand change.

The 2014 National Defense Authorization Act (NDAA), the federal law that governs the budget and expenditures for the DoD, has brought additional support to the issue of military sexual assault care by increasing the requirements for programs in the service branches.

New to the 2014 NDAA were the following pronouncements (U.S. House of Representatives Committee on Armed Forces, 2013; June 7):

- Command discretion on court martial findings has been eliminated. The convening authority is *not required* to take action based upon court martial findings, but any action that is taken cannot be overturned later.
- If charges of sexual assault are dropped, or if authorities decline to prosecute, a written explanation will be required. The decision will be investigated by a civilian authority and become part of the permanent record.
- The statute of limitations has been removed.
- A service member will face mandatory dishonorable discharge or dismissal if found guilty of the most serious offenses.
- Anyone accused of military sexual trauma (MST), pending an investigation, is allowed to be transferred to another command.
- A need exists for additional training mandates, legal assistance for victims, and a complete review of policies and procedures currently in place regarding MST.
- Trained and certified Sexual Assault Nurse Examiners-Adult/Adolescent are to be assigned at the brigade level or other unit level subject to the discretion of the Secretary of Defense.

- At least one full-time sexual assault nurse examiner is required for a medical facility that has a 24-hour emergency department and nurse examiners must be made available to other medical facilities.
- The Secretary of Defense is required to report on the adequacy of training, qualifications, and experience of those assigned to positions involving sexual assault prevention and response in the Armed Forces.

Senator Barbara Boxer (D-CA) subsequently introduced an amendment to effectively standardize training and program management requirements across all the services of DoD by creating a baseline expectation for acceptable standards (American Nurses Association, 2014).

Congress passed the 2015 NDAA, which President Obama signed into law in December 2014. The law now directs all military sexual assault forensic examination training to be standardized across the services. The DoD is awaiting guidance on implementation of this new requirement.

FUTURE ISSUES

The DoD is beginning to realize the commitment and the human resources required to address the issue of sexual assault in the ranks and meet the NDAA. As with any new paradigm, adjustments will be necessary along the course to balance the need for services, the mode of care delivery, and the resources available. As military nurses seek to expand their forensic knowledge and skills, this will translate to having a trained, competent, mobile resource that can respond to any platform to deliver forensic care, and truly embrace the motto "World Class Care – Anytime, Anywhere."

REVIEW QUESTIONS

1. What are some of the unique environments in which military members serve that challenge the delivery of forensic care?

2. What reporting options are available to service members?

3. Does the Department of Defense currently recognize the specialty of forensic nursing?

4. Name one high visibility case of sexual misconduct in the United States military.

REFERENCES

American Nurses Association. (2014). *Sexual assault forensic examinations in the military: The Boxer amendment.* Retrieved from http://www.nursingworld.org/BoxerAmendment-IssueBrief

Department of Defense, Task Force on Care for Victims of Sexual Assault. (2004). *Task force report on care for victims of sexual assault.* Washington, DC: Department of Defense. Retrieved from http://www.defense.gov/news/may2004/d20040513satfreport.pdf

Department of Justice. (2013). *A national protocol for sexual assault medical forensic exams: Adults/adolescents* (2nd ed.). Washington, DC: Department of Justice. Retrieved from www.ncjrs.gov/pdffiles1/ovw/2065534.pdf

Ferguson, C. T. (2008). Caring for sexual assault patients in the military: Past, present, and future. *Journal of Forensic Nursing, 4,* 190–198.

Lynch, V. A., & Duval, J. B. (2011). *Forensic nursing science* (2nd ed.). St. Louis, MO: Elsevier/Mosby.

Ortiz, M. (2008). Standing by, ready to serve: The case for forensic nurses in uniform. *Military Medicine, 173,* 42–46.

U.S. House of Representatives Committee on Armed Forces. (2013). *National Defense Authorization Act for fiscal year 2014 (NDAA).* Report Number 113–102. Washington, DC: U.S. Government Printing Office. Retrieved from http://www.gpo.gov/fdsys/pkg/CRPT-113hrpt102/pdf/CRPT-113hrpt102.pdf

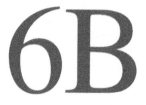

CHAPTER

6B

Emerging Issues: Human Trafficking

Donna Sabella

OBJECTIVES

At the completion of this chapter, the learner will be able to:

- Explain what human trafficking is and describe different types of trafficking.
- Describe how victims are trafficked.
- Discuss who trafficked persons are and where they come from.
- Describe the physical and emotional consequences of being trafficked.
- List common health problems of this population.
- Describe how to recognize and identify victims and signs and symptoms of trafficking.
- List sample questions to ask possible trafficking victims.
- Discuss intersecting systems and services available to trafficking victims.
- List appropriate nursing practices and interventions for working with suspected victims.
- Provide examples of preventive measures to combat human trafficking.

KEY TERMS

Human trafficking: A form of exploitation and control in which someone is forced to provide a service or engage in a behavior against his or her will with no remuneration. It involves some measure of force, fraud, and/or coercion against the individual being trafficked, who often is unable to leave the situation under threat of harm.

Human trafficking victim: Refers to anyone who has been trafficked and exploited against his or her will to work or provide any number of services through force, fraud, or coercion. Victims are often held against their will, unable to leave on their own under threat of personal harm or harm to their family and loved ones. Trafficking victims can be of any age, male or female, and come from every country.

Labor trafficking: A form of trafficking whereby individuals are forced to provide services as domestics, general laborers, farm workers, factory workers, and restaurant employees with little to no compensation for their services.

Sex trafficking: A form of trafficking in which individuals are forced to provide sexual services against their will with little or no remuneration.

Traffickers: Those who exploit others for personal gain and profit anywhere along the process. Traffickers include anyone who recruits, transports, harbors, sells, or is involved in making any arrangements to exploit another. Traffickers can include family members, loved ones, and friends, as well as strangers. Traffickers are frequently male, but female traffickers exist as well, and it is not unusual for a trafficker to have been a former human trafficking victim.

Trafficking Victims Protection Act (TVPA): First enacted in 2000 to grant prosecutors the power to punish traffickers and protect trafficking victims, it focused on prevention, protection, and punishment. Since then, the TVPA has been reauthorized several times, with each new version providing more authority to prosecute and address more aspects of human trafficking.

HISTORY AND THEORY

Human trafficking, also known as modern day slavery, has existed for many years both in the United States and abroad. For many countries, the practices of slavery, which go back to the earliest times, consisted of denying certain groups of people, usually based on their race and/or ethnicity, the right to freedom, free will, and free speech. Typically, such practices were legal and even condoned by society. People were bought and sold and were viewed by those making such purchases as their personal property to do with as they pleased. Slaves had no voice, no rights, and no recourse. They were considered to be less than human and unworthy of membership in the human race.

Many countries, such as Iceland, France, Sweden, Germany, Spain, and Japan, early on passed bills or took stands to abolish and make illegal such practices, but some countries took longer to condemn and outlaw slavery. In the United Kingdom, slavery was abolished through all of the British Empire in 1833 with the passage of the Slavery Abolition Act. The United States took a bit longer. In the December of 1865, the Thirteenth Amendment, which Congress had passed in January of that year, was ratified by the states (About Slavery, 2004). This amendment abolished slavery throughout the country, or so it seemed.

No one is sure where slavery ended and human trafficking began. Both are driven by similar social desires, wants, and needs, and have a number of things in common. Chief among the commonalities for those purchasing services is the need and desire for cheap labor and cheap goods. Human trafficking is an international and global phenomenon. Every year, the American government publishes a *Trafficking in Persons Report*, which summarizes the nature and extent of human trafficking in more than 180 countries (U.S. Department of State, 2014).

Definition and Characteristics of Human Trafficking

- Article 3, paragraph (a) of the Protocol to Prevent, Suppress and Punish Trafficking in Persons defines trafficking in persons as "the recruitment, transportation, transfer, harboring or receipt of persons, by means of the threat or use of force or other forms of coercion, of abduction, of fraud, of deception, of the abuse of power or of a position of vulnerability or of the giving or receiving of payments or benefits to achieve the consent of a person having control over another person, for the purpose of exploitation. Exploitation shall include, at a minimum, the exploitation of the prostitution of others or other forms of sexual exploitation, forced labor or services, slavery or practices similar to slavery, servitude or the removal of organs" (United Nations, 2000; p. 3).
- Human trafficking is a criminal activity. Although figures are difficult to estimate, some report that human trafficking is one of the top three forms of organized crime, which includes drugs and arms trafficking (United Nations Office on Drugs and Crime, 2014).
- To be labeled as human trafficking, US guidelines provide that the behavior must contain at least one of the following components, which are defined below (U.S. Department of Health and Human Services, 2012a):

- Force can involve the use of physical restraint or serious physical harm. Physical violence, including rape, beatings, and physical confinement, is often employed as a means to control victims, especially during the early stages of victimization, when the trafficker breaks down the victim's resistance.
- Fraud involves false promises regarding employment, wages, working conditions, or other matters. For example, individuals might travel to another country under the promise of well-paying work at a farm or factory only to find themselves manipulated into forced labor. Others might reply to advertisements promising modeling, nanny, or service industry jobs overseas, but be forced into prostitution once they arrive at their destination.
- Coercion can involve threats of serious harm or physical restraint against any person; any scheme, plan, or pattern intended to cause a person to believe that failure to perform an act would result in serious harm or physical restraint against any person; or the abuse or threatened abuse of the legal process.

Types of Human Trafficking and Definitions

Typically, human trafficking falls into two broad categories: sex trafficking and labor trafficking. However, other categories may include organ trafficking and child trafficking.

- Sex trafficking can have several variations and terms:
  - Sex trafficking is defined as "the recruitment, harboring, transportation, provision, or obtaining of a person for the purpose of a commercial sex act." Such an act is considered severe when the victim is under the age of 18 and when force, fraud, or coercion are involved (U.S. Congress, 2000).
  - The terms prostitution and/or commercial sexual exploitation (CSE) are also used when referring to sex trafficking. When CSE involves children, it is referred to as the commercial sexual exploitation of children (CSEC). If the victims are domestic and minors, the phenomenon is referred to as domestic minor sex trafficking (DMST).
  - Closely related to sex trafficking is sex tourism whereby mostly adult males, although female sex tourists exist as well, travel to other countries for the purpose of engaging in sexual activities with children. Many sex tourists are American citizens. Popular sex tourism destinations include Cambodia, Thailand, the Dominican Republic, and Brazil (Bender & Furman, 2004; de Chesnay, 2012; Malarek, 2011; Ward, 2010).
- Labor trafficking is defined as the "recruitment, harboring, transportation, provision, or obtaining of a person for labor or services, through the use of force, fraud or coercion for the purpose of subjection to involuntary servitude, peonage, debt bondage, or slavery" (U.S. Congress, 2000; U.S. Department of Health and Human Services, 2012b.)
- Debt bondage occurs when someone is being forced to work against his or her will, hence, trafficked. In such a case, traffickers demand labor of some form as a means of paying back either a real or alleged debt, which grows increasingly larger as the victim's wages are not appropriately applied to pay down the debt. Victims are continuously charged excessive fees for such items as clothing, housing, food, and transportation, with various fines added to the debt for different reasons. Essentially, the "debt" can become so large that it could never be repaid and the victim is trapped. Debt bondage can be found in both labor and sex trafficking (U.S. Department of Health and Human Services, 2012a, 2012b).
- Organ trafficking occurs when someone is forced or deceived into relinquishing an organ to traffickers, agrees to sell an organ but does not receive any money or less than what was agreed-upon or what the organ would be worth on the fair market, or unknowingly has an organ removed while undergoing a procedure for another health issue. Commonly harvested organs include the liver and kidneys (United Nations Office on Drugs and Crime, 2014).
- Child soldiering involves forcing children into armed combat. According to the Paris Principles (UNICEF, 2007), the internationally agreed-upon definition for a child associated with an armed force or armed group is any person under 18 years of age who is, or who has been, recruited or used by an armed force or armed group in any capacity, including but not limited

to children, boys and girls, who are used as fighters, cooks, porters, messengers, spies, or for sexual purposes. The term does not refer only to a child who is taking or has taken a direct part in hostilities (Child Soldiers International, 2014; UNICEF, 2007).

Where, Who, and How Many

- No country is immune to human trafficking; it occurs in any or all its forms in every country (U.S. Department of State, 2014).
- A given country can be considered as a source, transit, and/or destination country, or any combination thereof (U.S. Department of State, 2014).
- Precise numbers of victims are difficult to ascertain. Estimates on the number of victims range from 600,000 to 800,000 to 27 million globally every year (U.S. Department of State, 2007).
- An estimate of people trafficked within the United States ranges from 14,500 to 17,500 persons (U.S. Department of State, 2004).
- Within the United States, labor trafficking is the most prevalent form of trafficking of foreign nationals (U.S. Department of State, 2011).
- Within the United States, sex trafficking is the most prevalent form of trafficking of American citizens (U.S. Department of State, 2011).
- The majority of sex trafficking victims globally are women and children (U.S. Department of State, 2007, 2010).
- Between 40% and 50% of human trafficking victims are children (International Labour Conference, 2005) with some estimates for children trafficked into the United States internationally at greater than 50% (Center for Problem-Oriented Policing, n.d.).
- Victims of sex trafficking can be found working in brothels, the pornography industry, strip clubs, escort agencies, massage parlors, truck stops, and prostitution rings.
- Sex trafficking victims who are school-aged often can and do attend school on a regular basis and often look no different from their classmates (Flores, 2010; Smith, 2014).
- The United States has seen a recent increase in gang involvement in domestic minor sex trafficking whereby, aside from dealing in drugs, gangs recruit young girls into prostitution (Kashino, 2013; Lederer, 2011).
- Labor trafficking victims can be found working in restaurants, factories, as domestic servants or nannies in private homes, on farms, in nail salons, and in construction.
- For traffickers, human trafficking can be a lucrative endeavor. A low risk of being caught and prosecuted exists and the profit margin is quite high in most cases.
- Trafficking victims include individuals of all ages, genders, nationalities, races, and educational and socioeconomic backgrounds.
- Those most vulnerable to being trafficked tend to be young, poor, powerless, and have no health problems (de Chesnay, 2012).
- The 2011 *Trafficking in Persons Report* has identified that within the United States, US citizens are more often exploited for sexual purposes than for forced labor, and that foreign workers are more often exploited for labor purposes than for sexually exploitative purposes (U.S. Department of State, 2011).
- Internationally trafficked victims in the United States come from all over the world, including Africa, Asia, India, Central America, South America, Russia, and Eastern Europe (Center for Problem-Oriented Policing, n.d.). It is estimated that about 1,500 to 2,200 people are trafficked from other countries into Canada before reaching the United States (UNICEF-Canada, 2014); likewise, victims are trafficked from Mexico into the United States (Ditmore, Maternick, & Zapert, 2012).
- Aside from internationally trafficked victims, any given country also has domestic victims, those who are born and raised in the country where they are trafficked. In the United States, a majority of domestic victims are reportedly children involved in sex trafficking, which is referred to as domestic minor sex trafficking (DMST) (U.S. Department of State, 2010).

INTERSECTING SYSTEMS AND SERVICES

Human trafficking involves a number of different players, facilitators, and disciplines. Numerous systems are involved in the investigation and prosecution of human trafficking cases and of those who traffick, as well as providing support and services to those who have been trafficked. It is not unusual for systems and services to overlap, particularly when the focus is on working with victims to remove them from harm's way, to prosecute their traffickers, and to provide them with a variety of services to help in their recovery and healing. For example, after removing a victim from his or her trafficking situation, law enforcement personnel may contact healthcare providers to continue to examine the individual to ensure his or her safety and well-being, and both disciplines may begin the task of collecting evidence to be used by the courts to prosecute the alleged traffickers. In general, a team effort exists among many individuals and disciplines.

Systems and Services

- Local law enforcement agencies are often the first to be involved in cases of suspected trafficking. Their role is to collect evidence, determine if the case involves human trafficking, and distinguish between victim and victimizer.
- The criminal justice system, including the courts and lawyers, are involved in prosecuting suspected traffickers and sentencing them and/or defending trafficking victims.
- Correctional and forensic institutions are where those convicted of trafficking are often sent to serve out their time. Unfortunately, victims who are misidentified may also be incarcerated.
- The Federal Bureau of Investigation (FBI) or other international law enforcement agencies, such as the International Criminal Police Organization (INTERPOL), the Canadian Border Service, or the Royal Canadian Mounted Police, may become involved in cases, especially those involving trafficking of minors or cases crossing state or international borders.
- Local, state, provincial, national, and federal government agencies are often involved in developing policy and laws and in funding resources related to human trafficking prosecution and victim services, respectively.
- Child protective agencies may be called in to provide protection, shelter, and services for minors who have been trafficked until such time that they can be turned over to appropriate family members or sanctioned guardians.
- The US Immigration and Customs Enforcement (ICE) agency investigates cases of alleged human trafficking.
- The US Department of Homeland Security (DHS) is responsible for investigating human trafficking, arresting traffickers, and protecting victims.
- Medical and healthcare agencies and professionals provide medical care to trafficking victims and, in some cases, collect evidence.
- Behavioral healthcare agencies and professionals provide mental health services to those who have been trafficked.
- Shelters and community programs offer residential treatment for victims, especially for unattended minors who are brought into the United States from other countries and have no family in the United States.
- Interpreters are called in when traffickers or victims do not speak English.
- Victim advocate agencies provide advocates to help victims through the legal process, especially if a victim is to testify against his or her traffickers, and help the victim to access services for which he or she may be eligible.
- The US Congress has been involved in the fight against human trafficking. In 2000, Congress passed the bipartisan Trafficking Victims Protection Act (TVPA), which President Clinton signed in October (U.S. Congress, 2000). The TVPA 2000 was created to ensure that traffickers would be justly and effectively punished and that victims would be protected. The three main components focus on prevention, protection, and punishment. The TVPA has been reauthorized in

2003, 2005, 2008, and 2013, with each reauthorization targeting different aspects of human trafficking and adding provisions to expand its reach (ATEST, 2014).

- The 2013 Trafficking Victims Protection Reauthorization Act (TVPRA) includes the following provisions (ATEST, 2014; U.S. Congress, 2013):
  - Provides invaluable resources to support holistic services for survivors and to enable law enforcement agencies to investigate cases, hold perpetrators accountable, and prevent slavery from happening in the first place.
  - Prevents US foreign aid from going to countries that use child soldiers.
  - Penalizes the confiscation of identity documents, a prevalent form of coercion that traffickers use to exploit victims.
  - Creates a grant-making program to respond to humanitarian emergencies that result in an increased risk of trafficking, such as the situation in Haiti after the 2010 earthquake when children's vulnerability to re-trafficking escalated sharply.
  - Authorizes the Office to Monitor and Combat Trafficking in Persons (J/Tip office) to form local partnerships in focus countries to combat child trafficking through Child Protection Compacts.
  - Enhances law enforcement's capacity to combat sex tourism by extending jurisdiction under the 2003 PROTECT Act to prosecute US citizens living abroad who commercially sexually exploit children.
- Many other countries, such as Canada and Mexico, have developed laws and policies to prevent human trafficking, protect victims, and prosecute offenders. In 2002, Canada enacted a law aimed specifically at human trafficking; a number of amendments to the Criminal Code of Canada have since followed. In Mexico, early anti-trafficking provisions were directed at child trafficking. In 2007, however, the country adopted a law which criminalizes all aspects of human trafficking (Cawley, 2014; Mexico, 2014; Public Safety Canada, 2014; United Nations Office on Drugs and Crime, 2014).

Table 6B.1 lists resources and organizations that provide information and services to victims and information to those who seek to learn more about human trafficking.

TABLE 6B.1 Resources

Amnesty International
Stop Violence Against Women
www.amnestyusa.org/violence-against-women/end-human-trafficking/organizations-working-to-stop-human-trafficking/page.do?id = 1108431
Information on human trafficking, including an extensive list of organizations working to stop it

Catholic Charities Community Services
Developing Individual Growth and New Independence Through Yourself (DIGNITY)
www.catholiccharitiesaz.org/catholiccharities/dignity.aspx
Assistance to victims of sex trafficking in Arizona

Children of the Night
www.childrenofthenight.org
Founded by Dr. Lois Lee
Assistance to American children involved in prostitution

Coalition Against Trafficking in Women
www.catwinternational.org
Assistance to women who are victims of sex trafficking worldwide

Dawn's Place
http://ahomefordawn.org/index.php
A residential program in Philadelphia that supports women who are trafficked and prostituted

(continued)

TABLE 6B.1 Resources (continued)

Free the Slaves
www.freetheslaves.net
Resources and targeted actions aimed at combating all forms of trafficking worldwide

GEMS
Girls Educational and Mentoring Services
www.gems-girls.org
A program in New York that helps girls and young women aged 12 to 24 who have been sexually trafficked

Humantrafficking.org
www.humantrafficking.org
Country-specific information on national laws and government agencies, as well as nongovernmental organizations

International Justice Mission
www.ijm.org
Legal investigation and representation for victims of human trafficking

Not For Sale
www.notforsalecampaign.org
Campaign to stop global slave trade and end human trafficking

Polaris Project
www.polarisproject.org
Information on national and local programs; operates the National Human Trafficking Resource Center hotline (1–888–3737–888) (often aligned in this manner to make the number easier to remember)/text message: "BeFree" at 233733

Prevent Human Trafficking
http://preventhumantrafficking.org/16zr2l1ijdwbdlnwmimtzsdn11rs70
Offers a variety of solutions and programs to help combat and prevent human trafficking

Prostitution Research and Education
www.prostitutionresearch.com
Conducts research on prostitution, pornography, and trafficking; offers education and consultation to researchers, survivors, the public, and policymakers

Salvation Army International
Combating Human Trafficking
www.salvationarmyusa.org/usn/www_usn_2.nsf/vw-text-dynamic-arrays/8081A4079639D55A802573E00 0530965?openDocument
Program to oppose and prevent sexual trafficking in women and children worldwide

Shared Hope International
www.sharedhope.org
Focuses on preventing conditions that foster sex trafficking, restoring victims of sex slavery, and bringing justice to vulnerable women and children

Stop the Traffik
www.stopthetraffik.org
International efforts to end trafficking; site provides information in several languages

U.S. Department of Health and Human Services
Administration for Children and Families Campaign to Rescue and Restore Victims of Human Trafficking
www.acf.hhs.gov/trafficking
Various resources, including toolkits for healthcare providers

POPULATIONS AT RISK

- Theoretically, anyone could become a trafficking victim. Victims, whether they are international or domestic, can be fraudulently deceived into being trafficked with false promises of a good job, a better life, or a chance to receive an education, make good money, or be a model. Unfortunately, once they agree to take advantage of such opportunities, they find that they are now far from home and that nanny job they were promised turns out never to have existed. Instead, they are forced into something far worse.
- Parents may entrust a child to someone who promises that the child will be well cared for and have a better life and education elsewhere, never suspecting that the child will be sold into slavery once out of the parents' reach (Aronowitz, 2009; Grumiau, 2012; ILO, 2009; International Federation of Social Workers, 2014; Skinner, 2008).
- Aside from fraud, it is not uncommon for victims to be forced into human trafficking through physical means, such as kidnapping, physical assault, or restraint. At times, victims are threatened with bodily harm to themselves, their loved ones, and/or family members if they do not do what they are told (United Nations Office on Drugs and Crime, 2009; U.S. Department of Health and Human Services, n.d., 2012a).
- A number of social, environmental, and/or personal factors place people at risk, including living in an area or a society where the following conditions exist or occur (Batstone, 2007; Polaris Project, 2014a; Sabella, 2011).

Environmental and Social Factors

- Civil and political unrest
- Armed conflicts
- Poverty
- Lack of employment opportunities
- Lack of education
- Lack of marketable job skills
- A rapid increase in population growth
- Rapid industrialization
- High demand for cheap goods
- High demand for sex
- Naval and military bases
- Large-scale sporting events
- Large-scale conventions, conferences, and concerts
- The subordination of women and girls
- A government's lack of support of human rights
- Natural disasters, such as earthquakes or tsunamis

Personal Factors

- Being in foster care
- Being a runaway
- Coming from a dysfunctional family
- Having a parent who is incarcerated or addicted
- Having a history of sexual abuse
- Being a member of an oppressed or marginalized group
- Being undocumented
- Not having a birth certificate
- Having an addiction
- Paying off a debt incurred by a family member; debt bondage

PRACTICE AND PREVENTION

- Nurses can and do play an important role both in detecting possible cases of human trafficking as well as in treating victims of human trafficking. In addition, at times they may collect evidence in cases of sexual and/or physical assault and abuse to help support a possible conviction of traffickers.
- Although nurses working in any healthcare arena may encounter possible victims, nurses who work in emergency departments (EDs), correctional facilities, and schools likely will encounter possible victims. Regardless of the setting in which a nurse works, he or she should be well-informed about human trafficking. Once well-informed, the nurse is prepared to move forward with practice involving first, knowing how to identify a possible human trafficking victim, and second, how to treat and care for the individual who is now a patient.

Identifying Possible Victims

- A number of signs may signal that an individual is being trafficked. A nurse's primary duty is to provide health care that is related to what prompts the patient to seek care. Aside from a patient's healthcare needs, however, the patient could also be a victim of human trafficking. By being alert to this possibility, the nurse could help save someone's life or at the very least remove the person from an untenable situation and provide information for law enforcement officers to bring the possible traffickers to justice.
- Nurses are not law enforcement officers and should never assume the role of interrogator or law enforcement authorities. The importance of being able to identify possible victims is to forward any suspicions to the appropriate personnel and agencies. It is important to note that the signs provided below may have other explanations beside human trafficking. It is up to law enforcement officers to make that determination.
- According to the United Nations Office on Drugs and Crime (2008, 2014), victims may exhibit a number of clues suggesting the possibility of human trafficking. Some general indicators are that these persons:
  - Believe that they must work against their will
  - Are unable to leave their work environment
  - Show signs that their movements are being controlled
  - Feel that they cannot leave
  - Show fear or anxiety
  - Are subjected to violence or threats of violence against themselves or their family members and loved ones
  - Suffer injuries that appear to be the result of an assault
  - Suffer injuries or impairments that are typical of certain jobs or control measures
  - Suffer injuries that appear to be the result of the application of control measures
  - Are distrustful of authorities
  - Are afraid of revealing their immigration status
  - Are not in possession of their passports or other travel or identity documents, as those documents are being held by someone else, usually the trafficker, as a means of control over the victim's movement and ability to move freely
  - Have false identity or travel documents
  - Are found in or connected to a type of location likely to be associated with exploiting people
  - Are unfamiliar with the local language
  - Do not know their home or work address
  - Allow others to speak for them when addressed directly in their primary language
  - Act as if they were instructed by someone else
  - Are forced to work under certain conditions
  - Are disciplined through punishment
  - Are unable to negotiate working conditions

- Receive little or no payment for the work they do
- Have no access to their earnings
- Work excessively long hours over long periods with no days off
- Live in poor or substandard accommodations
- Have no access to medical care
- Have limited contact with their families or with people outside their immediate environment
- Are unable to communicate freely with others
- Perceive that they are bonded by debt
- Are in a situation of dependence
- Come from a place that is known to be a source of human trafficking
- Some trafficking victims, often minors who are commercially sexually exploited, may present with some of the following (United Nations Office on Drugs and Crime, 2008, 2014):
  - Unexplained and frequent absences from school
  - Unduly tired when at school
  - Sporting new clothes, jewelry, and electronics, although the student has no job
  - Decline in grades and enjoyment of prior activities
  - Relationships with people, especially men, considerably older than he or she is
  - Tattoos, which may indicate belonging to someone
  - Suspicion of drug abuse where none existed before
  - Increased time away from home spent with "friends," often at the mall or other places
  - Increased time spent on the phone, Facebook, and/or the computer
  - Change in dress to a more revealing style of clothing
  - Change in mood
- In addition, the United Nations Office on Drugs and Crime (2008, 2014) suggests that some possible indicators are unique for sex or labor trafficking, regardless of age. For those who have been sexually trafficked, possible indicators include that these persons:
  - Are of any age, although the age may vary according to the location and the market
  - Move from one brothel to the next or work in various locations
  - Are escorted when they travel to and from work and other outside activities
  - Have tattoos or other marks indicating "ownership" or branding by their exploiters
  - Work long hours or have few days off, if any
  - Sleep where they work
  - Live or travel in a group, sometimes with other people who do not speak the same language
  - Possess few items of clothing
  - Have clothes that are typically worn for performing sex work
  - Only know sex-related words in the local language or in the language of the client group
  - Have no cash of their own
  - Are unable to show an identity document
- For those who have been trafficked for labor, possible indicators include that these individuals:
  - Live in groups in the same place where they work and leave those premises infrequently, if at all
  - Live in degraded, unsuitable places, such as in agricultural or industrial buildings
  - Are not dressed adequately for the work they do; for example, they may lack protective equipment or warm clothing
  - Receive only leftovers to eat
  - Have no access to their earnings
  - Have no labor contract
  - Work excessively long hours
  - Depend on their employer for a number of services, including work, transportation, and accommodation
  - Have no choice of accommodation
  - Never leave the work premises without their employer

- Are unable to move freely
- Are subject to security measures designed to keep them on the work premises
- Are disciplined through fines
- Are subjected to insults, abuse, threats, or violence
- Lack basic training and professional licenses
- Notices are posted in languages other than the local language
- Absence of workplace health and safety notices, and limited or no access to healthcare providers or services
- Employer or manager is unable to show the documents required for employing workers from other countries
- Employer or manager is unable to show records of wages paid to workers
- Health and safety equipment is of poor quality or absent
- Equipment is designed or has been modified so that children can operate it
- Evidence exists that labor laws are being breached
- Evidence suggests that workers must pay for tools, food, or accommodation or that those costs are being deducted from their wages
- Children are also exploited in numerous ways. The United Nations Office on Drugs and Crime (2008, 2014) lists the following as possible indicators of child labor trafficking related to begging and criminal activity. These children:
  - Tend to beg in public places and on public transportation
  - Carry and/or sell illicit drugs
  - Have physical impairments that appear to be the result of mutilation
  - Are of the same nationality or ethnicity and move in large groups with only a few adults
  - Are unaccompanied minors who have been "found" by an adult of the same nationality or ethnicity
  - Move in groups while travelling on public transportation; for example, they may walk up and down the length of trains
  - Participate in the activities of organized criminal gangs
  - Are a part of large groups of children who have the same adult guardian
  - Are punished if they do not collect or steal enough
  - Live with members of their gang
  - Travel with members of their gang to the country of destination
  - Live as gang members with adults who are not their parents
  - Move daily in large groups and over considerable distances
- The following might also indicate that people have been trafficked for begging or for committing petty crimes:
  - New forms of gang-related crime appear in a locale or region
  - Evidence suggests that the group of suspected victims has moved over a period of time through a number of countries
  - Evidence suggests that suspected victims have been involved in begging or in committing petty crimes in another country
- General indicators in a healthcare setting:
  - Nurses in many areas of nursing may encounter victims. Nurses in the ED may interface with victims, but nurses in any setting should be aware that the following could signal human trafficking (United Nations Office on Drugs and Crime, 2008, 2014):
    - The individual is not allowed to speak for him/herself and is accompanied by someone who dominates the interactions.
    - The person accompanying the individual refuses to leave the person alone with the healthcare staff.
    - The individual may defer to the person accompanying him or her.
    - The individual is accompanied by a man or woman who is much older.
    - The individual appears nervous, anxious, and afraid.

- The individual exhibits evidence of self-mutilation or branding.
- The individual is not properly dressed for the weather or dressed in a provocative style.
- The information provided seems suspicious and/or inconsistent.
- Aside from the above, a number of physical, medical, and behavioral signs and injuries could indicate that someone has been trafficked (de Chesnay & Greenbaum, 2013; Sabella, 2011, 2013; Taylor & Blake, 2013, U.S. Department of Health and Human Services, n.d.):
  - Sex trafficking:
    - Genital injuries, such as vaginal and rectal tears, abrasions, swelling, and lacerations
    - Urinary tract infections
    - Evidence of sexual assault with a foreign object
    - Vaginal fistulas, lacerations, and perforations
    - Venereal and sexually transmitted infections, including trichomoniasis; hepatitis A, B, and C; syphilis; gonorrhea; human papillomavirus (HPV); genital herpes; chlamydia; human immunodeficiency virus (HIV); acquired immunodeficiency syndrome (AIDS); and pelvic inflammatory disease (PID)
    - Evidence of repeated abortions
    - Injuries such as broken bones, missing teeth, sprains and bruises, stab wounds, and burns related to being beaten and/or tortured
    - Bite marks
    - Hearing loss from being beaten about the head
    - Temporal mandibular joint disease from providing oral sex
    - Dermatological problems, such as scabies, lice, rashes, and various infections
    - Gunshot wounds
    - Tattoos and brandings that indicate being the property of the pimp or trafficker
    - Bald spots related to hair being pulled
    - Backaches related to wearing high heels
    - Dental problems
    - Indications of addiction, such as track marks
    - Gastrointestinal and nutritional problems, and eating disorders
    - Headaches
    - Respiratory infections, including pneumonia
    - Anxiety
    - Depression and suicide attempts
    - Difficulty sleeping
    - Posttraumatic stress disorder (PTSD)
  - Labor trafficking (U.S. Department of Health & Human Services, 2012b):
    - Various physical problems, such as chronic back pain, muscle strains, and sprains
    - Cardiovascular problems
    - Respiratory conditions
    - Visual problems
    - Malnutrition
    - Dehydration
    - Exhaustion
    - Communicable diseases, such as scabies and tuberculosis
    - Poor personal hygiene
    - Stunted growth in children and failure to thrive
    - Psychological problems, such as anxiety, depression, and PTSD
- Practice
  - Human trafficking victims may have no or limited access to healthcare services for a number of reasons. On their own, they may not know how to access services, may experience financial and linguistic obstacles in procuring care, or may fear any contact with authority figures due to mistrust based on past experiences or what their traffickers have told them

about authorities of any kind. In addition, if traffickers are involved, they may minimize the individual's problem, not wish to spend money on the individual, and choose not to risk presenting for care and coming under suspicion. A nurse's first priority in working with either a suspected or known victim of human trafficking is to ensure that the patient is safe and to address whatever healthcare and medical issues he or she has. Although each case and situation is different, the following are general guidelines on what to do and how to work with a patient who is suspected or known to be a victim:

- The individual should be separated from the person who brought the individual to the healthcare setting. A victim is unlikely to report being trafficked when the trafficker is present. Some agencies have policies that patients are to be questioned alone. If the facility lacks such a policy, the nurse is encouraged to think of a reason to take the suspected victim elsewhere, such as to the restroom, to question him or her alone.

- If trafficking is suspected and the victim's primary language differs from the care provider, the person who brought the patient to the facility should not serve as an interpreter. The nurse should arrange for a professional interpreter or, if necessary, work with an interpreter by phone. The interpreter must speak the same language and dialect as the victim.

- The nurse should try to develop a rapport with the individual, but recognize that the patient may be reluctant to disclose. Although the nurse is a healthcare professional, he or she is a stranger to the person who may have been deceived in the past and has no reason to trust anyone. Perhaps the first and most important question for the nurse to ask is whether the person feels safe speaking to the nurse at that moment.

- The nurse must maintain confidentiality at all times.

- The nurse should refrain from asking the suspected victim whether he or she is being trafficked. Many victims, both domestic and international, are unfamiliar with that term. Instead, below are some key questions the nurse may ask to assess and screen for possible trafficking (U.S. Department of State, 2009), keeping in mind that he or she is conducting an assessment, not an interrogation:
  - Where are you from?
  - What brings you here?
  - Where do you live now?
  - What city are we in?
  - What type of work do you do?
  - Are you getting paid? Is anything taken out of your pay?
  - Can you leave your job if you want to?
  - Can you come and go as you please? Are you afraid to leave? Why?
  - Have you or your family been threatened?
  - What are your working and living conditions like? How are you treated?
  - Do you have to ask permission to eat/sleep/go to the bathroom?
  - Are there locks on your doors/windows so you cannot get out?
  - Has your identification or documentation been taken from you?
  - Would you like some help?
    - The nurse should never ask a suspected or known victim for details about the trafficking experience, the traffickers' identity, or about what is being done about him or her. That line of questioning usually falls to law enforcement officials.
    - If the nurse suspects trafficking, it is recommended that he or she notify hospital security or the appropriate personnel as per hospital or agency policy. It is not the nurse's role to determine that this is a case of human trafficking.
    - Unless the law in that area or jurisdiction states otherwise, an adult victim who does not want to acknowledge that he or she is being trafficked or to press charges has the right to refuse help.
    - A person who is being trafficked cannot be forced to report it and press charges. As with intimate partner violence, reporting may confound the situation and further endanger the victim.

- If the suspected or known victim is a minor, the nurse must report the case to a law enforcement agency or child protective services in accordance with mandatory reporting policies.
- The nurse is advised to never directly confront a suspected or known trafficker, but instead, report that information to law enforcement officials.
- The nurse should have small, palm-size cards with information in several languages about human trafficking, including the national hotline number and local numbers, which a suspected victim can easily take and hide.
- Posters should be displayed, especially in women's bathrooms. These posters can contain resources and contact information, such as, in the United States, the National Human Trafficking Resource Center (NHTRC) hotline number. Both those who suspect human trafficking and victims in the United States may call this number to access help. Healthcare providers in other countries with similar hotline numbers can post them as appropriate and needed.
- If the country or jurisdiction offers access to help through other means, the posters should also state this information. For instance, in the United States, both victims and those who suspect human trafficking can access help via the text message: "BeFree." The same can be done in other countries if this option exists.
- The nurse should understand if the suspected or known victim refuses to speak or share information. Many victims experience high levels of trauma and may be reluctant to trust or fear consequences if they do so.
- If necessary and appropriate, and with the patient's permission, the nurse may collect an evidence kit, obtain photographic imaging, document injuries, and turn this information over to law enforcement officials to help build a case against those suspected of trafficking.
- Cultural factors need to be considered, particularly when working with patients from other countries and cultures.
- The nurse's demeanor should convey patience and a nonjudgmental attitude, and never reveal shock, horror, or dismay when working with a suspected or known victim.
- Nurses may assess for human trafficking, but protective services and law enforcement officers are responsible for providing additional care for victims and for prosecuting perpetrators.
- Although nurses are charged with treating healthcare problems with which victims present, only professionals who are appropriately trained in interviewing victims as well as providing mental health services should be charged with those duties.
- Prevention
  - One of the most vexing aspects of human trafficking is prevention. Just as slavery continued to exist in many parts of the United States after Lincoln signed the Emancipation Proclamation, no law, policy, or public reaction is likely to stop or completely eradicate human trafficking. Internationally, human trafficking is a complex and multilayered phenomenon with numerous causes, many of which are difficult to address and treat.
  - Primary prevention, which is optimal and sorely needed, is difficult to attain. However, secondary and tertiary prevention measures exist and include efforts to:
    - Educate parents, teachers, and students about human trafficking—what it is, what it looks like, and the warning signs that indicate one is being groomed to be trafficked
    - Educate teachers, parents, and the public about risk factors for human trafficking
    - Provide education and increase public awareness about the connection between the Internet and human trafficking
    - Post information in hotels, malls, schools, public restrooms, public transportation, and sporting stadiums about human trafficking
    - Research companies to learn whether the products they sell and buy are only from those that provide decent wages and treatment to their employees
    - Promote positive images of women and girls in the community so they are valued as other than objects of sexual pleasure
    - Encourage local media to provide free public service announcements about human trafficking and the national hotline number

- Talk to family members and friends about not buying or paying for sex
- Find an organization that works with people in the community providing education, training, and support to those at risk of being trafficked and donate money to help that entity continue its work

CONCEPTS AND ISSUES

- Driving factors: Human trafficking is indeed a form of slavery where people, the goods they make, and/or the services they provide are the product. It is a product that the world not only wants, but demands at the cheapest cost possible. The concepts and motivations that underlie this phenomenon consist of the trifecta of the seller, the product, and the buyer.
  - For traffickers, the motivation is the opportunity to make a large profit with a low risk of deterrence. Even if apprehended, traffickers are not easily prosecuted. Traffickers are also motivated by:
    - The need to survive and earn a living
    - The need to control others and be in power
    - Modeling: Having been raised in a household where a parent or adult was a pimp or a trafficker
    - The opportunity to no longer be a victim by becoming a trafficker and helping to recruit new victims
  - For victims, several routes and motivations exist for being trafficked:
    - Coming from a poverty-stricken background and needing to survive
    - Hope and desire for a better life and opportunity elsewhere
    - False promise of a romantic relationship or marriage proposal that becomes a bondage situation
    - Being a runaway
    - Being sold into either sex or labor trafficking by parents, husbands, or boyfriends
    - Being given away by parents who were led to believe that the child would be cared for
    - As repayment for a family debt
    - Being raised in a household where other family members were involved in prostitution
    - Coming from a culture where women and girls are powerless and have no voice
    - Coming from a location or country that benefits from human trafficking, such as areas where sex tourism is high
    - Victims are often recruited through:
      - A friend or loved one
      - False advertisements for modeling or other forms of employment, such as domestic work (e.g., nannies, maids), construction work, or food service
      - Dating and marriage agencies
  - For consumers, the motivation is the opportunity to employ cheap labor, purchase products as inexpensively as possible, and/or consume various legal and illegal services.
- Characteristics:
  - Human trafficking is a universal occurrence.
  - Trafficking often goes undetected because victims can be isolated, drugged, threatened, and beaten.
  - Actual numbers of victims and types of human trafficking victims are difficult to ascertain and many of the numbers cited regarding victims are outdated and of questionable validity. In addition, a lack of evidenced-based and high-quality research exists to support a number of claims made related to human trafficking, which many regard as problematic (Weitzer, 2014).
  - Although many places worldwide have laws against human trafficking, the laws vary and the definitions and elements of human trafficking can widely differ, creating confusion (Heinrich & Sreeharsha, 2013).
  - Human trafficking is a covert and dangerous business that is often sanctioned by and involves those in authority who choose to ignore it for financial gain or personal benefit.

- Cases of human trafficking are often difficult to prosecute because of a lack of evidence, including the reluctance of victims to come forward to testify against their traffickers for fear of reprisal to themselves and/or their loved ones.
- One study showed that human trafficking is rarely prosecuted in the United States, despite the proliferation of laws (Farrell, McDevitt, Pfeffer, Fahy, Owens, Dank, & Adams, 2012). The study also found:
  - Labor trafficking is often ignored as the focus is heavily on sex trafficking.
  - State laws differ not only in how they define human trafficking, but also how each state should respond to the problem.
  - Local criminal justice officials tend not to be informed about human trafficking and have limited experience investigating cases of human trafficking.
  - There exists a lack of properly prepared and specialized interviewers to gather evidence and statements from victims.
- Most interventions occur at the secondary or tertiary level and consist of working with someone after he or she has been victimized. Although human trafficking is unlikely ever to cease, much more can and should be done at the primary level to prevent human trafficking and lessen its occurrence.
- Few residential treatment programs exist for adult victims, and even fewer for minor victims.

FUTURE ISSUES

Why Does Demand Thrive?

- According to the Polaris Project (2014b), labor trafficking and sex trafficking of US citizens and foreign nationals persist and thrive for a number of reasons, including:
  - Low risk: When the community is unaware of the issue, when government and community institutions are not trained to respond, when ineffective or dormant laws exist to address the crime, when safety nets for victims do not exist, and when law enforcement does not investigate and prosecute the crime, human traffickers perceive little risk or deterrence to affect their criminal operations.
  - High profits: When individuals are willing to buy commercial sex, they create a market and make it profitable for traffickers to sexually exploit children and adults. When consumers are willing to buy goods and services from industries that rely on forced labor, they create a profit incentive for labor traffickers to maximize revenue with minimal production costs.
- Although these reasons explain its continued presence, it is important to address what can be done to prevent and combat human trafficking and what can be done to lessen the number of cases that occur globally every day. Watching a movie or attending a lecture about human trafficking is a positive step in increasing awareness, but it does not stop human trafficking from occurring. The US Department of State (n.d.) offers 20 ways the public can help fight human trafficking, as provided in Table 6B.2.
- Aside from these suggestions, a nurse can:
  - Become educated about human trafficking and share this knowledge with colleagues, family, and friends. Table 6B.3 provides a list of recommended readings and links to websites for healthcare professionals who want to learn more about the issue and what they can do.
  - Speak to employers and agencies about developing policies in the workplace for treating and dealing with suspected or known victims.
  - Request that continuing nursing education contact hours be offered for trainings on human trafficking.
  - Lobby academic programs to include courses or training about human trafficking for students at both the graduate and undergraduate levels.
  - Provide training to school and camp nurses and all nurses who work with children and adolescents to be able to recognize the signs that a child is being trafficked.

TABLE 6B.2 Twenty Ways to Fight Human Trafficking

1. Learn the red flags that may indicate human trafficking and ask followup questions so you can help identify a potential trafficking victim. Human trafficking awareness training is available for individuals, businesses, first responders, law enforcement, and federal employees.
2. In the United States, call the National Human Trafficking Resource Center at 1–888–373–7888 (24/7) to get help and connect with a service provider in your area; report a tip with information on potential human trafficking activity; or learn more by requesting training, technical assistance, or resources. Call federal law enforcement directly to report suspicious activity and get help from the Department of Homeland Security at 1–866–347–2423 (24/7), or submit a tip online at www.ice.gov/tips, or from the U.S. Department of Justice at 1–888–428–7581 from 9:00 am to 5:00 pm (EST). Victims, including undocumented individuals, are eligible for services and immigration assistance.
3. Be a conscientious consumer. Discover your Slavery Footprint, and check out the Department of Labor's List of Goods Produced by Child Labor or Forced Labor. Encourage companies, including your own, to take steps to investigate and eliminate slavery and human trafficking in their supply chains and to publish the information for consumer awareness.
4. Incorporate human trafficking information in your professional associations' conferences, trainings, manuals, and other materials as relevant example.
5. Join or start a grassroots anti-trafficking coalition.
6. Meet with and/or write to your local, state, and federal government representatives to let them know that you care about combating human trafficking in your community, and ask what they are doing to address human trafficking in your area.
7. Distribute public awareness materials available from the Department of Health and Human Services or the Department of Homeland Security.
8. Volunteer to perform victim outreach or offer your professional services to a local anti-trafficking organization.
9. Donate funds or needed items to an anti-trafficking organization in your area.
10. Organize a fundraiser and donate the proceeds to an anti-trafficking organization.
11. Host an awareness event to watch and discuss a recent human trafficking documentary. On a larger scale, host a human trafficking film festival.
12. Encourage your local schools to partner with students and include the issue of modern day slavery in their curriculum. As a parent, educator, or school administrator, be aware of how traffickers target school-aged children.
13. Set up a Google alert to receive current human trafficking news.
14. Write a letter to the editor of your local paper about human trafficking in your community.
15. Start or sign a human trafficking petition.
16. Businesses: Provide internships, job skills training, and/or jobs to survivors of human trafficking. Consumers: Purchase items made by survivors of trafficking, such as from Jewel Girls or Made by Survivors.
17. Students: Take action on your campus. Join or establish a university or secondary school club to raise awareness about human trafficking and initiate action throughout your local community. Consider writing a research paper on a topic concerning human trafficking. Professors: Request that human trafficking be an issue that is included in the academic curriculum. Increase scholarship about human trafficking by publishing an article, teaching a class, or hosting a symposium.
18. Law Enforcement Officials: Join or start a local human trafficking task force.
19. Mental Health or Medical Providers: Extend low-cost or free services to victims of human trafficking assisted by nearby anti-trafficking organizations. Train your staff how to identify the indicators of human trafficking and help victims.
20. Attorneys: Look for signs of human trafficking among your clients. Offer pro bono services to trafficking victims or anti-trafficking organizations. Learn about and offer human trafficking victims the legal benefits for which they are eligible. Assist anti-trafficking NGOs with capacity-building and legal work.

U.S. Department of State. (n.d.). *20 ways you can help fight human trafficking.* Retrieved from http://www.state.gov/j/tip/id/help/

- Volunteer services as appropriate to local agencies.
- Join a local anti-human trafficking coalition.
- Provide financial support to an agency that supports victims and survivors of human trafficking.
- Collaborate with other healthcare professionals either on the job and/or in the community and lobby local policymakers to strengthen laws and increase punishments.

TABLE 6B.3 Recommended Readings

Bales, K. (2005). *Understanding global slavery.* Berkeley, CA: University of California Press.

Bales, K., & Soodalter, R. (2010). *The slave next door.* Los Angeles, CA: University of California Press.

Clawson, H. J., Dutch, N. M., & Williamson, E. (2008). *National symposium on the health needs of human trafficking: Background document.* Washington, DC: Office of the Assistant Secretary for Planning and Evaluation, U.S. Department of Health and Human Services.

de Chesnay, M. (Ed.). (2013). *Sex trafficking: A clinical guide for nurses.* New York, NY: Springer Publishing.

Estes, R., & Weiner, N. (2001). *The commercial sexual exploitation of children in the U.S., Canada, and Mexico.* Philadelphia, PA: University of Pennsylvania.

Family Violence Prevention Fund, World Childhood Foundation. (2005). Turning pain into power: *Trafficking survivors' perspectives on early intervention strategies.* San Francisco, CA: Family Violence Prevention Fund. Retrieved from http://www.futureswithoutviolence.org/user files/file/ImmigrantWomen/Turning%20Pain%20intoPower.pdf

Farley, M., Cotton, A., Lynne, J., Zumbeck, S., Spiwak, F., Reyes, M., Alvarez, D., & Sezgin, U. (2003). Prostitution and trafficking in nine countries: An update on violence and posttraumatic stress disorder. *Journal of Trauma Practice, 2*(3/4), 33–74.

Fernando, B. (2005). *In contempt of fate: The tale of a Sri Lankan sold into servitude who survived to tell it.* Meerimac, MA: BeaRo Publishing.

Kara, S. (2009). *Sex trafficking: Inside the business of modern slavery.* New York, NY: Columbia University Press.

Lloyd, R. (2011). *Girls like us.* New York, NY: Harper Collins.

Rodriguez, A. (2009). *Labor trafficking.* Bonita Springs, FL.

Sage, J., & Kasten, L. (2006). *Enslaved: True stories of modern day slavery.* New York, NY: Palgrave Macmillan.

Shelley, L. (2010). *Human trafficking: A global perspective.* New York, NY: Cambridge University Press.

Zimmerman, C., Hossain, M., & Watts, C. (2011). Human trafficking and health: A conceptual model to inform policy, intervention and research. *Social Science and Medicine, 73,* 327–335.

- Advocate for more support and services for victims in the nurse's state, especially for children.
- Sign up for free newsletters and emails from any of the numerous organizations combating human trafficking to stay informed.
- Challenges and future progress
  - Traditionally, healthcare providers have been one of the least represented groups of professionals to address human trafficking and participate in the identification, assessment, and care of trafficked patients. Human trafficking is globally recognized as a public health issue that has negative consequences on victims' physical, medical, and psychological well-being, all areas that are within the purview of healthcare providers. Yet, little time and effort is devoted to educating students and professionals about the phenomenon. Healthcare professionals should receive training on all aspects of human trafficking and be given the tools to effectively screen and treat those who need services. Because they serve in a variety of areas and settings and work with many different people and populations, often on the frontlines, healthcare providers are uniquely well-positioned to take a more active and necessary role in combating this universal threat to people's health and well-being.
  - Much work needs to be done to prevent and combat human trafficking, identify and provide support and services for victims, and arrest and prosecute perpetrators. Yet, progress is being made, for example, regarding state human-trafficking laws in the United States (Heinrich & Sreeharsha, 2013):
    - The Uniform Law Commission is developing a uniform human-trafficking law that would be the same for all states.
    - The *Uniform Crime Report* will collect nationwide data on human trafficking instead of from agencies that selectively volunteer this information. Such an approach will help keep law enforcement agencies better informed about human trafficking.

- Increased interest and effort exist in passing laws that prohibit the arrest of victims, that expunge prior records, and that recognize the need for victim assistance, especially for mental health issues.
  - Some laws now mandate training on human trafficking at police academies and a move exists to foster interdisciplinary participation of agencies in supporting victims.
- Another area to be addressed is the validity of prevalence data on human trafficking. A review of the use and misuse of research in books on sex trafficking suggests a need for more rigorous and methodologically sound research, including the prevalence statistics repeated in much of the literature (Fedina, 2015). Although this does not apply directly to nurses, the implications of using questionable data affect what nurses do because this information impacts practice, research, policy, and support for victims.

CASE STUDY

Nina, a 16-year-old adolescent female, lives with her mother and her mother's boyfriend in a middle-class neighborhood. She is the oldest of three children and in tenth grade. Nina had been a good student and active in sports at her high school until about a year ago. Her father, with whom she was quite close, suffered a sudden, fatal myocardial infarction. In the year since his death, Nina has become withdrawn, depressed, and tearful. She has lost interest in her friends and in socializing, and attending school is a struggle. During the school year, Carl, an 18-year-old male senior at her school, has begun to take an interest in her and tells her that he knows how she feels as his father also died when he was in tenth grade. The two develop a rapport and she feels he is the only person who understands her and what she is going through. She resents that her mother has found a new partner and that her two sisters are moving on from the loss of their father. Carl has money, a car, and is a popular among the party crowd. He is also attractive and Nina is flattered that he likes her. She is eager to please him and allows Carl to make the decisions in their budding relationship. She begins spending increasing time with him, and coming home late, even during school nights. He has bought her a cell phone so he can call her whenever he wants. He often suggests that she join him and his friends at parties he has at his house when his parents are away. On nights when his parents are home, Carl takes her to parties at other people's houses or to hotel rooms rented by some of his older friends. One night, her mother catches Nina coming home after 2 am, sneaking into the house through an open window. When her mother asks where she has been, Nina states she was at Carl's house and fell asleep, thereby missing her curfew. Her attire becomes more provocative, and she begins wearing makeup, which is out of character for her. She suddenly seems to have new items, including expensive jewelry and clothes. When her mother asks Nina how she is acquiring these items, she says that they are gifts from her boyfriend, yet she tells her friends at school that she has a job and is purchasing these items with the money she makes. Several months into her relationship with Carl, Nina reports not feeling well "down there" to her 14-year-old sister, who tells their mother. The mother takes Nina to the physician who shares with her and her mother that Nina has chlamydia. The physician also discovers that Nina has a tattoo that says "Li'l C" on her left hip.

REVIEW QUESTIONS

1. What is your initial assessment of this situation?
2. What could be evidence of trafficking?
3. Aside from trafficking, what are some possible explanations for this situation?
4. What are some questions the healthcare provider could ask Nina and/or her mother to determine if this patient might be a trafficking victim or a victim of domestic violence?

5. What are some questions to ask about the boyfriend?

6. Since the patient is in high school, what role might the school nurse play in assessing what is occurring?

7. Were it possible to conduct a complete examination, what healthcare problems might the staff expect to find or anticipate in a patient with a history of being trafficked?

8. What would you do in this situation if you were caring for this patient?

9. How does Nina's age affect your actions?

10. What are some things you might not do if you were caring for this patient?

11. What do healthcare professionals need to know that would help them recognize victims of human trafficking?

12. What are some resources in your area that you could contact for this patient and/or her family should she prove to be a trafficking victim?

13. What might be the expected outcome for Carl should he prove to be her boyfriend? And what might be the outcome should he prove to be her trafficker?

REFERENCES

ATEST. (2014). *Relevant authorization statutes.* Retrieved from http://www.endslaveryandtrafficking.org/fy2014/Relevant-Authorization-Statutes.php

Aronowitz, A. A. (2009). *Human trafficking, Human misery: The global trade in human beings.* Westport, CT: Praeger Publishers.

Batstone, D. (2007). *Not for sale: The return of the global slave trade and how we can fightback.* San Francisco, CA: Harper Collins Publishers.

Bender, K., & Furman, R. (2004). The implications of sex tourism on men's social, psychological and physical health. *Qualitative Report, 9*(2), 176–191. Retrieved from http://www.nova.edu/ssss/QR/QR9-2/bender.pdf

Cawley, M. (2014). *Extent of Mexico human trafficking obscured by lack of info.* Retrieved from http://www.insightcrime.org/news-analysis/extent-of-mexico-human-trafficking- obscured-by-lack-of-info

Center for Problem-Oriented Policing. (n.d.). Look beneath the surface: Role of health care providersin identifying and helping victims of human trafficking [PowerPoint presentation]. Retrieved from http://www.popcenter.org/problems/trafficked_women/PDFs/toolkit/Role_of_Health_Care_Providers.pdf

Child Soldiers International. (2014). *Who are child soldiers?* Retrieved from http://www.child-soldiers.org/about_the_issues.php

de Chesnay, M. (2012). Sex trafficking and sex tourism. In M. de Chesnay & B. Anderson (Eds.). *Caring for the vulnerable: Perspectives in nursing theory, practice and research* (pp. 385–392). Sudbury, MA: Jones & Bartlett, Inc.

de Chesnay, M., & Greenbaum, J. (2012). Physical trauma. In M. de Chesnay (Ed.). *Sex trafficking: A clinical guide for nurses* (pp. 263–280). New York, NY: Springer Publishing Company.

Ditmore, M., Maternik, A., & Zapert, K. (2012). *The road north: The role of gender, poverty and violence in trafficking from Mexico to the U.S.* New York, NY: Urban Justice Center. Retrieved from http://sexworkersproject.org/downloads/2012/swp-2012-the-road-north-en.pdf

Farrell, A., McDevitt, J., Pfeffer, R., Fahy, S., Owens, C., Dank, M., & Adams, W. (2012). *Identifying challenges to improve the investigation and prosecution of state and local human trafficking cases.* Washington, DC: National Institute of Justice. Retrieved from https://www.ncjrs.gov/pdffiles1/nij/grants/238795.pdf

Fedina, L. (2015). Use and misuse of research in books on sex trafficking: Implications for interdisciplinary researchers, practitioners, and advocates. *Trauma, Violence & Abuse, 16*(2), 188–198.

Flores, T. (2010). *The slave across the street: The true story of how an American teen survived the world of human trafficking.* Boise, ID: Ampelon Publishing Company.

Grumiau, S. (2012). *UNICEF aids Restavek victims of abuse and exploitation in Haiti.* Retrieved from http://www.unicef.org/adolescence/haiti_61518.html

Heinrich, K., & Sreeharsha, K. (2013). The state of state human trafficking laws. *The Judges' Journal, 52*(1), 28–31.

International Federation of Social Workers. (2014). *Human trafficking.* Retrieved from http://ifsw.org/publications/human-rights/human-trafficking/

International Labour Conference. (2005). *A global alliance against forced labour: Global report under the follow up to the ILO Declaration on Fundamental Principles and Rights at Work 2005.* Geneva, Switzerland: International Labour Office. Retrieved from http://www.ilo.org/wcmsp5/groups/public/@ed_norm/@declaration/documents/publication/wcms_081882.pdf

International Labour Organization (ILO). (2009). *Training manual to fight trafficking in children for labour, sexual and other forms of exploitation: Understanding child trafficking.* Retrieved from http://www.unicef.org/protection/Textbook_1.pdf

Kashino, M. M. (2013). You're pretty: You could make some money. *Washingtonian.* Retrieved from http://www.washingtonian.com/articles/people/youre-pretty-you-could-make-some-money/

Lederer, L. J. (2011). Sold for sex: The link between street gangs and trafficking in persons. *Protection Project Journal of Human Rights and Civil Society, 4,* 1–20. Retrieved from http://www.protectionproject.org/wp-content/uploads/2011/11/The-Protection-Project-Journal-of-Human-Rights-Civil-Society-Volume-IV.pdf

Library of Congress. (2014). Mexico: Federal Senate approves of law against human trafficking. *LAW.gov.* Retrieved from http://www.loc.gov/lawweb/servlet/lloc_news?disp3_l205403877_text

Malarek, V. (2011). *The johns: Sex for sale and the men who buy it.* New York, NY: Arcade Publishing.

Polaris Project. (2014a). *Human trafficking.* Retrieved from http://www.polarisproject.org/

Public Safety Canada. (2014). *National action plan to combat human trafficking.* Retrieved from http://www.public-safety.gc.ca/cnt/rsrcs/pblctns/ntnl-ctn-pln-cmbt/index-eng.aspx

Sabella, D. (2011). The role of the nurse in combating human trafficking. *American Journal of Nursing, 111*(2), 28–39.

Sabella, D. (2013). Health issues and interactions with adult survivors. In M. de Chesnay (Ed.). *Sex trafficking: A clinical guide for nurses* (pp. 151–166). New York, NY: Springer Publishing Company.

Skinner, E. B. (2008). *A crime so monstrous: Face-to-face with modern-day slavery.* New York, NY: Free Press.

Smith, H. A. (2014). *Walking prey: How America's youth are vulnerable to sex slavery.* New York, NY: Palgrave MacMillan.

Taylor, G., & Blake, B. (2013). Sexually transmitted infections. In M. de Chesnay (Ed.). *Sex trafficking: A clinical guide for nurses* (pp. 239–262). New York, NY: Springer Publishing Company.

U.S. Congress. (2000). Pub. L. No. 106–386. Victims of Trafficking and Violence Protection Act of 2000. Retrieved from http://www.state.gov/documents/organization/10492.pdf

U.S. Congress. (2013). Pub. L. No. 113–4. Violence Against Women Reauthorization Act of 2013. Retrieved from http://www.gpo.gov/fdsys/pkg/PLAW-113publ4/html/PLAW-113publ4.htm

U.S. Department of Health and Human Services. (2012a). *Fact sheet: Human trafficking.* Washington, DC: U.S. Department of Health and Human Services. Retrieved from http://www.acf.hhs.gov/programs/orr/resource/fact-sheet-human-trafficking

U.S. Department of Health and Human Services. (2012b.). *Fact sheet: Labor trafficking.* Retrieved from http://www.acf.hhs.gov/programs/orr/resource/fact-sheet-labor-trafficking-english

U.S. Department of State. (2004). *Trafficking in persons report 2004.* Washington, DC: U.S. Department of State. Retrieved from http://www.state.gov/g/tip/rls/tiprpt/2004

U.S. Department of State. (2007). *Trafficking in persons report 2007.* Washington, DC: U.S. Department of State. Retrieved from http://www.state.gov/g/tip/rls/tiprpt/2007

U.S. Department of State. (2010). *Trafficking in persons report 2010.* Washington, DC: U.S. Department of State. Retrieved from http://www.state.gov/g/tip/rls/tiprpt/2010

U.S. Department of State. (2011). *Trafficking in persons report 2011.* Washington, DC: U.S. Department of State. Retrieved from http://www.state.gov/g/tip/rls/tiprpt/2011

U.S. Department of State. (2014). *Trafficking in persons report 2014.* Washington, DC: US Department of State. Retrieved from http://www.state.gov/j/tip/rls/tiprpt/2014/index.htm

U.S. Department of State. (n.d.). *20 ways you can help fight human trafficking.* Retrieved from http://www.state.gov/j/tip/id/help/

UNICEF. (2007). *The Paris principles: Principles and guidelines on children associated with armed forces or armed groups.* Paris, France: UNICEF. Retrieved from http://www.unicef.org/emerg/files/ParisPrinciples310107English.pdf.

UNICEF-Canada. (2014). *Protecting children from trafficking.* Retrieved from http://www.unicef.ca/en/policy-advocacy-for-children/children-from-trafficking

United Nations (UN). (2000). *Protocol to prevent, suppress and punish trafficking in persons, especially women and children, supplementing the United Nations Convention Against Transnational Organized Crime.* New York, NY: UN. Retrieved from http://www.osce.org/odihr/19223;http://www.osce.org/odihr/19223?download=true; http://www.uncjin.org/Documents/Conventions/dcatoc/final_documents_2/convention_%20traffeng.pdf

United Nations Office on Drugs and Crime. (2008). *Toolkit to combat trafficking in persons* (2nd ed.). New York, NY: United Nations. Retrieved from http://www.unodc.org/unodc/en/human-trafficking/2008/electronic-toolkit/electronic-toolkit-to-combat-trafficking-in-persons—index.html

United Nations Office on Drugs and Crime. (2009). *Anti-human trafficking manual for criminal justice practitioners Module 4: Control methods in trafficking in persons.* New York, NY: United Nations. Retrieved from http://www.unodc.org/documents/human-trafficking/TIP_module4_Ebook.pdf

United Nations Office on Drugs and Crime. (2014). *Global report on trafficking in persons.* New York, NY: United Nations. Retrieved from http://www.unodc.org/documents/data-and-analysis/glotip/GLOTIP_2014_full_report.pdf

Ward, J. M. (2010). Rationalizing sexual tourism: How some countries benefit from selling sex. *Student Pulse, 2*(4), 1–4. Retrieved from http://www.studentpulse.com/articles/235/rationalizing-sexual-tourism-how-some-countries-benefit-from-selling-sex

Weitzer, R. (2014). New directions in research on human trafficking. *Annals of the American Academy of Political and Social Science, 653*(1), 6–24. Retrieved from http://ann.sagepub.com/content/653/1/6.full

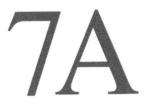

CHAPTER **7A**

Overarching Issues: Testifying

Judy Malmgren
Cyndi Leahy

OBJECTIVES

At the completion of this chapter, the learner will be able to:

- Describe the role of the forensic nurse in the judicial/legal system.
- Discuss professional practice issues that guide a forensic nurse's interaction with the judicial/legal system.
- Name steps the forensic nurse should take when preparing to testify in court.
- Describe the general principles involved in providing testimony as a fact or expert witness.

KEY TERMS

Court: "[A] governmental body consisting of one or more judges who sit to adjudicate disputes and administer justice" (Garner, 2005; p. 302).

Curriculum vitae (CV): Provides information that is specific to an individual's expertise, and includes education, work experience, awards, memberships, professional accomplishments, and prior experience testifying.

Expert witness: "[E]vidence about a scientific, technical, professional, or other specialized issue given by a person qualified to testify because of familiarity with the subject or special training in the field" (Garner, 2005, p. 474).

Fact-finder/trier of fact: "[T]he person or persons who will decide the case: the judge in a bench trial, or the jury in a jury trial" (Vukelic, 2005; p. 114).

Fact witness: A person who has personal knowledge about a particular case and testifies about what he or she has observed.

Hearsay: "[T]estimony that is given by a witness who relates not to what he or she knows personally, but what others have said" (Garner, 2005; p. 599).

Justice: "[T]he fair and proper administration of laws" (Garner, 2005; p. 718).

Objection: Meaning to put forth opposition (Garner, 2005).

Opposing counsel: "[A]ttorney for the other party" (Vukelic, 2005; p. 117).

Rule of law: "[T]he doctrine that every person is subject to the ordinary law within the jurisdiction" (Garner, 2005; p. 1104).

Subpoena: Meaning "under penalty"; a writ summoning a witness to appear in person before a court or tribunal under penalty of punishment.

Subpoena duces tecum: A writ instructing the recipient to present the court with items relevant to the case, such as medical records, laboratory results, forensic nursing reports, and photographs.

Voir dire: A series of questions to test the competence of a witness or potential juror (Garner, 2005).

Forensic nurses are provided with unique opportunities and experiences as they interact and navigate between two different systems: health care and law. As with other nursing specialties, nursing science provides the framework for knowledge and practice. However, linking the term "forensic" with "nurse" highlights additional sources of knowledge needed for this role. The word "forensic" denotes the application of scientific principles to legal investigation and public or legal debate, which may require testimony from the forensic nurse. The guiding principles of professional nursing practice are important concepts for the forensic nurse to convey to those within the legal community and throughout the legal and judicial system.

FORENSIC NURSING AND THE LEGAL SYSTEM

Violence is a global issue, which occurs on a local, state/provincial, national, and international level. The impact of violence threatens every segment of society. The culture of violence and in some cases its apparent acceptance impacts not only the legal system but the healthcare system as well. Forensic nurses provide a tailored solution; these nurses are specially educated to serve in a role that fulfills the needs of both the legal and healthcare systems. According to Markowitz (2007; p. 3), "Forensic nurses can be found at any point along the continuum where health care and the legal system intersect."

The presence of forensic nurses within the community enables patients and their families to have access to needed services, and can benefit the legal and court systems as well (Plichta, Clements, & Houseman, 2007). Although becoming an expert in the law is not the goal of the forensic nurse, the forensic nurse is expected to possess basic knowledge of legal processes and laws relevant to his or her practice. An understanding of legal principles will guide relevant factual and objective testimony as the nurse progresses along the novice-to-expert continuum (Benner, 1984).

Most countries have specific rules of law that prohibit violence and maltreatment, facilitating the development of the forensic nursing role. A primary focus of forensic nursing is the health consequences of violence and maltreatment. As García-Moreno (2013; p. 9) states, "[W]here violence persists, health is seriously compromised." By assisting patients' access to equitable and quality health care, the forensic nurse improves patient outcomes.

Interacting with the Judicial System

The amount of time and frequency with which the forensic nurse interacts with the legal and judicial system varies, and depends upon a number of factors. These factors include the population served, the nurse's caseload, and geographic location of the nurse's patient population (or practice). The presence of a community-level coordinated response to violent crime and maltreatment, such as a sexual assault response team (SART), a child advocacy multidisciplinary team (MDT), and a death review team may also play a factor in the nurse's level of involvement with the legal community. More often, forensic nurses are being called upon to assist these team members in making legal and investigative decisions by sharing knowledge of nursing care and the healthcare system.

Justice is an important concept to both the legal and the healthcare system. For the legal community, justice "is sometimes seen as synonymous with broad legal empowerment of the poor and disenfranchised" (Agrast, Botero, Martinez, Ponce, & Pratt, 2012–2013; pp. 9–10). In broad nursing terms, justice is considered to be fair and equitable access to quality care. Although the forensic nurse is specifically educated to apply scientific and legal principles in the identification and collection of evidence, it is incorrect to describe the forensic nurse as an arm of law enforcement or a prosecution team (Lawson & Rowe, 2009). The primary role of the forensic nurse in the legal and judicial system is to educate.

For the forensic nurse who is practicing at the basic level, areas in which to educate those in the legal and judicial system include the:

- Role of the forensic nurse
- Steps of the medical-forensic examination
- Identification, collection, and preservation of evidence
- Presence (or lack) of physical findings
- Limitations of the forensic evaluation

The information shared with the legal and judicial system depends on the forensic nurse's experience and education. For example, novice forensic nurses are educated to identify and document physical examination findings, and might speak to the presence of an injury, whereas the advanced forensic nurse would be better prepared to discuss mechanisms of injury.

Transitioning into Practice

The primary goals and objectives of the forensic nurse understandably differ from those of the legal community and judicial system. For nurses who are transitioning into forensic practice, fundamental nursing values, ethical principles, and professional integrity must remain at the forefront. Forensic nursing is based on nursing science and is regulated by regional and international laws and standards of care. The primary purpose of regulatory and governing bodies is to protect members of the public as they access professional nursing care, and to facilitate the nurse's ability to deliver effective, timely, safe, and competent nursing care (Russell, 2012). Forensic nurses integrate population-focused knowledge with their knowledge of patient rights, healthcare risks, ethics, and evidence-based practice standards (Doane & Varcoe, 2007). Population-focused care improves patient outcomes, which may ultimately assist the judicial system to achieve its desired outcomes as well.

JUSTICE SYSTEMS

Organized social systems have a set of rules, or codes of law, legal consequences, and proceedings to achieve and administer justice. Major forms of law include: common (British Empire, United States [US], Canada), civil (Anglo-American, Canadian, South American, African), socialist (mainly China), and religious (Muslim countries). In common and civil law countries, courts are arranged at different levels. Courts offer a legal setting for a fair debate between parties regarding criminal or civil matters.

Managing legal outcomes associated with violence and maltreatment while protecting freedom and human rights is complex and challenging. The World Justice Project (2014) evaluates how rules of law are enacted and enforced across the globe by using key principles to measure the strengths and weaknesses of the rules of law. The mere existence of law does not guarantee that justice will be achieved, and "in many countries . . . acts of violence against women are not investigated thoroughly or documented precisely, and . . . domestic violence continues to be regarded as a private matter and not a criminal offence, while complaints of sexual violence continue to be treated with skepticism" (UN, 2010; p. 19).

> "The rule of law is the foundation for communities of opportunity and equity – it is the predicate for the eradication of poverty, violence, corruption, pandemics, and other threats to civil society" W. H. Neukom, Founder, President and CEO of the World Justice Project (Agrast et al., 2012–2013; p. 1).

The issue of gender-based violence is well-recognized from an international human rights standpoint, as seen in international laws, treaties, and declarations. The World Health Organization (WHO) presents violence against women as a global epidemic, and a fundamental violation of women's human rights (Krug, 2002). Many states have incorporated these precepts into their laws, but gaps remain as international law is "not empowered to impose sanctions on noncompliant states" (Merry, 2003; p. 942). Specialized courts for gender-based violence exist in a number of countries, including Brazil, Spain, Uruguay, Venezuela, the United Kingdom, the United States, and Canada for the purpose of "decreasing court processing time; increasing conviction rates; providing a focal point for programs and services for victims and offenders; and, in some cases, allowing for the specialization of police, Crown prosecutors, and the judiciary in domestic violence matters" (DOJ of Canada, 2015).

In some countries, the rule of law addresses specific types of gender-based violence, such as:

- Domestic violence and intimate partner violence
- Sexual violence, including sexual assault and sexual harassment
- Harmful practices, including early marriage, forced marriage, female genital mutilation, female infanticide, prenatal sex-selection, virginity testing, HIV/AIDS cleansing
- Femicide/feminicide, so-called honor crimes, acid attacks, crimes committed in relation to bride-price and dowry, maltreatment of widows, forced pregnancy, and trying women for sorcery/witchcraft
- Trafficking and sexual slavery (UN, 2010).

COURT SYSTEMS

Courts are established to handle disputes involving laws of a particular territory, district, or jurisdiction. Each level of government has jurisdiction over an assigned region, and follows its own set of laws. In the United States, the federal government and its court system deals with disputes over federal laws, disputes between states, and civil complaints involving the Constitution and civil rights. The US Supreme Court is the highest court of the land. Lower US courts are the circuit courts (13 regional appellate courts), district courts (94 courts), as well as specialized courts that consider matters of international trade and bankruptcy. An appellate court reviews and has the authority to reverse decisions made by the district court, the court which first tries the matter. If the circuit court opinion does not satisfy a party, the case may be appealed and qualify for review by the Supreme Court, which is also an appellate court. The federal government shares power with the state governments, and the courts of the state deal with disputes over state laws and civil issues.

The two systems of justice – criminal and civil – differ in purpose and penalties.

- "The criminal justice system deals with the administration of criminal law or the law of crimes. In a criminal law proceeding, the parties are the prosecuting unit of government (local, state, or federal) that brings the criminal charges and the accused (or the defendant) against whom the charges are brought. A criminal justice proceeding begins when a person is accused by the government of the commission of a crime" (Wecht & Rago, 2006; p. 139).

- "The civil justice system is really a system of private justice. In the civil justice system, the parties are private individuals or companies or corporations who are either suing or being sued" (Wecht & Rago, 2006; p. 140). Civil matters may include breach of contract, violation of civil rights, failure to meet a social-welfare standard, and other disputes involving government.

In criminal matters, penalties include the loss of freedom, whereas with civil matters, the penalties may be monetary damages or the individual could be given permission to do something or directed to refrain from doing something. Military justice is another system that exists in the United States and Canada. These courts handle matters pertaining to laws that govern those serving in the military. Forensic nurse testimony may become necessary in any of these systems of justice.

TESTIMONY

A court provides a legal forum for public debate; this is an environment that most people would rather avoid. "Dread" and "uneasiness" are words that forensic nurses often use in describing their feelings about their first experiences when testifying. The challenge can be even more daunting for an individual who is unfamiliar with court process or who is unclear about the expectations others may have regarding his or her testimony.

Various individuals may participate in court proceedings, including:

- Lawyers (for each side)
- Judge
- Courtroom deputy
- Court reporter
- Witnesses
- Jury (in some cases)

The judge and jury are the fact-finders, also known as the triers of fact. Two parties are involved: the government and the defendant in criminal trials, and the plaintiff and the defendant in civil suits. Except where a defendant chooses to represent him/herself, each party is represented by an attorney (or lawyer or counsel). In some cases, each side may have more than one attorney who represents that party.

Trial by Jury

"Under the *Canadian Charter of Rights and Freedoms*, individuals accused of the most serious criminal offences generally have the right to choose to be tried by a jury or by a judge alone. A jury is a group of people, chosen from the community, who assess the facts of a case after a judge explains the law to them. They then make a decision based on their assessment. Sentencing, however, is left to the judge. Trial by jury is also available in some civil litigation, but is rarely used" (DOJ of Canada, 2015).

The judicial system can result in poor outcomes not only for the victim of violence, but also for the innocent and the wrongfully accused. The individual, family, and community can be positively or negatively affected by a verdict, underscoring the weighty responsibility of the forensic nurse as a witness in a court of law. Conviction of the innocent and miscarriages of justice are a systemic problem, and the risk is elevated when the rules of evidence are inadequately or poorly applied. A basic knowledge of the judicial system will help the forensic nurse to develop the necessary skills to effectively testify with confidence. Forensic nurses must have a basic understanding of the:

- Role of those involved in administering justice
- Process of presenting clear, accurate, objective testimony
- Rules of evidence
- Important legal precedents in the nurse's country or jurisdiction (i.e., in the United States, the cases of *Crawford v. Washington* (2004) and *Daubert v. Merrell Dow Pharmaceuticals* (1993), etc.)

Adapting to any new role takes time and experience. Testifying as a forensic nurse is no exception. When testifying or engaged in related interactions with the legal and judicial system, the nurse must consider the implications of what he or she says and does. Testimony offered by the forensic nurse must be clear, truthful, reliable, complete, and objective. These tenets are true regardless of which side seeks testimony from the forensic nurse (See Table 7A.1).

Types of Testimony

The two primary types of testimony are that of a fact witness, and that of an expert witness.

Fact Witness Testimony. The testimony of a fact witness is limited to that person's firsthand knowledge regarding a case, and might pertain to who, what, when, where, and how. Fact testimony tends to include sensory data related to sight, hearing, touch, smell, and taste. Fact witness testimony does not include what someone else experienced, felt, knew, or believed; that is considered hearsay.

A forensic nurse who testifies as a fact witness may be asked to provide information about healthcare procedures, treatments, vital signs, and the standards and protocols that he or she used when caring for the patient. In addition, the forensic nurse fact witness may be asked to verify the authenticity of certain packages of evidence as the ones that he or she collected, sealed, and labeled. The attorney may use this opportunity to introduce photographic images taken by the nurse. For instance, the attorney may ask the forensic nurse whether the photographic image being presented in court is a true and accurate representation of what the nurse observed at the time of the examination.

Expert Witness Testimony. In contrast, expert witness testimony is defined as "evidence about a scientific, technical, professional, or other specialized issue given by a person qualified to testify because of familiarity with the subject or special training in the field" (Garner, 2005; p. 474). Within the scope of the US federal rules of evidence, these "are not only experts in the strictest sense of the word, e.g., physicians, physicists, and architects, but also the large group sometimes called 'skilled' witnesses, such as bankers or landowners testifying to land values" (Fed. R. Evid. 702). An intelligent evaluation of facts is often difficult or impossible without the application of some scientific, technical, or other specialized knowledge, and the expert witness provides context for the trier of fact.

A person may be qualified to provide expert witness testimony based on his or her:

- Specific field
- Vocation
- Discipline
- Experience
- Background

Before attempting to introduce a witness to the court as an expert, the attorney conducts a voir dire, meaning to speak the truth. Voir dire involves the attorney asking the witness a series of questions about the witness' occupation, education, licensing, experience, and other details provided in the expert's curriculum vitae (CV) (Sapir, 2007), and is also the process used to select jurors. Even though the attorneys for both parties likely have a copy of the expert witness' CV, the witness answers the questions orally for the benefit of the court. In some circumstances, if the witness has testified previously as an expert in the same court, the judge may forgo the voir dire. The judge makes the ultimate decision as to whether the witness is deemed an expert.

The function of the expert witness is to provide "knowledge upon which others rely," and the knowledge must be justified (Sanders, 2007; p. 1542). Forensic nurses practicing in the United States should be aware of the *Daubert* standard, which is applied to determine whether an opinion or something about which the expert plans to testify is relevant, sufficiently reliable, and based upon scientific principles, methods, or knowledge (*Daubert v. Merrell Dow Pharmaceuticals*, 1993). As previously stated, the main purpose of expert testimony is to educate the trier of fact, who determines the ultimate outcome of the legal proceeding.

TABLE 7A.1 Tips for Effective Testimony

- Be prepared. Review the medical records and reports prior to court.
- Listen carefully to the entire question before answering. Ask for clarification, when needed. Do not interrupt the questioner.
- Pause briefly before answering; it allows for consideration of the response.
- Make eye contact with the trier of fact (the judge or the jury).
- Maintain good posture while on the witness stand and be cautious of nonverbal body language.
- Avoid using terms such as "always," "never," or "with 100% certainty."
- Responding with "I don't know" or "I don't recall" is acceptable when the expert does not know the answer.

(Vukelic, 2005)

The role of an expert witness is to provide a balanced and objective opinion at all times (Working Group on the Prevention of Miscarriages of Justice of Canada, 2011). Delivering objective testimony is essential; forensic nurse expert witnesses "who appear biased in favor of the prosecution or the victim will simply not be as effective when they testify as experts" (Canaff, 2009; p. 92), and will justifiably lose credibility. The loss of credibility by the forensic nurse in one case may affect his or her subsequent credibility as an expert witness.

Due to the expert witness' specialized knowledge and expertise, he or she may be asked to render an opinion that goes beyond that to which the fact witness may testify. This opinion might include commentary on what the findings may mean or suggest. Any opinion, however, should be grounded in the scientific method and should focus "on the nature of documented injury and other obtained evidence, not the believability of the victim," for example (Campbell, Long, Townsend, Kinnison, Pulley, Adames, & Wasco, 2007; p. 12). Finally, in most jurisdictions, forensic nurses and other expert witnesses cannot render an opinion on the ultimate issue at trial; that task is reserved for the trier of fact. (31A *Am. Jur. 2d*, 2015).

Legal Terminology

Just as medical terminology is foreign to lawyers and judges, terms used during judicial proceedings may be confusing to the forensic nurse. A few commonly used terms during the court proceedings include "object," "overrule," and "sustain." Attorneys will use the phrase "I object," meaning to put forth opposition (Garner, 2005). When an objection is made, the forensic nurse must stop speaking until the judge makes a ruling on the matter. The judge will either allow the question to be answered (overrule) or prevent the testimony (sustain).

A complex issue regarding testimony is known as hearsay, which is defined as "testimony that is given by a witness who relates not to what he or she knows personally, but what others have said" (Garner, 2005; 599). Hearsay evidence creates confusion even among legal professionals (Spencer, 2008). The witness may believe the information to be true, but the court may not permit it based on the inability to verify it as fact, making it unreliable (Law Reform Commission, 2010). Testifying to what someone else said, thought, or felt (outside of court, in the past) is generally considered hearsay evidence. Exceptions exist to the hearsay rule, such as allowing admission of some statements made by the patient to the healthcare provider for purposes of medical diagnosis and treatment. A full discussion of hearsay and its exceptions, however, is beyond the scope of this curriculum.

PREPARATION FOR TESTIFYING

The first steps in preparing for court begin with the initial interaction with the patient, client, inmate, or as with the nurse death investigator, the decedent. Preparation starts with providing nursing care, which aligns with accepted professional standards and is within the forensic nurse's scope of practice. The use of the nursing process (assessment, diagnosis, outcome identification, planning, implementation, and evaluation) cannot be overstated. In addition to the nursing process, thorough and detailed documentation by the forensic nurse is critically important. Documentation should be completed with the following data collection in mind:

- Identification and management of the patient's healthcare needs
- Collection of data for evidentiary purposes
- A record that is useful to the parties and fact-finders in a court of law
- A record that is useful to the forensic nurse in preparing for and providing accurate and meaningful testimony in court

The forensic nurse should not rely on memory; pertinent details should be clearly documented. Statements of evidentiary relevancy made to the forensic nurse should be entered into the report as close to verbatim as possible (Canaff, 2009).

Forensic nurses should be prepared to have their documentation be closely analyzed and scrutinized since it may be used in criminal or civil court proceedings. In some cases, an attorney may retain an outside forensic nurse expert to assess and evaluate the standard of care and documentation of the forensic nurse who conducted the examination.

Being Called to Testify

The forensic nurse may be subpoenaed by the prosecution, the defense, or both. The term subpoena is defined as "under penalty," and is a writ summoning a witness to appear in person before the court or tribunal under penalty of punishment. A subpoena is a paper that is served on the witness, and provides the date and time, the courtroom, the names of the parties, and sometimes basic instructions for the witness. In criminal cases, the names will be listed as government versus defendant (i.e., *State v. Jones*) and in civil cases, as plaintiff versus defendant. Most subpoenas name only the defendant. Therefore, the forensic nurse may need to contact the court or the individual who issued the subpoena to determine the name of the patient for whom the nurse has cared.

Another type of subpoena used in common law countries is the subpoena duces tecum, which is a writ instructing the recipient to present the court with items that are relevant to the case, such as medical records, laboratory results, forensic nursing reports, and photographs. Forensic nurses who are authorized by their organization to gather these items are legally bound to provide all the documents or materials requested; it is a violation of the order to redact, discard, or omit documents and extraneous material or notes. The forensic nurse should consult his or her facility's legal department and risk management office regarding policies on these matters.

Meeting with the Attorneys

Once a subpoena has been served for the forensic nurse to testify as a witness, the nurse and the attorney who issued the subpoena should plan to meet in advance of the court date for the purpose of preparing. The forensic nurse needs to know:

- The type of testimony that he or she is be expected to offer (i.e., fact or expert witness)
- Whether the case is criminal or civil
- Whether the trial is to be heard by a judge or a jury
- Where and what time to arrive

This encounter also permits the attorney an opportunity to discuss the nurse's experience and qualifications, the questions that the attorney plans to ask during the trial, and the forensic nurse's responses. The attorney may also ask the forensic nurse to educate the attorney on aspects of forensic nursing, the process of the forensic examination and evidence collection, the findings, and if the forensic nurse may have an opinion that may be relevant to the case. The opposing counsel may also contact the forensic nurse to request a meeting in preparation for the trial. When a meeting is requested in the absence of a subpoena, the forensic nurse should refer to organizational policy. Meetings are usually scheduled ahead of time and occur at a mutually agreed-upon time and location.

Additional Considerations

In addition to carefully reviewing the documentation, at least two other considerations are important when preparing for court. First, the nurse should compile and bring to court at least two copies of his or her curriculum vitae (CV). A CV differs from a résumé in that the former provides information that is specific to the individual's expertise, and includes education, work experience, awards, memberships, professional accomplishments, and prior experience testifying. The CV must be carefully maintained, reviewed for accuracy, and regularly updated.

Because forensic nursing is practiced at the intersection of nursing and the law, a forensic nurse can reasonably expect to interact with the legal and judicial system. A foreseeable interaction is being asked – or summoned – to appear in court as an expert or fact witness. By preparing adequately – knowing the nurse's applicable Nursing Practice Act, and scope and standards of practice; providing high-quality care; becoming familiar with the laws and regulations in the nurse's country, state, province, or jurisdiction; learning about the court system and its rules; reviewing information regarding the details of the patient's care and case – and testifying truthfully and objectively, the forensic nurse is uniquely positioned to make a valuable and compelling contribution in a court of law.

REFERENCES

31A *American Jurisprudence 2d* (2015).

Agrast, M. D., Botero, J. C., Martinez, J., Ponce, A., & Pratt, C. S. (2012–2013). *World justice project: Rule of law index, 2012–2013*. Washington, DC: World Justice Project. Retrieved March 10, 2015, from http://worldjusticeproject.org/sites/default/files/WJP_Index_Report_2012.pdf

Benner, P. (1984). *From novice to expert: Excellence and power in clinical nursing practice*. Menlo Park, CA: Addison-Wesley.

Campbell, R., Long, S. M., Townsend, S. M., Kinnison, K. E., Pulley, E. M., Adames, S. B., & Wasco, S. M. (2007). Sexual assault nurse examiners' experiences providing expert witness court testimony. *Journal of Forensic Nursing, 3*(1), 7–14.

Canaff, R. (2009). Nobility in objectivity: A prosecutor's case for neutrality in forensic nursing. *Journal of Forensic Nursing, 5*(2), 89–96.

Crawford v. Washington, 541 U.S. 36, 124 S. Ct. 1354, 158 L. Ed.2d 177 (2004).

Daubert v. Merrell Dow Pharmaceuticals, Inc., 509 U.S. 579, 113 S. Ct. 2786, 125 L. Ed. 2d 469 (1993).

Department of Justice (DOJ) of Canada. (2015). *Canada's court system: How the courts are organized*. Retrieved March 10, 2015, from http://www.justice.gc.ca/eng/csj-sjc/ccs-ajc/page3.html

Doane, G. H., & Varcoe, C. (2007). Relational practice and nursing obligations. *Advances in Nursing Science, 30*(3), 192–205.

Fed. R. Evid. 702, advisory comm. n. Retrieved March 10, 2015, from http://www.uscourts.gov/uscourts/rules/rules-evidence.pdf

García-Moreno, C. (2013). *Global and regional estimates of violence against women: Prevalence and health effects of intimate partner violence and non-partner sexual violence*. Geneva, Switzerland: World Health Organization, London School of Hygiene and Tropical Medicine & South African Medical Research Council. Retrieved from http://apps.who.int/iris/bitstream/10665/85239/1/9789241564625_eng.pdf

Garner, B. A. (Ed.). (2005). *Black's law dictionary* (8th ed.). Eagan, MN: West Publishing.

Krug, E. G. (2002). *World report on violence and health*. Geneva, Switzerland: World Health Organization. Retrieved March 10, 2015, from http://whqlibdoc.who.int/hq/2002/9241545615.pdf

Law Reform Commission. (2010). *Consultation paper: Hearsay in civil and criminal cases*. Dublin, Ireland: Law Reform Commission. Retrieved March 10, 2015, from http://www.lawreform.ie/_fileupload/Hearsayfull.pdf

Lawson, L., & Rowe, S. (2009). The scientific foundations of SANE education. *Journal of Forensic Nursing, 5*(2), 115–118. doi: 10.1111/j.1939-3938.2009.01043.x

Markowitz, J. (2007). *The role of the sexual assault nurse examiner in the prosecution of domestic violence cases*. Alexandria, VA: National District Attorneys Association.

Merry, S. E. (2003). Constructing a global law: Violence against women and the human rights system. *Law and Social Inquiry, 28*(4), 941–977.

Plichta, S., Clements, P., & Houseman, C. (2007). Why SANEs matter: Models of care for sexual violence victims in the emergency department. *Journal of Forensic Nursing, 3*(1), 15–23.

Russell, K. A. (2012). Nurse Practice Acts guide and govern nursing practice. *Journal of Nursing Regulation, 3*(3), 36–42.

Sanders, J. (2007). Expert witness ethics. *Fordham Law Review, 76*(3), 1539–1584.

Sapir, G. I. (2007). Qualifying the expert witness: A practical voir dire. *Forensic Magazine, 4*(1), 1–5.

Spencer, J. R. (2008). *Hearsay evidence in criminal proceedings.* Oxford, England: Hart Publishing. Retrieved from http://lawcommission.justice.gov.uk/docs/lc245_evidence_in_criminal_proceedings_hearsay_and_related_topics.pdf

Vukelic, J. M. (2005). *Testifying under oath: How to be an effective witness.* Volcano, CA: Volcano Press.

Wecht, C., & Rago, J. T. (2006). *Forensic science and law: Investigative applications in criminal, civil, and family justice.* Boca Raton, FL: Taylor & Francis.

Working Group on the Prevention of Miscarriages of Justice (Canada) & Public Prosecution Service of Canada. (2011). *The path to justice: Preventing wrongful convictions.* Ottawa, Canada: Public Prosecution Service of Canada.

World Justice Project. (2014). *Rule of law index 2014.* Washington, DC: World Justice Project. Retrieved from http://worldjusticeproject.org/publication/rule-law-index-reports/rule-law-index-2014-report

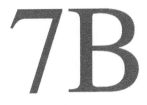

CHAPTER

Overarching Issues: Vicarious Trauma

Cyndi Leahy

OBJECTIVES

At the completion of this chapter, the learner will be able to:

1. Define vicarious trauma (VT).
2. Discuss at least three factors that increase the risk of experiencing negative effects of VT.
3. Identify at least three strategies for managing VT and promoting resiliency.

KEY TERMS

Burnout: A gradual loss of energy and ambition brought on by chronic stress; usually work-related or associated with the care of a dependent family member. The person may complain of difficulty concentrating, completing tasks, and focusing on responsibilities. Symptoms often include exhaustion with an increase in absenteeism or missing work-related meetings or deadlines and a decrease in work performance, goal-setting, and participation in activities that promote professional growth.

Compassion fatigue (CF): Changes characterized by a diminished capacity for empathy and compassion when carrying out expected actions and responsibilities; a normal, preventable, and reversible consequence of expending oneself to mitigate the suffering and related negative outcomes in others; also known as empathy fatigue (Boscarino, Figley, & Adams, 2004; Figley, 1995a; Stebnicki, 2008).

Countertransference: The clinician's inner experience and a subsequent transformative effect that occurs due to interaction with a person who is suffering from a trauma (Stamm, 1997).

Empathy: The ability to understand and relate to a person's experience (suffering or joy) by putting yourself in his or her place. Controlled empathy is the mindful application of empathy integrated with knowledge of VT and self-awareness while taking inventory of inner responses (intra-post patient encounter). The clinician balances empathy with professional boundaries and uses barriers and techniques that promote therapeutic outcomes while minimizing countertransference.

Posttraumatic stress disorder (PTSD): "[C]linical syndrome in which an initial fear response does not abate" after 1 month following exposure (Yehuda & LeDoux, 2007; p. 23). The diagnosis is based on symptoms, duration of the symptoms, and exclusion of other causes. The coexisting clinical symptoms are re-experiencing (intrusive thoughts, flashbacks, nightmares); avoidance (withdrawing, isolation, avoiding reminders); hyperarousal (insomnia, irritability, exaggerated startle response, hypervigilance, difficulty concentrating, and gaps in memory); and negative changes in cognition and mood (APA, 2013).

Vicarious resilience: The ability to cope with and maintain a positive outlook on one's effectiveness and role in mitigating suffering. Resilience and compassion satisfaction are positive outcomes that often occur when working with individuals who have experienced trauma.

Vicarious traumatization (VT): Also referred to as secondary trauma or secondary traumatic stress. A phenomenon that affects those in a position of "helper" who, due to bearing witness to trauma material and traumatic suffering of victims, experience neurobiologic reactions, emotions, and temporary or long-lasting changes in their own life, health, or worldview perspective. Signs and symptoms parallel those seen in PTSD; however, VT and PTSD are not the same. Often VT effects are gradual, result from a cumulative toll, and can have a contagion effect on others in the clinician's support system (Saakvine & Pearlman, 1996; Tabor, 2011).

Worldview: How a person perceives him/herself and makes sense of the world; is created by the person's experiences, beliefs, values, ideals, and knowledge about morality; good and evil; the purpose and meaning of life; and the origin, function, and future of the world (Aerts et al., 1994; Vidal, 2008).

DEFINING VICARIOUS TRAUMA

A "vicarious" experience is created by a neurobiological reaction to "bearing witness" through seeing, hearing, or reading about something that occurred in the life of another individual. When a human being witnesses powerful events, a complex chain of physiological and neurobiological responses prompts vicarious emotions, feelings, sensations, or thoughts. The experience and responses may be negative, positive, or a mixture of both, and may resolve spontaneously or lead to changes and long-term effects.

Bearing witness to someone's direct trauma or suffering can lead to vicarious traumatization, a term coined by McCann and Pearlman (1990). Vicarious trauma refers to an exposure to trauma material and a countertransference during the interaction that results in subsequent experience, schema, or outcome (Jenkins & Baird, 2002; Saakvine & Pearlman, 1996; Tabor, 2011). Repeated or chronic unmanaged exposures can overwhelm one's ability to cope, demonstrate compassion or empathy, or find personal or professional satisfaction. Aside from nurses, members of other at-risk professions include emergency providers, first responders, therapists, counselors, social workers, journalists, attorneys, judges, teachers, clergy, and humanitarian and other aid workers (Aiken, Clarke, Sloane, Sochalski, & Siber, 2002).

Vicarious trauma was first defined by Saakvitne and Pearlman (1996; p. 151) as "the transformation in the inner experience...that comes about as a result of empathic engagement with clients' trauma material." Five ideological areas of belief about self, others, or the world that may be negatively affected are safety, trust, esteem, intimacy, and control (Maslow, 1954; McCann & Pearlman, 1990). A range of potential behavioral, physical, interpersonal, personal, and professional outcomes may result from VT, including a shift in beliefs and worldview; a decreased capacity to cope with stress or emotional situations; decreased contentment and joy; withdrawal; decreased capacity for empathy and compassion; and difficulty in forming or maintaining personal relationships.

WHAT VT IS AND IS NOT

Vicarious trauma is not a disease, syndrome, or illness; its outcomes may be positive or negative. Moreover, vicarious trauma is not the same as posttraumatic stress disorder (PTSD), but may produce

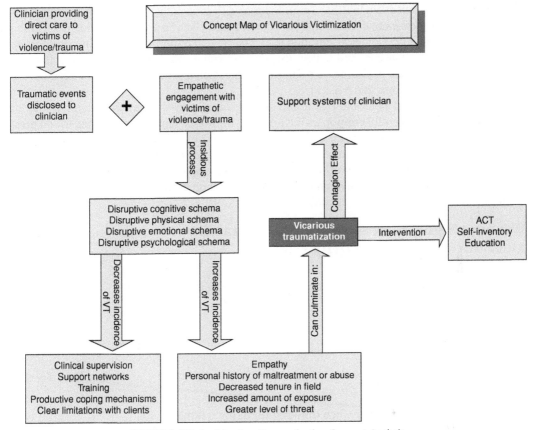

FIGURE 7B.1 Vicarious Traumatization Concept Analysis.

A nonnursing example of vicarious trauma that causes a change in worldview and an inability to separate from the trauma:

A father receives a distressing call from his son, who discloses that he is being bullied by his college roommate through social media. The father feels sorry for his son, and finds it difficult to control his emotions of rage and shock. The father strongly relates to this incident, recalling his own maltreatment during childhood. He does not think he can say or do anything to help. The son's problem worsens. Over time, the father begins drawing away from his son and others, and loses interest in activities he once enjoyed. He feels the world is evil, and he becomes distrustful of others.

An example of VT that is well-managed in a nonnursing occupation:

An experienced high school teacher is concerned about one of her senior students. The student is not completing her assignments on time and she seems disinterested and irritable. The teacher meets with the student privately after school. The student explains that her mother was recently diagnosed with a terminal illness, and she talks about how difficult life has become. The teacher offers words of comfort and helps the student formulate a plan to meet the requirements for graduation. The teacher offers to work with the student on the missing work and refers her for free tutoring through the school. She also provides information on other important resources in the school and community. The teacher is pleased the student benefits from the meeting, and the encounter reminds the teacher how much she values her professional knowledge and experience. The student leaves feeling understood and supported.

symptoms similar to those seen in PTSD. Trauma stories with content that includes serious threat, terror, intense fear, physical pain, or emotional suffering are more likely to prompt emotional mirroring and produce profound physiological, emotional, and perceptual responses. Past history, personality, female gender, genetic makeup, and beliefs also increase vulnerability to VT. It is widely accepted that "healthy persons elicit physiological responses to threatening stimuli that are processed unconsciously" (Yehuda & LeDoux, 2007; p. 22).

Signs or symptoms of neurobiological and subcortical responses to trauma material may or may not be present. Perceptible responses include uncomfortable sensations; elevated blood pressure, and heart and breathing rates; and changes in mood or emotion. Vicarious trauma can trigger or exacerbate depression, anxiety, substance abuse, and self-neglect, as well as preexisting PTSD, and contribute to shifts in worldview. Fatigue, disinterest, apathy, stress, hopelessness, and emotional pain may occur, as well as changes in the ability and desire to satisfy personal needs or the needs of others (Darr & Johns, 2008).

Warning Signs of Neurobiological Irritability and Subcortical Overactivity

- Hyperarousal
  - Sleep disturbances (difficulty falling/staying asleep; nightmares)
  - Irritability
  - Inability to relax
  - Increased startle response
- Re-experiencing
  - Waking disturbances
  - Flashbacks
  - Intrusive thoughts
  - Sensations and changes felt when thinking about the trauma
- Avoidance (Emotional Numbing)
  - Feeling the need to numb oneself
  - Isolation
  - Avoiding intimacy
  - Pretending to be interested, hear, or pay attention to friends/family
  - Losing connections with others
  - Substance abuse
  - Negative changes in cognition and mood
  - Distorted worldview
  - Persistent or recurrent emotions from primary exposure
  - Detachment
  - Loss of interest in activities once enjoyed

EFFECTS OF VT

Researchers are only beginning to understand VT, its effects, and the importance of preventive care for clinicians (Pearlman & Caringi, 2009). Vicarious trauma can lead to the development of compassion fatigue (CF) and burnout, and contributes to workforce dropout. Although CF and burnout are interrelated and can overlap, the terms are not interchangeable.

Compassion fatigue is called the "cost of caring" for others (Figley, 1995b), or an evolving consequence of caring. Also known as empathy fatigue, compassion fatigue is a consequence of VT. Compassion and empathy are therapeutic modalities that benefit individuals who experience direct trauma. However, the inner transformative effect of empathic engagement raises vulnerability, prompting one author to note that "empathy is the helper's greatest asset and also possibly his/her greatest liability" (Meichenbaum, n.d.; p. 3).

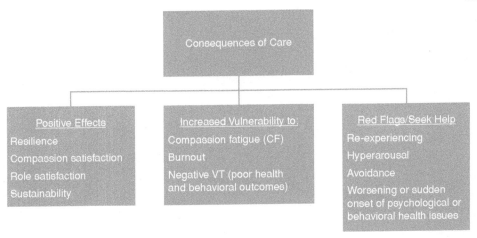

FIGURE 7B.2   Consequences of Care.

When empathy is uncontrolled, the inner response to trauma material can be greater and the clinician is more vulnerable to over-identify with the person or family, mirror the person's emotions, and become preoccupied with the trauma (American Counseling Association, 2011). Those who lack knowledge about VT, self-awareness, and skills that are protective and improve recovery and resiliency are more vulnerable to: disruptions in health; personal, interpersonal, and professional life; and poor physical and psychological health outcomes.

Negative changes in work performance may be manifested by irritability, horizontal violence, withdrawal, decreases in quality of performance and effectiveness, time management issues, increased absenteeism, and changing jobs.

It is important to note that long-term negative effects from disruptions in cognitive, physical, emotional, and psychological schema are not an inevitable consequence of working with victims of trauma and carrying trauma stories (Figley & Roop, 2006; Pearlman & Caringi, 2009; Stamm, 2005, 2010; Stamm, Figley, & Figley, 2010; ProQOL, 2015b; Tabor, 2011). Stamm (2005, 2010) highlights possible positive effects of VT, such as trauma growth, vicarious resiliency, and compassion satisfaction (CS). Compassion satisfaction and CF are influenced by three distinct environments (see Figure 7B.3): "the actual work situation itself, the environment of the person or people with whom we are providing care or assistance, and the personal environment that we bring to the work we do" (ProQOL.org, 2015a). Trauma work experience, knowledge of VT, and continuing education; self-awareness and coping skills; organizational, leadership, and peer support; setting boundaries; and preplanning for VT are all preventive and protective modalities (Tabor, 2011). Increased resiliency, compassion satisfaction, stress-exposure tolerance, capacity to demonstrate compassion, and clinical effectiveness are other examples of desirable outcomes.

SOURCES OF VT

Vicarious trauma in the forensic nursing role originates from empathic engagement during exposure to trauma material related to physical and/or sexual assault, maltreatment, abandonment, exploitation, death, or other traumatic events. Physical signs of injury may also contribute. The inner experience created by these exposures are transformative in nature, and can precipitate strong feelings, emotions, and sensations in response to the physical examination findings, the patient's or family's emotional reaction, and the trauma story. Increased vulnerability to VT can result when the nurse mirrors the facial affect and body posture of the patient, and pictures or imagines the story. These are a normal part of the empathic engagement process, and can help improve shared meaning during communication, yet self-constraint through controlled empathy

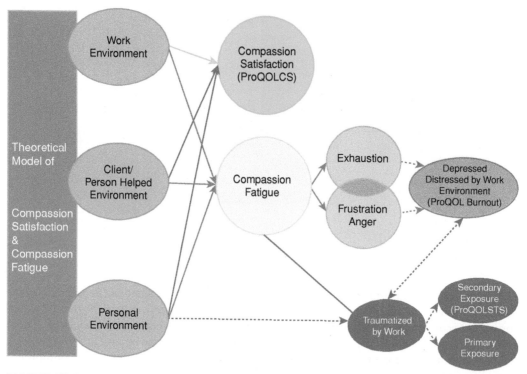

FIGURE 7B.3 Theoretical Model of Compassion Satisfaction and Compassion Fatigue. Copyright Beth Hudnall Stamm, 2009.

is protective. Vulnerability factors for negative VT include a lack of forensic nursing experience, a lack of current practice knowledge and education, having a past history of a major trauma, and ignoring telltale evidence-based physical and behavioral warning cues (Bride, Hatcher, & Humble, 2009; Pross, 2006).

Major Sources of Trauma Material Exposure in Forensic Nursing

- Violence: Situations where threat and imminent danger are present (interpersonal, domestic/family, intimate partner; violence child/elder maltreatment; perpetration by stranger; armed violence; and gang-related violence)
- Intense fear: Related to a near-death experience, maiming, disfigurement, or life-altering traumatic injury (accidental or nonaccidental)
- Natural disaster
- War-related combat
- Torture
- Terrorism

No one is immune to negative effects from trauma. Negative issues that arise in response to VT do not signify personal weakness or a flawed personality. Becoming informed about VT to strategize a plan to manage or recover from a negative VT experience is the responsibility of the forensic nurse. Informing forensic nurses and improving VT outcomes is also the responsibility of leadership the organization in which the nurse works, and the profession of forensic nursing. All levels are accountable to mitigate the potentially damaging effects of chronic exposure to traumatic life experiences of the forensic nurse's patient population.

Warning Signs and Symptoms

- Problems with judgment, safe and appropriate decision-making, concentration, and memory
- Mood swings, outbursts, changes in relationships, lack of interest in intimacy
- Decreased ability to cope; decreased reliance on healthy or effective coping skills

- Increased crying or sadness
- Changes in eating and/or sleeping patterns
- Increased reliance upon alcohol to cope or relax
- Emotional exhaustion
- Feeling alone
- Forgetting one's accomplishments and successes
- Lowered job satisfaction
- Decreased job performance
- Feelings of powerlessness, anger, guilt, and being overwhelmed
- Dread of being called out for a case; lowered compassion or empathy toward patients/others; avoidance
- Changes in beliefs and worldview (safety, trust, intimacy, esteem, and control)

As noted, forensic nurses who work with death, child or elder maltreatment, victims of domestic and intimate partner violence, and sexual assault are especially vulnerable to negative VT responses. Responses may be further intensified for forensic nurses who have a past or current history of violence or maltreatment, are experiencing other types of family-related stress or trauma, or encounter patients who share the same or similar characteristics of a loved one.

> "We have not been directly exposed to the trauma scene, but we hear the story told with such intensity, or we hear similar stories so often, or we have the gift and curse of extreme empathy and we suffer. We feel the feelings of our clients. We experience their fears. We dream their dreams. Eventually, we lose a certain spark of optimism, humor and hope. We tire. We aren't sick, but we aren't ourselves" (Ochberg, n.d.).
>
> Cathy spent the entire night taking care of her 17-year-old patient who presented with a chief complaint of sexual assault involving penile-vaginal, penile-anal, and penile-oral penetration by several gang members while at a party last night. The patient's description in combination with the examination findings distressed Cathy. The patient reminded Cathy of her own daughter who was the same age, and Cathy felt the mother's anguish and anger. For the next week, Cathy found herself dwelling on the patient and her mother. She had trouble sleeping, and she used alcohol to help her stop thinking about the assault. She and her daughter began arguing more. Cathy stopped letting her daughter drive herself to and from her evening job, or even go to visit her friends. Others, including her coworkers, noticed that Cathy was more irritable than usual and was less communicative.

Although the nurse can take personal steps to reduce the risk VT, external factors may exist that are beyond his or her immediate control. Inadequate or absent professional or organizational resources may exist, including a lack of effective multidisciplinary team effort and support, high staffing needs or shortage, failure to recognize achievements, and unrealistic job performance expectations.

PERSONAL – PROFESSIONAL DYNAMIC

Forensic nursing is trauma-based; VT should be considered a potential occupational hazard. Emotionally laden stories of trauma create a level of vulnerability that may be new to the nurse. Stress from working with traumatized patients and families can deplete reserves normally used for other areas of the nurse's life. Caseload, hours worked, work demands, and lack of leadership support can impede natural VT recovery and resiliency, and lead to burnout early in the forensic nursing career.

Besides role-related responsibilities and demands, nurses must also manage important aspects of their personal life. For some, unexpected events in life, such as sickness, accident, death, and/or tragedy can become realities of day-to-day life that are added to existing responsibilities. Difficulties in balancing personal and professional responsibilities can compound the challenge of maintaining well-being and one's quality of life.

PROTECTIVE FACTORS

Advanced knowledge and specialized skills in nursing practice reduce the nurse's vulnerability to VT. Protective factors in professional nursing include:

- Professional development
- Patient-centered care
  - Caring behaviors and therapeutic communication
  - Controlled empathic engagement
  - Patient advocacy
  - Patient education
  - Familiarity with and availability of resources for patients and families
  - Basing healthcare decisions on the patient's values, beliefs, and preferences
  - Informed consent-refusal
- Evidence-based practice (EBP)
- Nursing ethics; professionalism; nursing standards and principles; nursing process
- Objectivity and professional boundaries
- Inter/intradisciplinary collaboration, teamwork, and collegiality
- Integration of evidence in practice; using evidence to solve practice problems

Even though the forensic nurse and the patient have been brought together by trauma, when the nurse maintains self-awareness during therapeutic communication, he or she can remain focused on the health, safety, and well-being of the patient. When the nurse does not direct feelings of empathy toward a nursing goal, he or she is more likely to experience secondary trauma and personal distress, and more apt to compromise pre-established professional boundaries. Further, the forensic nurse's professional role may shift from one applying specialized knowledge to identify and improve health outcomes to the role of a peer, victim companion, or victim advocate.

Establishing clear professional boundaries early in one's forensic nursing career is an important step to managing therapeutic behaviors and communication. Maintaining boundaries in the nurse–patient relationship is the nurse's job and helps the nurse to objectively analyze the patient's trauma and to solve clinical problems, mitigate suffering, and provide patient-centered care.

The nurse's use of controlled empathy facilitates shared meaning and benefits the care of the patient, but also offers the nurse protection against harmful VT. Controlled empathy is mindful and reflects the concept of understanding the individual's trauma, but with the purpose of identifying interventions and resources to treat, relieve suffering, render aid, and promote healing. The nurse considers the patients' point of view, taking into consideration their values and preferences. Standardizing the approach to care by using the nursing process in combination with evidence-based knowledge and systematic methods of practice will protect the nurse.

An effective, collaborative multidisciplinary team (MDT) can provide protective benefits during the patient care period and following the encounter. Each member of the team has or is developing experience in working with victims of trauma and their families and is equally vulnerable to the negative effects of VT. When teams are comprised of individuals who know and have developed trust in one another, open and honest dialogue is more likely, which can help reduce the VT burden and toll on any one team member.

Poor team interactions compromise the forensic nurse's ability to effectively process trauma and effectively minimize the impact of VT. Forensic nurses who have a negative, critical, and judgmental attitude toward other disciplines or persons serving in those roles are at an increased risk for experiencing harmful effects from VT. The forensic nurse must have a clear understanding of his or her role, and its limitations. Every team member is responsible for fulfilling his or her role to the best of that person's ability; it is not the forensic nurse's responsibility to critique or perform the roles of others. Education about VT encourages a trusting and supportive atmosphere, strengthens the team, and encourages a culture of acceptance and support.

Key Points

- Researchers are only beginning to understand VT and its effects.
- Negative consequences from VT are more likely when perceptions are based on the nurse's own preferences, values, and beliefs, rather than those of the patient.
- Vicarious trauma often alters a person's view about self, and his or her outlook and perspective on life. Alterations in worldview are a distinct feature of VT.
- Vicarious trauma produces changes that may be positive, negative, or a combination of both.
- Multidisciplinary teams that foster collegiality and trust and are educated about VT are more likely to be understanding and supportive of team members.

Work Environment

The work environment should be designed or redesigned to reflect an awareness of VT and communicate appreciation for the nurse (e.g., in that the nurse's actions make a difference to the organization, the community, and vulnerable patient populations). The nurse is more likely to sense that the organization values his or her role in promoting patient outcomes when a private, secure, safe, clean, and pleasant patient care and staff environment exists. Access to needed services and resources, technology, equipment, supplies, assistance from others, and support are also necessary. Optimally, nurse leaders and supervisors demonstrate VT awareness as evidenced by their expectations of nurses (time, workload, and other job performance demands). A culture of collaboration and teamwork is also important, as is the ability to request time off without guilt or fear of compromising patient care. Organizational culture should reflect acceptance and understanding of how working with victims of trauma can impact providers and should encourage providers to access preventive and treatment resources (Bell, Kulkarni, & Dalton, 2003; Tabor, 2011). Staying current in practice, pursuing professional growth and advancement, and seeking project- or work-related opportunities also protect against VT; forensic nurse leaders and supervisors should encourage and value these endeavors (Pross, 2006).

When working with a patient who has experienced trauma, the forensic nurse is encouraged to note his or her own habits in meeting personal needs, the number of cases he or she performs, and the ratio of uninterrupted hours worked to the number of breaks taken. It is important for the forensic nurse to develop a habit of taking regular and adequate time away from the immediate work environment in cases where VT is perceived as unavoidable or when VT signs and symptoms are experienced. Professional growth and sustainability are at risk when the nurse ignores his or her own needs or symptoms of negative VT.

Stacey was excited about her new forensic nursing role. Although she had a full-time job in the hospital's emergency department, she signed up for forensic nurse call on many of her days and weekends off. When called in to work, she would be so focused on her case that she would ignore her needs for hydration, nutrition, bathroom breaks, and breaks from the trauma encounter. It was not unusual for her to have several consecutive cases involving patients who had experienced a major trauma. Her manager did not notice this, and her colleagues did not offer to take her shifts of call. Over time, she began to struggle with feelings that she was incompetent and powerless to create any type of meaningful social change. She dreaded being called in and felt chronically drained, both physically and emotionally. She was unable to relax, preoccupied with her patients' trauma, and lost connections with friends outside of work.

Mary knew that she could work long shifts without taking a break, but she forced herself to take time away from the clinical area and the patients. Every few hours she would take a 10- to 15-minute break, and she appreciated that her work environment made it possible and safe for her to step away when it was needed. She found this helped her feel psychologically and emotionally recharged. She also began to protect her scheduled time off to be with friends and family and to engage in activities she enjoyed outside of work. Her manager supported Mary's efforts to balance her work with her personal life and values. Mary also accepted opportunities for professional growth, and read literature and attended conferences that helped her stay current in her practice.

Personal Environment

Stress from fatigue, hunger, health problems, job burnout, or life situations can lower the nurse's threshold for VT. After an intense trauma exposure, the forensic nurse should make extra effort to connect with other people, rest, exercise, and enjoy recreation. Developing habits that incorporate these activities can contribute to the nurse's sense of well-being and quality of life. If good habits already exist, those areas of life require sustained nurturing.

> Tina knew that her life was enriched by exercise and spending time with friends. She felt refreshed for hours following her Pilate class and aerobic workout. Now that Tina is a forensic nurse, she wants to learn all she can and she feels energized by the intriguing cases. However, she has stopped going to the gym and no longer feels she has time to talk with or see her friends. Tina is dealing with emotions she does not recall struggling with in the past, especially guilt, sadness, fear, and anger. She also feels worthless and that nothing she does is making any real difference.
>
> Sharon noticed that she seems far more resilient to trauma exposure now than when she first began her forensic nursing career a decade ago. She recognized that VT was not always easy to manage, but her determination to lead a full and meaningful life outside work helped her to advance and grow in her role as a forensic nurse. The advice, support, and example that Sharon's mentor set helped Sharon establish clear personal and professional boundaries.

Possessing self-awareness not only optimizes personal health outcomes, wellness, and quality of life, but also improves the ability to recognize when outside help is needed or is necessary for recovery. The presence of one or more warning signs can prompt a predetermined action to counteract VT. Vulnerability to negative VT can stem from the individual, the role, the patient population, others in the nurse's personal and professional life, and the organization for which the nurse works (Pearlman & Caringi, 2009). Examples include the following.

Individual Factors

* Chronic illness or disease, PTSD, depression, anxiety, or poor general health
* Lack of an adequate or effective support system
* Losing connection with others, not working at relationships, not having relationships outside work
* Low self-esteem
* Lack of regular and aerobic exercise
* Lack of interests outside work
* Lack of a reliable support system and good relationships with loved ones and coworkers
* Caring for an aging or ill parent or family member
* Caring for an infant, or young or disabled child
* Substance abuse
* Major life changes or crises (e.g., divorce, relocation, tragedy, death of a family member)
* Lack of awareness of VT, self, and personal triggers of dysfunctional coping behaviors
* A tendency to feel sympathy or to have uncontrolled empathy

Forensic Nursing Role Factors

* Limited forensic nursing experience, education, and professional development
* Consecutive and cumulative exposures to trauma stories
* Witnessing human suffering, grief, or crises
* Demanding and long shifts at work
* Back-to-back forensic cases
* Role confusion or unrealistic expectations of oneself:
  * Always giving, caring, compassionate, empathic, self-sacrificing at the expense of self
  * Placing the needs of everyone else above self and self-care needs

Organizational Factors

- Demanding workload and hours
- Unrealistic expectations that exceed the nurse's capabilities, or results in the nurse ignoring self-care, comfort, or health-related needs
- Lack of recognition of VT as a serious and potential outcome
- Lack of resources for nurses to obtain rest, nourishment, and support
- Environment that does not adequately provide safety for patient and staff, emergency response, comfort care supplies, sanitation, up-to-date and accessible supplies, technology, equipment
- Lack of policies and systems in place to handle the needs of the nurse in crisis or experiencing VT
- Failure to recognize nursing accomplishments or to empower autonomy

When signs of negative vicarious trauma become self-evident or are detected by others, intervention is the next step to improve outcomes, and to avoid a contagion effect on members of the nurse's support system. Intervention is a proactive response involving mindfulness that takes inventory of the biopsychosocial cues (signs, symptoms, sensations, behaviors, changes in patterns) and the mental timeline that traces the response to a specific versus cumulative encounter(s). Initiation of healthy coping tools – both those built into the vicarious resiliency strategy and those that have proven to be personally effective in past circumstances – are essential.

SELF-CARE PLANNING

"Self-care is a skillful attitude that needs practice throughout the day" (Meichenbaum, n.d.; p. 14, quoting Mahoney, 2003; p. 25). Establishing and maintaining a personal self-care plan that includes daily habits and activities that promote posttrauma recovery help mitigate damaging emotional and health effects. An evidence-based self-care strategy includes friendships and regular connections with people outside work, and daily habits and routines that address the mind, body, and spirit (Stebnicki, 2008). Posttrauma recovery involves quality time away from the trauma or stimulus to process the trauma and address one's needs. Forensic nurses have a responsibility to themselves to take a proactive and preventive approach to achieve resiliency, wellness, quality of life, and a sense of well-being.

Skills that Nurture Resilience

- Self-monitoring one's thinking processes;
- Avoiding "thinking traps," such as blaming oneself or others, jumping to conclusions, making unfounded assumptions, and ruminating;
- Detecting "icebergs" or deeply held beliefs that lead to emotional overreactions;
- Engaging in problem-solving that is "realistically optimistic";
- Placing events in perspective;
- Learning ways to stay calm and focused; and
- Practicing skills in real life to change counterproductive thoughts and behaviors into more resilient thoughts and behaviors (Reivich & Shatte, 2002).

Mind, Body, and Spirit Recovery

- Rest
- Nutrition
- Hydration
- Skin and body care/pampering
- Quality sleep
- Attending to health needs (including preventive health screenings)
- Regular and meaningful recreation

- Exercise
- Spiritual activities
- Caring for important relationships; making time for loved ones and close friends
- Hobbies and interests outside work
- Friendships outside work
- Having an effective support system

Sustainable and satisfying forensic nursing practice includes a well-planned strategy of maintaining a strong sense of purpose and well-being and activities that contribute to quality of life. The plan should take into account needs, preferences, and vulnerabilities of the mind, body, and spirit.

Specific evidence-based choices, responses, and actions exist that mitigate the effects of detrimental and/or chronic exposure to trauma. Early identification of the signs and symptoms of VT and appropriate interventions improve outcomes.

Prevention

The ABCs of VT primary prevention are: awareness, balance, and connections (Rothschild & Rand, 2006). Awareness refers to self-knowledge regarding limitations, stress, triggers, available support sources, and outside resources. Balance applies to priority-setting in a manner that permits an equal distribution of quality time between one's personal and professional life. Connections pertain to the individual, other people, and personal interests. It involves staying connected and forming new connections outside of work. These areas support positive VT outcomes, such as nurse-resiliency and job satisfaction. Self-care involves integrating knowledge about VT, skills, and tools to reduce risks and improve resiliency.

Preventive and Care Resources

- Vicarious trauma education and knowledge
- Regular self-evaluation and reflection
- Maintaining professional boundaries
- Healthy coping styles
- Personal support systems
- Peer meetings and case review

Expert Help and Resources

Vicarious traumatization is a natural, predictable, preventable, and manageable consequence of forensic nursing and other helping professions. Those entering such a profession often do so because they see themselves as "givers" and find personal satisfaction in making a difference in the lives of others. Knowledge of VT and self-awareness are essential to remaining effective in the forensic nursing role, and to sustaining role satisfaction. Nurses, as a group, are known as self-sacrificing, trustworthy, caring, and compassionate. By way of these attributes, they are often willing to set aside their own needs, overextend themselves, and ignore serious signs in response to VT. Forensic nurses have specialized education in the care and treatment of victims and perpetrators of trauma; however, nurses must also be informed and well-educated regarding VT to minimize poor health outcomes and other damaging effects, including compassion fatigue and professional burnout. The work environment, organization, team, and the nurse all play an important part in promoting forensic nurse resiliency, health and well-being, quality of life, and role satisfaction. Forensic nurses must strategize and implement their own VT prevention, resiliency, and self-care plan, listen to concerns expressed by members of their support system, and reach out for professional help when sustained VT effects are present. Vicarious traumatization prevention involves an ongoing effort by the nurse, nurse leaders, colleagues, the organization, and the forensic nursing profession.

CASE STUDIES

CASE STUDY #1

Mary has been a registered nurse for 9 years, working 4 days a week on a busy obstetrics/gynecological unit. Five years ago, she began taking call 7 days a month for a sexual assault response team (SART) program, 24-hour on-call shifts. She averages four forensic examinations a month.

The SART nurses are independently contracted, and all have other full-time nursing jobs outside of SART. The examinations are performed at a free-standing site, and little opportunity exists for collegiality. For those who have the time to attend, opportunities exist for peer review and occasional in-services.

Mary prided herself on her ability to do what others considered "tough work." Other nurses at her hospital often told her, "I don't know how you do it; it must be so sad to do that work." Mary replied that she did not consider it as sad, and that this work was what she signed on to do.

Lately, Mary has been calling in sick more often at her hospital job, disorganized in her SART examinations, and increasingly critical of her peers. She has voiced frustration to her colleagues about the patients she has been seeing: "I can't believe how stupid some of these women are, walking alone at night, taking rides from strange guys, getting drunk." She told her partner that she "dreads" her cell phone ringing on the days she is on-call, because "getting a call means I have to hear all those stories, and I just don't think I can care about that anymore."

Mary feels guilty about this, and has begun drinking "to feel better" when she is not on-call. She has not shared these feelings with her nurse colleagues, for fear of being judged as "weak"; no one else has said they feel like this, so there must be something wrong with her.

Review Questions

1. What are the concerning feelings that Mary is experiencing?

2. What are the concerning behaviors that Mary is exhibiting?

3. Who is Mary's support?

4. What are some ways that Mary could address this issue with other nurses?

5. What are some ways to address these issues in your work setting? Ways in which this issue could be normalized? Ways to pull forensic nurses together?

CASE STUDY #2

Jessica is a 36-year-old forensic nurse who has worked in the domestic violence (DV) unit of a large inner-city hospital for 13 years, seeing an average of 12 patients per week. She has not received education about VT. During the past 3 years, her colleagues and family members began noticing changes in Jessica's attitude about life and her increasingly negative mood and health behaviors, but no one has addressed these concerns with her directly.

Jessica often complains that she feels extremely tired and overwhelmed. She is irritable and does not seem happy or interested in professional development opportunities. Her supervisor and coworkers have noticed that she takes twice as long as everyone else to finish the same work, and she is frequently late for work and meetings. Jessica shares personal experiences and complaints about her husband with anyone who will listen, including her patients.

Jessica says that she is too busy to take a vacation. Jessica's thinking and concerns are constantly focused on the lives of her patients and friends at work. On her days off, she will check in by text or phone with clients from the shelter. The only friends Jessica has are colleagues at work.

In addition to working full-time and taking call with the forensic nursing program, Jessica started volunteering at a women's shelter a year ago. "I can do more to help victims," she explained when her family expressed concern. She uses alcohol to help her relax when she is not working and avoids socializing outside of work. When Jessica thinks about the loss of relationships she once enjoyed with others, she reasons, If only others did their job the way they should, I wouldn't need to work so hard.

She feels tremendous guilt and recognizes that she is not the same person she was in the past. She recalls her life early in her marriage; her family was the most important thing. She remembers how much she used to enjoyed dance, painting, and running.

Review Questions

1. What is Jessica's support system?

2. What does Jessica demonstrate regarding self-awareness or a balance between her personal and professional life?

3. What do you notice about Jessica's professional boundaries?

4. What does Jessica do to relieve stress when she is not at work?

5. What new activities and habits might Jessica find helpful?

REFERENCES

Aerts, D., Apostel, L., Moor, B., Hellemans, S., Maex, E., VanBelle, H., & Van der Veken, J. (1994). *World views: From fragmentation to integration*. Brussels, Belgium: VUB Press. Retrieved from http://www.vub.ac.be/CLEA/pub/books/worldviews.pdf

Aiken, L. H., Clarke, S. P., Sloane, D. M., Sochalski, J., & Silber, J. H. (2002). Hospital nurse staffing and patient mortality, nurse burnout, and job dissatisfaction. *Journal of the American Medical Association, 288*(16), 1987–1993.

American Counseling Association. (2011). *Vicarious trauma: Fact sheet #9*. Retrieved from http://www.counseling.org/docs/trauma-disaster/fact-sheet-9—vicarious-trauma.pdf

Bell, H., Kulkarni, S., & Dalton, L. (2003). Organizational prevention of vicarious trauma. *Journal of Contemporary Human Services, 84*(4), 463–470.

Boscarino, J. A., Figley, C. R., & Adams, R. E. (2004). Compassion fatigue following the September 11 terrorist attacks: A study of secondary trauma among New York City social workers. *International Journal of Emergency Mental Health, 6*(2), 57–66.

Bride, B. E., Hatcher, S. S., & Humble, M. N. (2009). Trauma training, trauma practices, and secondary traumatic stress among substance abuse counselors. *Traumatology, 15*(2), 96–105.

Darr, W., & Johns, G. (2008). Work strain, health, and absenteeism. A meta-analysis. *Journal of Occupational Health Psychology, 13*(4), 293–318.

Figley, C. R. (1995a). Compassion fatigue as secondary traumatic stress disorder: An overview. In C. R. Figley (Ed.), *Compassion fatigue: Coping with secondary traumatic stress disorder in those who treat the traumatized* (pp. 1–20). New York, NY: Routledge.

Figley, C. R. (Ed.). (1995b). *Compassion fatigue: Coping with secondary traumatic stress disorder in those who treat the traumatized*. New York, NY: Routledge.

Figley, C. R., & Roop, R. G. (2006). *Compassion fatigue in the animal-care community*. Washington, DC: Humane Society Press.

Jenkins, S. R., & Baird, S. (2002). Secondary traumatic stress and vicarious trauma: A validation study. *Journal of Traumatic Stress, 15*(5), 423–432.

Mahoney, M. J. (2003). *Constructive psychotherapy: A practical guide*. New York, NY: Guilford Press.

Maslow, A. H. (1954). *Motivation and personality*. New York, NY: Harper & Row.

McCann, L., & Pearlman, L. A. (1990). Vicarious traumatization: A framework for understanding the psychological effects of working with victims. *Journal of Traumatic Stress, 3*(1), 131–149.

Meichenbaum, D. (n.d.). *Self-care for trauma psychotherapists and caregivers: Individual, social and organizational interventions*. Miami, FL: Melissa Institute for Violence Prevention and Treatment of Victims of Violence. Retrieved March 18, 2015, from http://www.melissainstitute.org/documents/meichenbaum_selfcare_11thconf.pdf

Ochberg, F. M. (n.d.). PTSD resources for survivors and caregivers: When helping hurts. *GiftfromWithin.org*. Retrieved March 18, 2015, from http://www.giftfromwithin.org/pdf/helping.pdf

Pearlman, L. A., & Caringi, J. (2009). Living and working self-reflectively to address vicarious trauma. In C. A. Courtois & J. D. Ford (Eds.), *Treating complex traumatic stress disorders: An evidence-based guide* (pp. 202–224). New York, NY: Guilford Press.

ProQOL.org. (2015a). *Full CS-CF model*. Retrieved from http://www.proqol.org/Full_CS-CF_Model.html

ProQOL.org. (2015b). *Professional quality of life: CS and CF: Understanding a theory and creating a model of compassion satisfaction and compassion fatigue: What we began in the 1990s we understand more in the 2010s*. Retrieved from http://www.proqol.org/CS_and_CF.html

Pross, C. (2006). Burnout, vicarious traumatization and its prevention. *Torture: Quarterly Journal on Rehabilitation of Torture Victims and Prevention of Torture, 16*(1), 1–9.

Reivich, K., & Shatte, A. (2002). *The resilience factor: Seven keys to finding your inner strength and overcoming life's hurdles*. New York, NY: Broadway Books.

Rothschild, B., & Rand, M. (2006). *The psychophysiology of compassion fatigue and vicarious trauma. Help for the helper: Self-care strategies for managing burnout and stress*. New York, NY: W. W. Norton & Company.

Saakvitne, K. W., & Pearlman, L. A. (1996). *Transforming the pain: A workbook on vicarious traumatization*. New York, NY: W. W. Norton & Company.

Stamm, B. H. (1997). Work-related secondary traumatic stress. *PTSD Research Quarterly, 8*(2), 1–3.

Stamm, B. H. (2005). *The ProQOL manual*. Pocatello, ID: Idaho State University.

Stamm, B. H. (2010). *The concise ProQOL manual* (2nd ed.). Pocatello, ID: ProQOL.org. Retrieved from http://www.proqol.org/uploads/ProQOL_Concise_2ndEd_12-2010.pdf

Stamm, B. H., Figley, C. R., & Figley, K. R. (2010). *Provider resiliency: A train-the-trainer mini course on compassion satisfaction and compassion fatigue*. Montreal, Canada: International Society for Traumatic Stress Studies.

Stebnicki, M. A. (2008). *Empathy fatigue: Healing the mind, body, and spirit of professional counselors*. New York, NY: Springer Publishing Company.

Tabor, P. D. (2011). Vicarious traumatization: Concept analysis. *Journal of Forensic Nursing, 7*(4), 203–208.

Vidal, C. (2008). Wat is een wereldbeeld? [What is a worldview?]. In H. Van Belle & J. Van der Veken (Eds.), *Nieuwheid denken. De wetenschappen en het creatieve aspect van de werkelijkheid* [Novel thoughts: Science and the creative aspect of reality]. Acco Uitgeverij.

Yehuda, R., & LeDoux, J. (2007). Response variation following trauma: A translational neuroscience approach to understanding PTSD. *Neuron Review, 56*, 19–32. doi 10.1016/j.neuron.2007.09.006

Vision of Ethical Practice

INTRODUCTION

The International Association of Forensic Nurses expects its members to aspire to the highest standards of ethical nursing practice. This vision of ethics is a framework for approaching professional decisions and stimulating ethical dialogue based on the ideals of our organization.

Forensic nurses acknowledge the importance of membership in a global society. This includes providing forensic nursing care in a manner that respects the uniqueness of the patient or client. Forensic nurses collaborate with nurses, healthcare providers, and other professionals throughout the world to promote ethically informed and culturally competent practices.

When faced with ethical choices, forensic nurses should use recognized ethical frameworks for decision making. The guiding principles of ethical decision making are autonomy, justice, beneficence, and nonmaleficence. Forensic nurses should consult and collaborate with appropriate ethical resources.

SCOPE

Fidelity to Patients and Clients

Forensic nurses serve patients and clients faithfully and incorruptibly. Forensic nurses respect confidentiality and advise patients and clients about the limits of confidentiality as determined by their practice setting.

Responsibility to the Public

Forensic nurses have a professional responsibility to serve the public welfare. Forensic nurses should be actively concerned with the health and welfare of the global community. Forensic nurses should recognize their role in preventing violence, which includes understanding the societal factors, such as oppression, that promote violence. Forensic nurses acknowledge the value and dignity of all human beings and strive to create a world where violence is not accepted.

Obligation to Science

Forensic nurses should seek to advance nursing and forensic science, understand the limits of their knowledge, and respect the truth. Forensic nurses should ensure that their research and scientific contributions are thorough, accurate, and unbiased in design and presentation. Forensic nurses should incorporate evidence-based knowledge in practice decisions.

Conflicts of interest should be disclosed. Scientific misconduct, such as fabrication, falsification, slander, libel, and plagiarism are incompatible with this Vision of Ethical Practice. Public comments regarding scientific matters should be made with care and precision, devoid of unsubstantiated claims, exaggeration, and/or premature conclusions.

Dedication to Colleagues

Forensic nurses perform work honestly and competently, fulfill obligations, and safeguard proprietary information. Forensic nurses should regard the tutelage of students as a trust conferred by society for the promotion of the student's learning and professional development. Forensic nurses should treat colleagues with respect, share ideas honestly, and give credit for their contributions.

The Vision of Ethical Practice was revised by the Ethics Committee in 2008, reviewed by Members, and approved by the Board in November of 2008.

Educational Preparation and Credentialing of the Forensic Nurse

Educational Preparation		
	Description/Definition	**References/Information**
Undergraduate Nursing Education	Includes: Diploma (typically hospital-based programs), Associate degree (e.g., community college programs), and baccalaureate (e.g., 4-yr college/ university programs). Following program completion, individual takes the NCLEX examination and may work as an RN. Undergraduate academic programs in accredited schools of nursing offer electives, minors, or concentrations in forensic nursing that can contribute to a degree in nursing.	American Nurses Association. Retrieved from http://www.nursing-world.org/MainMenuCategories/ANAMarketplace/ANAPeriodicals/OJIN/TableofContents/vol132008/No3Sept08/CareerEntryPoints.html International Association of Forensic Nurses, American Nurses Association. (2009, 2nd ed. forthcoming). *Forensic nursing: Scope and standards of practice.* Silver Spring, MD: Nursesbooks.org.
Graduate Nursing Education	May pursue a master's or doctoral degree. A master's degree prepares the nurse for an administrative, teaching, or research role or a leadership or consulting role in a clinical or health policy setting. A doctoral degree (PhD or DNP) educates a nurse for a leadership or advanced and specialized role. Enhances the knowledge and skills acquired in baccalaureate and pre-licensure nursing programs. Following matriculation and completion of the forensic core content and prescribed forensic clinical experiences, the forensic nurse can receive a master's or doctoral degree in the specialty of forensic nursing.	American Association of Colleges of Nursing. Retrieved from http://www.aacn.nche.edu/publications/brochures/GradStudentsBrochure.pdf International Association of Forensic Nurses, American Nurses Association. (2009, 2nd ed. forthcoming). *Forensic nursing: Scope and standards of practice.* Silver Spring, MD: Nursesbooks.org.

(continued)

Educational Preparation

	Description/Definition	References/Information
Doctoral Nursing Education	Doctor of Philosophy in Nursing • Represents the highest level of formal education for a career in research and scholarship • Prepares nurse scientists and scholars for the expression and communication of the knowledge base in the profession • Focus is on mastering and extending the knowledge of the discipline through research • Prepares graduates in a breadth of the discipline, and in depth in a particular area (AACN, 2010)	Doctor of Nursing Practice • Prepares nurse specialists at the highest level of advanced nursing practice • Designed for nurses committed to a practice career • Oriented toward improving outcomes of care • Incorporates integrative practice experiences and an intense practice immersion • Graduates support healthcare improvements through practice, policy change, and scholarship (AACN, 2006, 2010)
Postdoctoral Education or Fellowships	These studies allow a nurse to work as an independent researcher. The nurse gains skills and knowledge in a specific area of science and learns how to communicate knowledge through clinical practice. The specific content and skills acquired in terminal nursing degree programs are enhanced by formal forensic nursing core content and prescribed forensic clinical experiences. The programs may award diplomas.	American Association of Colleges of Nursing. Retrieved from http://www.aacn.nche.edu/publications/brochures/GradStudentsBrochure.pdf International Association of Forensic Nurses, American Nurses Association. (2009, 2nd ed. forthcoming). *Forensic nursing: Scope and standards of practice.* Silver Spring, MD: Nursesbooks.org.

Credentialing

	Description/Definition	References/Information
Competency Coursework	Teaching and learning completed to establish competency in a skill or set of skills; Competency can be developed through formal coursework, webinars, continuing education, professional conferences, and other mechanisms.	American Association of Colleges of Nursing. Retrieved from http://www.aacn.nche.edu/elnec/publications/peaceful-death
Continuing Education	Continuing education is a pathway to enhancing knowledge, building and maintaining competency, and preparing for career advancement. Furthers professional development through participation in activities that expand a nurse's professional role in providing quality health care to the public. Forensic nurses can gain additional skills and knowledge about topics of interest through continuing education offerings.	American Nurses Association. Retrieved from http://www.nursing-world.org/MainMenuCategories/ThePracticeofProfessionalNursing/NursingEducation/Continuing EducationforNurses International Association of Forensic Nurses, American Nurses Association. (2009, 2nd ed. forthcoming). *Forensic nursing: Scope and standards of practice.* Silver Spring, MD: Nursesbooks.org.

Credentialing

Description/Definition	References/Information
Assessment-Based Certificate Programs	Testing that allows a nurse to specialize in a specific area; Does not replace higher education, and may be paired with a master's degree. Forensic nursing-related certificate programs include content relevant to the forensic nurse, establish entrance and completion requirements, and may provide clinical internships; Results in a certificate that details successful completion.	American Nurses Association. Retrieved from http://www.nursing-world.org/MainMenuCategories/ ANAMarketplace/ANAPeriodicals/ OJIN/TableofContents/Vol21997/ No3Aug97/LicensureCertificationan-dAccreditation.html International Association of Forensic Nurses, American Nurses Association. (2009, 2nd ed. forthcoming). *Forensic nursing: Scope and standards of practice.* Silver Spring, MD: Nursesbooks.org.

Certification

Description/Definition	References/Information
Certification	Certification is a process used by organizations and agencies to ensure that the nurse in practice is qualified; Verifies education, training, and skills in a specific nursing specialty. The individual is awarded the certification following a review of requirements and in some cases, testing, which verifies an extensive base of knowledge, education, experience, and commitment to excellence for a specific nursing practice, including forensic nursing practice. For example, IAFN offers certification for sexual assault nurse examiners: Sexual Assault Nurse Examiner – Adult/ Adolescent (SANE-A®) and Sexual Assault Nurse Examiner – Pediatric (SANE-P®) Portfolio: Offers an alternative to examination-based certification programs; Involves review of a collective record of a professional's work and achievements. The American Nurses Credentialing Center in collaboration with IAFN offers a portfolio certification in Advanced Forensic Nursing (AFN-BC).	American Nurse Credentialing Center (ANCC) Advanced Forensic Nursing Certification. See eligibility requirements at http://www.nursecredential-ing.org/AdvForensicNursing-Eligibility. aspx American College of Forensic Examiners Institute. Certified Forensic Nursing Program (CFN). See eligibility requirements and information at http://www.acfei.com/forensic_certi-fications/cfn/ International Association of Forensic Nurses (IAFN). (2015). *Sexual Assault Nurse Examiner Adult/Adolescent (SANE-A) and SANE-P Certification Examination Handbook.* Commission for Forensic Nursing Certification. Available at: http://iafn.org/ American Nurses Credentialing Center. Retrieved from http://www. nursecredentialing.org/Forensic Nursing-Advanced

Appendix C

Answers to Review Questions

Chapter 1

1. Correct answer: a.

   A forensic nurse is a nurse who applies forensic science concepts while providing nursing care.

2. Correct answer: c.

   Recognition of a patterned injury; bruising consistent with a belt mark on a child is an action that demonstrates the assessment phase of the nursing process for a forensic client.

3. Correct answer: d.

   A conceptual model is defined as an organized representation of complex concepts.

4. Correct answer: d.

   Three ethical values of forensic nurses are objectivity, confidentiality, and boundaries.

5. Correct answers: a. 4, b. 6, c. 2, d. 5, e. 3, f. 1.

   a. Evaluates causes of accidents and injuries 4. Workers' compensation office

   b. Provides education on violence prevention 6. Public health department

   c. Collects evidence from the deceased 2. Coroner's office

   d. Writes policy briefs and recommendations 5. City council

   e. Collects epidemiological research data 3. Board of Health

   f. Consults legally on forensic issues 1. Attorney's office

Chapter 2

1. Correct answer: b.

   Rationale: The patient is not a minor and typically assault of adults does not require mandatory reporting.

2. Correct answer: b.

   Rationale: Injuries, if present, are often subtle and the patient may not be aware of them. Inspection and palpation are recommended, as well as use of toluidine blue dye and/or colposcopy.

3. Correct answers: b, c, f.

   Rationale: The patient does not recall all the events and often men will suck nipples during a frontal assault. Semen can leak on to external genitalia and downward toward the anus so both external and anal swabs are recommended. Since vaginal penetration is reported, a vaginal wall and cervical swab are recommended. No penetration of the rectal area was reported.

It could be argued that the patient may not remember, but the collection of this evidence is invasive – the nurse may ask if the patient wants to have a swab taken but otherwise would not typically obtain one.

4. Correct answer: d.

Rationale: The patient should still be offered treatment for STIs even if she has been in a relationship with her boyfriend; it is unknown if he is monogamous. Most emergency contraception still can be safely administered even if the patient is on birth control. Until more information is obtained about risk, it is unknown whether the patient needs HIV medication.

5. Correct answer: c.

Rationale: Using the term "story" (versus "history") and the term "alleged" both imply disbelief. This can worsen the risk for PTSD and is a form of secondary victimization.

6. Correct answer: a.

Rationale: Symmetrical patterned burns are more often nonaccidental injuries. Lacerations are blunt injury wounds and incised wounds are penetrating; the two types of wounds have different characteristics. Ecchymoses and bruises are not the same, although they may appear to be similar.

7. Correct answer: b.

Rationale: Although the nurse's opinion is important, he may have a skewed experience (e.g., seeing patients with a specific finding within his community). Ideally, the nurse would consult both his or her experience and the literature. Although quasi-experimental studies are typically small samples and not controlled, similar findings across studies will strengthen the findings and the nurse's opinion.

Chapter 3

1. Correct answer: c.

To be viable for transplant, organs must be perfused and used within 72 hours.

2. Correct answer: a.

The Model Post-Mortem Examination Act (1954) recommends a forensic examination in all of the following types of cases except the death of an older adult.

3. Correct answer: a.

Child protective services is the entity that is responsible for conducting a civil investigation of child abuse and neglect.

4. Correct answer: d.

A coroner can (usually) do all of the following except perform an autopsy.

5. Correct answer: c.

Toddlers are at an increased risk of death from all of the following except fire.

6. Correct answer: d.

Examples of asphyxia include all of the following except sudden infant death syndrome.

7. Correct answer: a.

Under specific guidelines, an autopsy can be performed without permission from the next-of-kin.

8. Correct answer: d.

Livor mortis is the pooling and settling of blood in dependent areas.

9. Correct answer: d.

   The triggering event that initiates a continuous sequence of events resulting in death is referred to as the proximate cause of death.

10. Correct answer: b.

    "Intentional" is not a manner of death.

Index

Note: The letters f or t following a page number indicate a figure or a table.